COLOR ATLAS of Real-Time Two-Dimensional Doppler Echocardiography

SECOND EDITION

COLOR ATLAS of Real-Time Two-Dimensional Doppler Echocardiography

SECOND EDITION

Edited by
RYOZO OMOTO, M.D.
Professor, Department of Surgery, Saitama Medical School

Shindan-To-Chiryo Co., Ltd.
Tokyo 1987

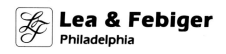 **Lea & Febiger**
Philadelphia

First Edition, 1984

Published by
SHINDAN-TO-CHIRYO CO., LTD.
  406. MARUNOUCHI BUILDING
  MARUNOUCHI CHIYODA-KU TOKYO JAPAN
ISBN : 4-7878-0123-6 C 0231

Distributed by
LEA & FEBIGER
600 SOUTH WASHINGTON SQUARE
PHILADELPHIA, PENNSYLVANIA 19106-4198
U.S.A.
ISBN 0-8121-1116-8

Printed and bound in Japan

Contributors

RYOZO OMOTO, M. D.

Professor, Department of Surgery, Saitama Medical School

YUJI KONDO, B. S.

Engineer, Medical Ultrasound Department, Aloka Co., Ltd.

CHIHIRO KASAI, Rh. D.

Manager of Research Institute, Aloka Co., Ltd.

KOROKU NAMEKAWA, B. S.

Chief Engineer of Research Institute, Aloka Co., Ltd.

YOSHIHIRO YOSHIKAWA, B. S.

Manager, Medical Ultrasound Department, Aloka Co., Ltd.

AKIRA KOYANO, B. S.

Exective Director, Aloka Co., Ltd.

KANJI MIURA, B. S.

Chief, Medical Ultrasound Department, Aloka Co., Ltd.

SHINICHI TAKAMOTO, M. D.

Assistant Professor, Department of Surgery, Saitama Medical School

SHUNEI KYO, M. D.

Assistant Professor, Department of Surgey, Saitama Medical School

MAKOTO MATSUMURA, M. D.

Assistant in Surgery, Department of Surgery, Saitama Medical School

YUJI YOKOTE, M. D.

Associate Professor, Department of Surgery, Saitama Medical School

Preface to the Second Edition

It seems difficult to believe that four years have passed since real-time two-dimensional Doppler echocardiography, color flow mapping, was first developed and commercialized in 1982. In many heart centers, wide-ranging and enthusiastic basic studies into the clinical significance of this new technique have been carried out, and of late, a considerable amount of clinical data has been accumulating. The results of these studies have established the diagnostic usefulness of the technique. We may say that it has made a significant impact on clinical cardiology. The rapid introduction and use of the technique both in Japan and overseas is astonishing.

The first edition of this text was published in December, 1983, which coincided exactly with the launching of the system on the market. With transition from a prototype to a commercial system, the authors, who were involved in developing the new modality called 2-D Color Flow Doppler, produced the first edition of this color atlas textbook. The authors believed that the early publication of a text that combined a manual for use with a fundamental image atlas, was essential for widespread use of the technique. The main objectives for publication of a second edition are:

1. 2-D Color Flow Doppler systems on the market have already entered a second generation with improved performance and imaging. This makes it necessary to include images produced by the new device in the text.

2. Since publication of the first edition, a considerable amount of clinical data has been collected, which allows inclusion of studies of diseases which were omitted earlier.

3. Applications of continuous-wave Doppler have become widespread, which has necessitated the inclusion of special methods of using the system, such as combining the use of 2-D Color Flow Doppler with continuous-wave Doppler techniques.

The authors of the second edition are the same as those who wrote the first. However, additional writers have assisted by providing chapters on new techniques and clinical applications. Most of the material used for the fundamental image atlas were obtained from actual scanning in the authors' institute and the diagnoses were confirmed by surgery or angiography.

2-D Color Flow Doppler is presently undergoing rapid progression and proliferation and is expected to develop into a diagnostic technique with even greater potential for the future. It is my sincerest wish that this second edition will contribute towards providing accurate understanding and application of 2-D Color Flow Doppler techniques in clinical cardiology at the present time.

January, 1987
Ryozo Omoto

Acknowledgements

The editor wishes to express his sincere gratitude to many associates for their enthusiastic assistance and to many friends for their encouragement in the publication of this book. He also extends his thanks and respects to Mr. Tetchu Majima, Mr. Rokuro Uchida, and the late Mr. Kano Kashiwabara, executives of Aloka Co., Ltd., who contributed so much effort and knowledge to this study. It is the editor's great pleasure to have been involved in the research and development of this new diagnostic modality in cardiology. As with the first edition, thanks are due to Professor Yutaka Doi, the Second Department of Internal Medicine, Porfessor Kazuichi Maeda, the Department of Pediatrics, Saitama Medical School, and Dr. Tsurio Matsumura, Chief of Cardiology, Omiya Red Cross Hospital, for providing much of the clinical material for this study. Gratitude is also due to Drs. Keisuke Ueda, Hideo Adachi, Haruhiko Asano, the Department of Surgery ,Saitama Medical School and Dr. Eiko Takanawa, the Department of Pediatrics, and other co-workers for their kind collaboration in the investigation and recording of clinical cases, data filing and other practical procedures. The editor also thanks Dr. Maylene Wong, Associate Professor of Cardiology Section, West Los Angeles Veterans Administration Medical Center for her continuous encouragement and support throughout the work.

The editor is much indebted to Mr. Hiroyoshi Fujizane and Mr. Takeshi Hisatsugi of Shindan-To-Chiryo Co., Ltd. for their special consideration in relation to this difficult publication and to Mr. Mitsuhiro Igarashi of Seishinsha Printing Co., Ltd. and Mr. Tokuryo Shibata, the designer, for their management of the technical problems in printing the color atlas. The editor extends his appreciation to Mr. Ralph Winters, Corometrics Medical Systems, Inc., and Mr. Chris W. P. Reynolds, professional medical translator, for their assistance with the English translation.

Lastly, the editor would like to give special recognition to his secretary, Mrs. Takako Ito, who typed the entire manuscript and organized all of the references.

Ryozo Omoto

How to Use This Book For Maximum Benefit

Most readers of this text are likely to be physicians, surgeons, sonographers, nurses, clinical technicians, or medical students. To be frank, the engineering principles of the device may form an area of weakness for the medical personnel who will use it. For that reason, Chapter 2 and Chapter 3 provide an easy-to-understand explanation along with many relevant diagrams to aid basic technical understanding. Since real-time two-dimensional Doppler echocardiography is a completely new technique, it is highly recommended that a full understanding of this section be obtained before using the device. However, should the reader find Chapter 2 difficult to understand, the next chapter may be embarked upon, and the comprehension of Chapter 2 left until later. Chapters 4 and 5 deal with the basic aspects of clinical scanning operation, its role and skillful use. When imaging intracardiac blood flow, various conditions, such as the appropriate positioning of the transducer to achieve the purpose of scanning, are extremely important. When practicing the use of the device, refer to Chapter 5, where the importance of understanding the three-dimensional concept of intracardiac blood flow is emphasized. It is also extremely useful to learn in advance about artifacts that constitute pitfalls to accurate interpretation of the color flow images. Chapter 6 provides detailed examples of artifacts. When learning how to use the device, it is necessary to become fully familiar with the patterns that appear in normal adults and children before proceeding to the chapters concerning heart disease. These are given in Chapter 7.

Chapters 8-12 are entirely devoted to the presentation of the color photographs of clinical cases. The photographs are presented just as they were imaged, and the presence of any artifacts is pointed out in the text. It is our intention for the reader to use this atlas as a reference. It offers substantial information on the interpretative parameters of the 2-D Doppler techniques.

The color atlas, one of the key sections of this book, is divided into four parts for the sake of printing convenience. Careful consideration has been given to facilitating cross-referencing between the case description and the case number in the color atlas. Care has also been taken to allow image interpretation from the color atlas alone.

Detailed explanations of the numbering of figures, tables, charts and the color atlas, and of how to refer to these sections, are given below.

The number following the indications, Fig., Tab. and Chart, indicates the chapter, and the succeeding number indicates the order in which each figure, table or chart appears in the chapter. For example, Fig. 4-3 designates the third figure in Chapter 4, and Tab. 7-2 the second table in Chapter 7.

The color atlas is denoted in boldface type in order to make a clear distinction from the figures in the respective chapters. In addition, it is characterized by the index-title such as "**Color Velocity Function**" or "**Case 3**" encircled by blue lines and placed above the page number. "**Case 3**", for example, not only refers to the case itself described under the title but also indicates the designation of the photograph in the color atlas as in "**Case 3, B**" or "**Case 3, B and C**". When the page of the picture in the color atlas is identified, the letter alone is often used in boldface type. The page of the photograph in the color atlas corresponding to the index-title is shown by the index-marker (**O**) in the margin on the left of the main description.

Special consideration is given to the color atlas in the index, in which boldface type indicates the pages of a color atlas.

As mentioned, the main purpose of the book is to present the color atlas of 2-D Doppler findings. The authors have devoted the book exclusively to the practical applications of this new modality. Some readers may need more information on the traditional techniques, i.e., 2-D echocardiography, pulsed-wave Doppler, and contionuous-wave Doppler. For such information, please refer to textbooks already published.

Suggested readings 1) Kisslo. J. A.: Two-dimensional echocardiography, N. Y., Churchill Livingston, 1980.

2) Talano, J. V., Gardin, J. M.: Textbook of two-dimensional echocardiography, N. Y., Grune & Stratton, 1983.

3) Hagan, A. K., DiSessa, T. G., Bloos, C. M., Calleya, H. B. (eds): Two dimensional echocardiography, Boston, Little, Brown and Company, 1983.

4) Spencer, M. P. (ed): Cardiac Doppler Diagnosis, volume 2, Dordrecht, Martinus Nijhoff publishers, 1984.

5) Nanda, N. C. (ed): Doppler echocardiography, Tokyo, Igaku-shoin, 1985.

6) Hatle, L., Angelsen, B.: Doppler ultrasound in cardiology, 2nd ed., Philadelphia, Lea & Febiger, 1985.

7) Feigenbaum, H.: Echocardiography, 4th ed., Philadelphia, Lea & Febiger, 1986.

8) Rolendt, J. (ed): Color Doppler flow mapping, Dordrecht, Martinus Nijhoff Publishers, 1986.

Abbreviations and Symbols

Abd Ao	abdominal aorta
ACW	anterior chest wall
AML	anterior mitral leaflet
Ao (AO)	aorta
AoAW	anterior wall of aorta
AoPW	posterior wall of aorta
AoV	aortic valve
APM	anterior papillary muscle
Ar Ao	aortic arch
As Ao	ascending aorta
ATL	anterior tricuspid leaflet
BRA	brachiocephalic artery
CA	celiac artery
CS	coronary sinus
DAo	descending aorta
FA	femoral artery
FL	false lumen
FO	fossa ovalis
FV	femoral vein
HA	hepatic artery
HV	hepatic vein
IA	iliac artery
IAS	interatrial septum
IVC	inferior vena cava
IVS	interventricular septum
LA	left atrium
LAPW	posterior wall of left atrium
LCC	left coronary cusp
LMCA	left main coronary artery
LSCA	left subclavian artery
LV	left ventricle
LVIT	left ventricular inflow tract
LVOT	left ventricular outflow tract
LVPW	posterior wall of left ventricle
MO	mitral orifice
MPA	main pulmonary artery
MV	mitral valve
NCC	non coronary cusp
PA	pulmonary artery
PML	posterior mitral leaflet
PoV	portal vein
PPM	posterior papillary muscle
PTL	posterior tricuspid leaflet
Pulm V	pulmonary valve
PV (PVe)	pulmonary vein
RA	right atrium
RCC	right coronary cusp
RPA	right pulmonary artery
RPV	right pulmonary vein
RV	right ventricle
RVAW	anterior wall of right ventricle
RVe	renal vein
RVOT	right ventricular outflow tract
SA	splenic artery

SMA	superior mesenteric artery
STL	septal tricuspid leaflet
SVC	superior vena cava
TO	tricuspid orifice
TV	tricuspid valve

AN	aneurysm
Ao-prosthesis	aortic valve prosthesis
AR (AI)	aortic regurgitation (aortic insufficiency)
AS	aortic stenosis
AS·AR	aortic stenosis and regurgitation
ASD	atrial septal defect
AVR	aortic valve replacement
DORV	double outlet of right ventricle
ECD	endocardial cushion defect
En	entry
HOCM	hypertrophic obstructive cardiomyopathy
IE	infective endocarditis
IF	intimal flap
M-prosthesis	mitral valve prosthesis
MR (MI)	mitral regurgitation (mitral insufficiency)
MS	mitral stenosis
MS·MR	mitral stenosis and regurgitation
MVR	mitral valve replacement
OMC	open mitral commissurotomy
PA	pulmonary atresia
PDA	patent ductus arteriosus
PH	pulmonary hypertension
PS	pulmonary stenosis
regurg(flow)	regurgitation, regurgitant flow
REn	reentry
TAP	tricuspid annuloplasty
TOF	tetralogy of Fallot
TGA	transposition of great arteries
Th	thrombus
TL	true lumen
TR (TI)	tricuspid regurgitation (tricuspid insufficiency)
TS	tricuspid stenosis
Veg, VGE	vegetation
VSD	ventricular septal defect
VSP	ventricular septal perforation

AoP	systolic pressure of the aorta
AR-jet	aortic regurgitant jet
A wave	filling velocity following atrial systole
away(flow)	flow away from the transducer
B-mode	two-dimensional echocardiography
CWD (CW)	continuous-wave Doppler

LVEDP	left ventricular end-diastolic pressure
maxV	maximal velocity
meanV	mean velocity
max ΔP	maximal pressure gradient
mean ΔP	mean pressure gradient
MR-jet	jitral regurgitant jet
MVA	mitral vahe area
P	pressure
P 1/2 T	pressure half-time
PWD	pulsed-wave Doppler
Rev	reverberation
RVP	right ventricular systolic pressure
R wave	rapid diastolic filling velocity
sample	sample volume, sample site
T-inflow	inflow blood through tricuspid valve
toward(flow)	flow toward the transducer
TRjet	tricuspid regurgitant jet
2-D echo	two-dimensional echocardiography

Contents

Chapter 4　Cautions for Clinical Use of the Instrument
·· **Kanji Miura, Ryozo Omoto**

Chapter 5　Clinical Use of 2-D Doppler as the Third Generation of Technology in Echocardiography ···················· **Ryozo Omoto**

Chapter 6　Pitfalls and Artifacts ··························· **Shinichi Takamoto**

Chapter 7　2-D Doppler Images in Normal Hearts
·· **Ryozo Omoto, Shunei Kyo**

Index-titles of color atlas

X

Chapter 1 Clinical Significance and Prospects of "Real-Time Two-Dimensional Doppler Echocardiography"

1－1　Steps Toward Real-Time Blood-Flow Imaging

Various attempts have been made to achieve noninvasive imaging of intracardiac blood flow using ultrasound. One is contrast echocardiography first studied by Gramiak and co-workers[1]. This technique has been developed by improving contrast material, but it is not completely noninvasive and its use has generally been limited to imaging flow in the right heart. Another attempt at intracardiac blood-flow imaging is the application of multichannel or multigate pulsed-Doppler[2,3]. This method was developed by Fish[4], Tanaka[5], Reneman[6], Brandestini[7] and Matsuo et al[8]. Stevenson and Brandestini[9,10,11] added color-coding to a digital multigate Doppler system for visualization of intracardiac blood flow. All of these techniques have achieved real-time visualization of the velocity profile along only one ultrasound beam line of the M-mode echocardiogram. A number of studies have been reported by Kitabatake[12] and Chihara[13], on two-dimensional mapping of the intracardiac blood flow. The use of an off-line computer-based system[14,15] was attempted to obtain two-dimensional blood flow imaging, but it was still far from fulfilling the clinical requirement for real-time imaging of the intracardiac blood flow. The multichannel digital pulsed-Doppler method was inadequate to obtain real-time two-dimensional blood flow images mainly because the processing time required for spectral analysis was too long to handle the rate at which data were acquired. On the other hand, an application of the MTI[16] (moving target indication) method seemed to be a more effective approach for this purpose.

It was not until 1982 that a new technique for real-time imaging of the intracardiac blood flow that could be expected to meet the clinical requirements was developed. This technique was being studied separately by a group of the authors, that is, by Namekawa, Kasai and Koyano[17,18,19], as well as by Bommer's group[20,21]. Bommer's studies, as reported in 1982, showed that they were still at the stage of animal experiments and, in clinical cases, had succeeded in the imaging of tricuspid valvular regurgitation only through enhancement of signal levels by using contrast agents. The authors' group reported on the clinical application of real-time two-dimensional Doppler echocardiography (sometimes called 2-D Doppler, or color flow mapping) for visualization of intracardiac blood flow without the use of contrast agents in 1982, and within a short period had confirmed its practical value[22,23] and its diagnostic effectiveness in acquired valvular disease[24], congenital heart disease[25] and aortic aneurysms[26].

1－2　Prospects of "Real-Time Two-Dimensional Doppler Echocardiography"

In the short time since its introduction to the cardiovascular field, real-time two-dimensional Doppler echocardiography has demonstrably proved its usefulness in many cardiac centers[27-33].

Obtaining noninvasive real-time images of the intracardiac blood flow is of great clinical significance and may result in significant changes in the conventional diagnostic approaches in cardiology. Some examples of the specific diagnostic capabilities of this technique revealed by the authors' earlier investigation are: (1) imaging of valvular regurgitation and semi-quantitative evaluation of the severity of the regurgitation; (2) imaging of the intracardiac shunt; and (3) imaging of entry and/or reentry in dissecting aortic aneurysms. The information on blood flow is simultaneously pictured in a real-time image superimposed on the conventional two-dimensional echocardiogram. It is believed that information on blood flow which is easily and repeatedly obtained by a fully noninvasive method will undoubtedly exert influence on diagnostic steps in cardiology. The investigation by 2-D Doppler may yield the correct diagnosis on the first outpatient examination. It may, in some cases, permit diagnosis while omitting unnecessary ventriculography, or give an indication for cardiac catheterization or X-ray angiocardiography. In the case of a dissecting aortic aneurysm, for example, 2-D Doppler allows the possibility of a smooth progression from diagnosis to treatment. It offers the image of the dissecting aneurysm and entry on the ascending aorta, then immediately gives an indication for angiography under diagnosis of the DeBakey's type-1 dissection, and finally is used during the emergency operation. Under special circumstances, when a patient is in critically ill condition, 2-D Doppler findings alone may provide a sufficient indication for cardiac surgery without examination by cardiac catheterization.

In fact, the combined experience from many heart centers has convincingly shown the effectiveness of 2-D Doppler in the detection and diagnosis of valvular disease[24,35-39], and congenital defects[40-47]. The application of 2-D Doppler for evaluation of abnormal cardiovascular anatomy of the human fetus is another potentially important[48-51] application. Intraoperative use of 2-D Doppler with epicardial[52-55] and/or transesophageal[56,57] approaches has been found very useful especially in the immediate evaluation of the effect of cardiac surgery prior to chest closure.

The limitations of this technique must also be well understood. One limitation is that the present system is still ineffective on small arteries such as coronary arteries. In the limited areas of the surface of the heart, there is a good possibility of achieving the imaging of small arteries during surgery by the use of high-frequency ultrasound[58].

2-D Doppler is an entirely new modality in the sense that a variety of new ideas and techniques have arisen in the course of its development. It can, however, be used in almost the same way as conventional echocardiography. It appears to the user that intracardiac blood flow is simultaneously imaged using the same technique and method as used in conventional echocardiography. Continuous-wave Doppler as well as the spectral analysis that is done in the conventional pulsed-Doppler technique is of course available in the 2-D Doppler device. The 2-D Doppler system is equipped with all the functions of the conventional echocardiography and adds the unique capability of imaging intracardiac blood flow. If the intracardiac blood-flow image is poor or unnecessary, merely switch the function off; if it is helpful and necessary, it should be utilized. This system can be understood as a modality with a higher level of capability added to conventional Doppler echocardiography. One possible obstacle may be the cost.

2-D Doppler is an extension of echocardiography. For the time being, it is called "real-time two-dimensional Doppler echocardiography" but the authors expect that it will be simply called "echocardiography" in the near future without any mention of "real-time" or "Doppler". Just 12 or 13 years ago when real-time two-dimensional echocardiography was gaining in popularity, "real-time" and "two-dimensional" were necessary terms to distinguish it from the existing M-mode echocardiography. But now it has become commonly accepted that "echocardiography" includes both the M-mode and the two-dimensional echocardiography. The relationship between the pulsed Doppler and 2-D Doppler is considered analogous to that between "M-mode" and standard "two-dimensional imaging".

1-3 Terminology

As indicated the terms used seem to be greatly influenced by the historical background. It is absolutely necessary, however, to give a definite name to this technique as a new modality. The authors named it at the time of its first communication at the Japanese Circulation Society in April, 1983, like the title of this book, "Real-Time Two-Dimensional Doppler Echocardiography", and used, as its abbreviation, "2-D Doppler". Bommer and co-workers used the term "Real-Time Two-Dimensional Color-Flow Doppler" in 1982 when the technique of real-time imaging was still at the experimental level[20]. Brandestini and co-workers used the term "Color-coded Doppler" for the multigated pulsed Doppler method[10] at the same meeting. It is also well known that one of the conventional single sample volume methods with pulsed Doppler has been commonly referred to as "pulsed-Doppler Echocardiography"[3,58,59] or "Doppler Echocardiography". The survey of these usages show the difficulty of standardizing the term, but at present, the authors propose to adopt the terms introduced above, "Real-time two-dimensional Doppler echocardiography" and "2-D Doppler". Naturally, "color flow mapping (or imaging)", "color Doppler flow mapping (or imaging)", and "color Doppler Echocardiography" are understood to be synonymous with 2-D Doppler. Eventually there will be a need to standardize the term used.

1－4　Third Generation Echocardiography

It is well known that the development and rapid widespread application of 2-D Doppler have led to a third generation of technology in echocardiography. The first generation, M-mode echocardiography, appeared in the 1960s. In the 1970s, real-time two-dimensional echocardiography was developed, leading to the appearance of second generation systems. In the 1980s, real-time blood flow images have been obtained from third generation echocardiography systems. However, although the expression, "third generation echocardiography" is appropriate, it does not merely mean 2-D Doppler imaging: the term also implies the inclusion of all the Doppler technology developed previously.

These instruments are already being marketed by several manufacturers and within the next one to two years it can be expected that almost all of the standard echocardiography systems will have 2-D Doppler modes.

References

1) Gramiak, R., Shak, P. M. and Kramer, D. H.: Ultrasound cardiography: Contrast studies in anatomy and function. Radiology, 92: 939-948, 1969.

2) Baker, D. W.: Pulsed ultrasound Doppler blood-flow sensing. IEEE Trans. Sonics Ultrasonics, SU-17: 170-185, 1970.

3) Baker, S. W., Rubenstein, S. A., and Lorch, G. S.: Pulsed Doppler echocardiography: Principle and application. Am. J. Med., 63: 69-80, 1977.

4) Fish, P. J.: Multichannel, direction resolving Doppler angiography. 2nd European Congress of Ultrasonics in Medicine, 72: 1975. Abstract

5) Tanaka, M., Terasawa, Y., and Konno, K.: Measurement of the intracardiac blood flow velocity distribution and flow pattern by the M-sequence modulated ultrasonic Doppler method. Proceedings of the 30th Meeting of the Japan Society of Ultrasonics in Medicine, 231-232, 1976. Abstract

6) Reneman, R. S., Hoeks, A., Slot, H. B., and Merode, T.: The on-line recording of velocity profiles and its potential in the diagnosis of peripheral arterial lesions. In Noninvasive Assessment of the Cardiovascular System. Edited by Dietrich, E. B. PSG Inc., 1982.

7) Brandestini, M. A., Howard, E. A., Weile, E. B., Stevenson, J. G., and Eyer, M. K.: The synthesis of echo and doppler in M-mode and sector scan. Proceedings of Annual Meeting of the American Institute of Ultrasound in Medicine: 125, 1979.

8) Matsuo, H., Inoue, M., Kitabatake, A., Hayashi, T., Asao, M., Terao, Y., Mishima, M., Senda, S., Shimazu, T., Tanouchi, J., Morita, H., Abe, H., Chihara, K., Hirayama, M., Inokuchi, S., and Sakurai, Y.: Analysis of Doppler flow signal by winograd fourier transform algorithm-detection of intracardiac flow dynamics by computer-based ultrasonic multi-gated pulsed doppler flowmeter. Proceedings of the 34th Meeting of the Japan Society of Ultrasonics in Medicine, 34: 3-4, 1978. Abstract

9) Stevenson, J. G.: Aortic and pulmonic insufficiency, evaluated by pulsed doppler echocardiography, and digital multigate doppler echocardiography. Atti del Congress Internazionale di Ecocardiografia, Edizioni Cepi (Roma) 202-216, 1980.

10) Stevenson, J.G., Kawabori, I., and Brandestini, M.A.: A twenty-month experience comparing conventional pulsed-doppler echocardiography and color-coded digital multigate doppler, for detection of atrioventricular valve regurgitation, and its severity. In Echocardiography. Edited by

H. Rijsterborgh, 399-407, Hague, Martinus Nijhoff Publishes, 1981.

11) Stevenson, J. G., Kawabori, I., and Brandestini, M. A.: Color-coded vistualization of flow within ventricular septal defects: Implications for peak pulmonary artery pressure. Am. J. Cardiol., 49: 944, 1982. Abstract

12) Kitabatake, K., Inoue, M., Asao, M., Mishima, M., Tanouchi, J., Masuyama, T., Hori, M., Abe, H., Chihara, K., Sakurai, H., Senda, S., Morita, H., and Matsuo, H.: Non-invasive visualization of intracardiac blood flow in human heart using computer-aided pulsed doppler technique. Clinical Hemorheology, 1: 85-91, 1982.

13) Chihara, K.: A data processing of Doppler signal. Proceedings of the 40th Metting of the Japan Scociety of Ultrasonics in Medicine, 13-14, 1982. Abstract

14) Asao, M., Matsuo, H., Kitabatake, A., Mishima, M., Tanouchi, J., Shimazu, T., Senda, S., Morita, H., Masuyama, T., Inoue, M., and Abe, H.: Application of computer-based ultrasonic multigated pulsed doppler flowmeter to flow mapping in clinical case. Proceedings of the 38th Meeting of the Japan Society of Ultrasonics in Medicine, 13-14, 1982. Abstract

15) Morita, H., Senda, S., Matsuo, H., Kitabatake, A., Asao, M., Tanouchi, J., Masuyama, T., and Abe, H.: Intracardiac flow visualization of regurgitation by a computer-based ultrasound multigated pulsed Doppler flowmeter, Am. J. Cardiol., 49: 943, 1982.

16) Angelsen, B. A. J., Kristofferen, K.: On ultrasonic MTI measurement of velocity profiles in blood flow, IEEE transactions on biomedical engineering. BME-26: 665-671, 1979.

17) Namekawa, K., Kasai, C., Tsukamoto, M., and Koyano, A.: Imaging of blood flow using autocorrelation. Ultrasound in Medicine and Biology, 8: 138, 1982. Abstract

18) Kasai, C., Namekawa, K., Koyano, A., and Omoto, R.: Real-time two-dimensional flood flow imaging using an autocorrelation technique. EEE Tans. Sonics Ultrasonics, SU-32: 458-464, 1985.

19) Omoto, R. Kasai, C.: Basic principles of Doppler color flow imaging. Echocardiography, 3: 463-473, 1986.

20) Bommer, W., Miller, L.: Real-time two-dimensional color-flow Doppler flow imaging in the diagnosis of cardiovascular disease. Am. J. Cardiol., 49: 944, 1982. Abstract

21) Bommer, W. J.: Basic principles of flow imaging. Echocardiography, 2: 501-509, 1985.

22) Omoto, R., Yokote, Y., Takamoto, S., Tamura, F., Asano, H., Namekawa, K., Kasai, C., Tsukamoto, M., and Koyano, A.: Clinical significance of newly developed real-time intracardiac two-dimensional blood flow imaging system (2-D Doppler). Jpn. Circ. J., 47: 191, 1983. Abstract

23) Omoto, R., Yokote, Y., Takamoto, S., Kyo, S., Ueda, K., Asano, H., Yoshikawa, Y., Iijima, S., Katabami, T., and Hidai, T.: Study on clinical application of real-time intracardiac two-dimensional blood flow imaging system. Proceedings of the 42th Meeting of the Japan Society of Ultrusonics in Medicine, 305-306, 1983. Abstract

24) Omoto, R., Yokote, Y., Takamoto, S., Kyo, S., Ueda, K., Asano, H., Namekawa, K., Kasai, C., Kondo, Y., and Koyano, A.: The development of real-time two-dimensional doppler echocardiography and its clinical siginificance in acquired valvular disease with special reference to the evaluation of valvular regurgitation. Jpn. Heart J., 25: 325-340, 1984.

25) Kyo, S., Takamoto, S., Ueda, K., Emoto, H., Tamura, F., Asano, H., Yokote, Y., Omoto, R., and Takanawa, E.: Clinical significance of newly developed real-time two-dimensional doppler echocardiography (2-D Doppler) in congenital heart diseases with special reference to the assessment of the intracardiac shunts. Proceedings of the 43th Meeting of the Japan Society of Ultrasonics in Medicine, 465-466, 1983. Abstract

26) Takamoto, S., Asano, H., Kyo, S., Ueda, K., Omoto, R., and Kondo, Y.: Experimental analysis of doppler motion ghost signal by real time two-dimensional doppler echocardiography system. Proceedings of the 43th Meeting of the Japan Socity of Ultuasonics in Medicine, 43: 435-436, 1983. Abstract

27) Sahn, D. J.: Real-time two-dimensional doppler echocardiography flow mapping. Circulation, 71: 849-853, 1985.

28) Schoenfeld, M. R.: Color-coded, real-time, two-dimensional doppler echocardiographic mapping of intracardiac blood flow. Journal of Cardiovascular Ultrasonography, 4: 3-4, 1985.

29) Miyatake, K., Okamoto, M., Kinosita, N., Izumi, S., Owa, M., Takao, S., Sakakibara, H., and Nimura, Y.: Clinical applications of a new type of real-time two-dimensional flow imaging system. Am. J. Cardiol., 54: 857-868, 1984.

30) Sahn, D. J., Valdes-Cruz, L. M.: New advances in two-dimensional doppler echocardiography.

Progress in Cardiovascular Diseases, 18 : 367-382, 1986.

31) DeMaria, A. N., Smith, M. D., and Kwan, O. L. : Doppler flow imaging : Another step in the evolution of cardiac ultrasound. Echocardiography, 2 : 495- 500, 1985.

32) Stewart, W. J., Levine, R. A., Main, J., and King, M. E. : Initial experience with color-coded doppler flow mapping. Echocardiography, 2 : 511- 521, 1985.

33) Yoshikawa, J., Kato, H., Yoshida, K., Asaka, T., Yanagihara, K., Okumachi, F., Shiratori, K., and Koizumi, K. : Real-time two-dimensional doppler echocardiographic diagnosis of aortic regurgitation in the presence of a mitral prosthesis. Circulation, 70 : (Suppl. II), 39, 1984. Abstract

34) Referene deleted.

35) Miyatake, K., Izumi, S., Okamoto, M., Kinoshita, N., Asanuma, H., Nakagawa, H., Yamamoto, K., Takamiya, M., Sakakibara, H., and Nimura, Y. : Semiquantitative grading of severity of mitral regurgitation by real-time two-dimensional doppler flow imaging technique. J. Am. Coll. Cardiol., 7 : 82-88, 1986.

36) Suzuki, Y., Kambara, H., Kadoya, K., Tamaki, S., Yamazato, A., Nohara, R., Osakada, G., Kawai, C., Kubo, S., and Karaguchi, T. : Detection and evaluation of tricuspid regurgitation using a real-time, two-dimensional, color-coded, doppler flow imaging system : Comparison with contrast two-dimensional echocardiography and right ventriculography. Am. J. Cardiol., 57 : 811-815, 1986.

37) Helmcke, F., Nanda, N., Hsiung, M. C., Sato, B., Adey, C. K., Goyal, R. G., and Gatewood, Jr., R. P. : Color Doppler assessment of mitral regurgitation with orthogonal planes. Circulation, 75 : 175-183, 1987.

38) Bouchard, A., Yock, P. G., Schiller, N. B., Newlands, J. S., Massie, B. M., Botvinick, E. H., Greenberg, B., and Cheitlin, M. D. : Quantitation of chronic aortic insufficiency using color doppler flow mapping. Circulation, 72 : (Suppl. III), 100, 1985. Abstract

39) Nishimura, R. A., Tajik, A. J., Reeder, G. S., and Seward, J. B. : Evaluation of hypertrophic cardiomyopathy by doppler color flow imaging : Initial observations. Mayo Clin. Proc., 61 : 631-639, 1986.

40) Kyo, S., Omoto, R., Takamoto, S., Ueda, K., Emoto, H., Asano, H., and Yokote, Y. : Real-time two-dimensional doppler echocardiography in congenital heart disease. J. Cardiography, 14 : 785-801, 1984.

41) Swensson, R. E., Sahn, D. J., and Valdes-Cruz, L. M. : Color flow Doppler mapping in congenital heart disease. Echocardiography, 2 : 545-549, 1985.

42) Ortiz, E., Robinson, P. J., Degnfield, J. E., Franklin, R., Macartney, F. J., and Wyse, R. K. H. : Localisation of ventricular septal defects by simultaneous display of superimposed color doppler and cross sectional echocardiography images. Br. Heart J., 54 : 53-60, 1985.

43) Ito, K., Suzuki, O., Yano, S., Shiraishi, H., and Yanagisawa, M. : Detection of shunt flow in total anomalous pulmonary venous connection using 2D-doppler echocardiography. Angiology, 36 : 414-418, 1985.

44) Suzuki, Y., Kambara, H., Kadota, K., Tamaki, S., Yamazato, A., Nohara, R., Osakada, G., Kawai, C., Kubo, S., and Karaguchi, T. : Detection of intracardiac shunt flow in atrial septal defect using a real-time two-dimensional color-coded doppler flow imaging system and comparison with contrast two-dimensional echocardiography. Am. J. Cardiol., 56 : 347-350, 1985.

45) Vitarelli, A. : Two-dimensional, contrast, and doppler echocardiography in congenital heart disease-diagnosis possibilities and complementary roles. Journal of cardiovascular ultrasonography, 4 : 117-137, 1985.

46) Reeder, G. S., Currie, P. J., Hagler, D. J., Tajik, A. J., and Seward, J. B. : Use of doppler techniques (continuous-wave, pulse-wave, and color flow imaging) in the noninvasive hemodynamic assessment of congenital heart disease. Mayo Clin. Proc., 61 : 725-744, 1986.

47) Satomi, G., Takao, A., Momma, K., Mori, K., Ando, M., Touyama, K., Konishi, T., Tomimatsu, H., Nakazawa, M., and Nakamura, K. : Detection of the drainage site in anomalous pulmonary venous connection by two-dimensional doppler color flow-mapping echocardiography. Heart and Vessels, 2 : 41-44, 1986.

48) De Vore, G. R., Hornstein, J., and Siassi, B., Platt, L. D. : Doppler color flow mapping in use in the prenatal diagnosis of congenital heart disease in the human fetus. Echocardiography, 2 : 551-557, 1985.

49) Friedman, D. M., Rutkowski, M. : Color flow mapping in the fetus : A new two-dimensional doppler technique. Journal of cardiovascular ultrasonography, 4 : 171-174, 1985.

50) Redel, D. A. Wippermann, J. A. : Prenatal diagnosis of heart disease using Doppler flow imaging. Proceedings of International Symposium on Doppler Echocardiography (Munich), 34, 1986.

51) Motoyama, T., Kyo, S., Ishida, T., Chin, I., Muramatsu, T., Dohi, and Y., Koshizuka, H. : Real-time visualization of fetus cardiovascular blood flow by color flow mapping doppler echocardiography. Japanese Circulation J., 49 : 851, 1985. Abstract

52) Takamoto, S., Kyo, S., Adachi, H., Mastumura, M., Yokoto, Y., and Omoto, R. : Intraoperative color flow mapping by real-time two-dimensional doppler echocardiography for evaluation of valvular and congenital heart disease and vascular disease. J. Thorac Cardiovasc. Surg., 90 : 802-812, 1985.

53) Maurer, G., Czer, L., De Robertis, M., Kass, R., Lee, M., Chauu, A., Gray, R., and Matloff, J. : Intraoperative doppler color flow mapping in valvular and congenital heart disease. Circulation, 72 : (Suppl. III), 206, 1985. Abstract

54) Omoto, R. : Intraoperative Echocardiography. Presentation at the 10th World Congress of Cardiology, Washington, D. C., 1986.

55) Bogunovic, N., Phillippi, H., Mannebach, H., and Gleichmann, U. : Color coded two-dimensional Doppler echocardiography in disease of the aorta. Proceedings of International Symposium on Doppler Echocardiography, 42, Munich, 1986.

56) Goldman, M. E., Thys, D., Ritter, S., and Hillel, Z. : Trans-esophageal real time Doppler flow imaging; A new method for intraoperative evaluation. J. Am. Coll. Cardiol., 7(II) : 1, 1986. Abstract

57) Kyo, S., Takamoto, S., Matsumura, M., Yokote, Y., and Omoto, R. : Color flow mapping visualization of coronary blood flow using transesophageal transducer. Proceedings of the 49th Meeting of the Japan Society of Ultrasonics in Medicine, 247-248, 1986. Abstract

58) Young, J. B., Quinones, M. A., Waggoner, A. D., and Miller, R. R. : Diagnosis and quantification of aortic stenosis with pulsed Doppler echocardiography. Am. J. Cardiol., 45 : 987-994, 1980.

59) Ciobanu, M., Abbasi, A. S., Allen, M., Hermer, A., and Spellberg, R. : Pulsed Doppler echocardiography in the diagnosis and estimation of severity of aortic insufficiency. Am. J. Cardiol. 49 : 339-343, 1982.

Chapter 2   Principle

2—1   Introduction

In a conventional pulsed Doppler device, blood flow velocity is obtained by analyzing Doppler signals using frequency analysis. To do this, about 20ms are required for only one sample volume data, and therefore obtaining a two-dimensional flow image in real-time is not possible. However, in two-dimensional Doppler (2-D Doppler), the blood flow velocity is estimated directly from the echo signals successively. Fig. 2-1 shows the echo waveforms when electromagnetic waves are transmitted twice in succession. The basic principle of 2-D Doppler is almost the same as that of the radar system. In Fig. 2-1 echoes from a building and an airplane are shown for two wave transmissions, (a) shows the echoes for the first wave transmission and (b) shows those for the second transmission. The echo waveforms from the building are always the same because the building is stationary, while the echo waveform or the retardation time from an airplane is different every time a pulse is transmitted, because the airplane is moving. When echo signals (b) for the second transmission are subtracted from those (a) for the first transmission, signals from stationary targets become null and only the echoes from moving targets are extracted. The basic principle of 2-D Doppler is thus to estimate flow velocity directly from succeeding received signals[1,2,3]. Details are given in the following sections.

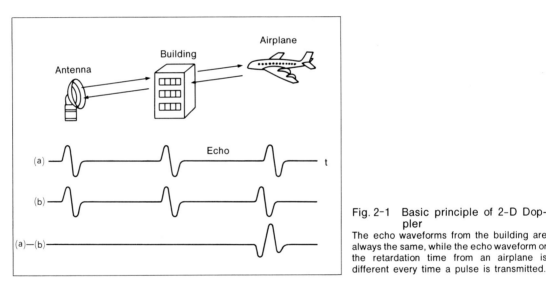

Fig. 2-1 Basic principle of 2-D Doppler
The echo waveforms from the building are always the same, while the echo waveform or the retardation time from an airplane is different every time a pulse is transmitted.

2—2   Basics of Pulsed Doppler System

1. Doppler effect*)
The Doppler effect is a phenomenon in which the sound wave frequency changes due to movements of the sound source and the observer. The frequency is expressed by the Eq. 2-1:

$$f_1 = f_0 \frac{c+v}{c-u} \qquad\qquad 2\text{-}1$$

where c is the sound velocity, f_0 is the frequency of transmission wave, v is the velocity of the observer's movement and u is the velocity of movement of the sound source. The

*) Johann Christian Doppler (1803-1853) was born in Salzburg. The Doppler effect was first presented in his paper "On the Colored Light of Double Stars and Some Other Heavenly Bodies" published in 1842[4].

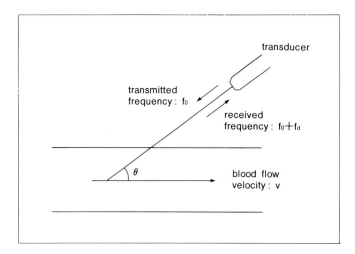

Fig. 2-2 Reflection of ultrasound from blood
The frequency of received wave is shifted by $2f_0v \cdot \cos\theta/c$.

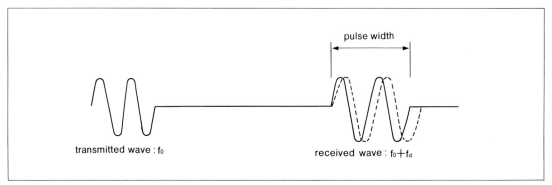

Fig. 2-3 Doppler effect in pulsed Doppler system
It is difficult to detect the frequency shift of less than 0.1% within a very short pulse width.

direction in which the sound source and the observer come closer is the positive direction. In a Doppler device using the echo method, a sound wave transmitted from a transducer reaches a blood cell as the observer and makes it vibrate. The vibrated blood cell acts as another sound source and generates a sound wave which can be detected by the same transducer. Therefore, when the sound wave reflected by the blood cell moving at velocity v is detected by the transducer, the frequency is determined by Eq. 2-1 where u=v. In general, the blood flow has a maximum velocity of a few m/s and the velocity of sound in the human body is about 1,500 m/s. Thus, applying the condition of c≫v to Eq. 2-1 results in the following equation :

$$f_d = f_1 - f_2 \approx 2f_0 \frac{v}{c} \qquad\qquad 2\text{-}2$$

The velocity v is the velocity in the direction of sound wave propagation. If the angle between the blood flow and the ultrasound beam is as shown in Fig. 2-2, Eq. 2-2 can be replaced with Eq. 2-3, which is a very important formula to show the basis of the Doppler effect :

$$f_d = 2f_0 \frac{v \cdot \cos\theta}{c} \qquad\qquad 2\text{-}3$$

Generally, in the CW (continuous wave) Doppler, the shift frequency f_d is obtained on the basis of the above-mentioned Doppler effect to allow calculation of the flow velocity. However, in the pulsed Doppler system, it is very difficult to detect Doppler frequency f_d from one transmission echo signal, because the pulse width is extremely short. This is shown in Fig. 2-3. For instance, the Doppler shift is only a few KHz at maximum in an ultrasonic wave frequency of a few MHz, which means that a shift of less than 0.1% must be detected. At present, it is very difficult to achieve detection at this level within a pulse width which contains only a few waves. Therefore, the pulsed Doppler system does not detect the Doppler frequency in the strict sense. However, apart from a discussion of its physical characteristics, a brief description of a mathematical explanation of the pulsed Doppler system, similar to that given for the CW Doppler system will be provided.

In the pulsed method, pulses of an ultrasound wave are transmitted at intervals of T sec. and the returned wave is received during the intermission of sound transmission. As the returned sound wave is delayed by the distance of travel from the sound source to the receiver, a two-dimensional image is available by scanning the sound beams in sequence. If the distance between the transducer and target is assumed to be R, the sound wave transmitted from the transducer is reflected by the target and received by the transducer again after traveling the distance of 2R. Therefore, the time which elapses from transmission to reception is expressed by 2R/c. If the target is moving at velocity v toward the transducer, the distance to the target at the nth transmission of the sound wave is expressed by R-vnT. Thus, the time between transmission and reception is 2(R-vnT)/c. If the transmission sound frequency is f_0, the phase delay of the received wave against the first transmission wave is expressed by the following equation:

$$\varphi_0 = 2\pi f_0 \left(-\frac{2R}{c}\right) \qquad\qquad 2\text{-}4$$

Similarly, the phase delay of the received wave for the nth transmission is expressed by:

$$\varphi_n = 2\pi f_0 \left(-\frac{2(R - v \cdot nT)}{c}\right)$$

$$= \varphi_0 + 2\pi f_d nT \qquad\qquad 2\text{-}5$$

Fig. 2-4 shows the relationship between the above two formulae. Because $2\pi f_0 nT = 2N\pi$ (N : integer) when f_0 is a multiple of the PRF (Pulse Repetition Frequency) $f_r = 1/T$, Eq. 2-5 can be rewritten as follows:

$$\varphi_n = 2\pi (f_0 + f_d)nT + \varphi_0 \qquad\qquad 2\text{-}6$$

Eq. 2-6 represents the phase delay of the nth recieved wave against the first transmission wave and this means that the same result is obtained as if f_0 is frequency-shifted by f_d.

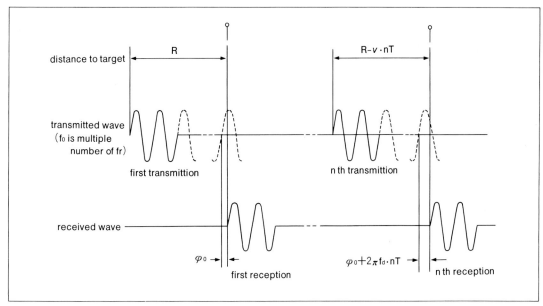

Fig. 2-4　Relation between transmission and reception
The phase of received wave is known by expanding the transmitted wave.

In Eq. 2-6, if nT is replaced with time t which continuously changes, the result is exactly the same as the case of a continuous wave. As the mathematical handling of the continuous wave is easier, the formula for a continuous wave is often used to analyze echo signals, even for the pulsed Doppler system.

2. Phase

In the previous section, it was explained that the measurment of Doppler signal is possible by examining the phases of received waves against that of each transmission wave. Let us consider this further. When a wave signal with amplitude A is considered, it can be taken as a point vector that rotates in a counterclockwise direction on the circumference of a circle with radius A. If the wave frequency is constant, the vector rotates at the same speed on the circumference. The abscissa (x-axis) is indicated by a real number and the ordinate (y-axis) is indicated by an imaginary number. A change of the imaginary number component of the rotating vector is expressed by a sinusoidal wave and that of the real number component is expressed by a cosine wave as shown in Fig. 2-5. In this case, the rotation angle φ of the rotating vector is called the phase angle or simply the phase. One cycle (period) of the sine wave or cosine wave corresponds to a complete vector rotation of the moving vector on the circle's circumference or it equals 2π as can be seen from Fig. 2-5. When the signal frequency is f, the angular frequency is $2\pi f$, and the phase angle at time t is $2\pi ft$. The phase difference between sine and cosine waves is $90°$.

When a signal frequency f is frequency-shifted by f_d by a Doppler effect, the rotation speed of the vector is different in angular frequency by $2\pi f_d$. The CW Doppler system directly detects the difference of rotation speed as previously described. In the pulsed Doppler system, the phase of a received wave against that of a transmission wave is expressed by the difference of the rotating vector as shown in Fig. 2-4. The angle difference corresponding to the positional difference is indicated by Eq.2-5. Fig. 2-6 shows the above condition. As n advances 1,2, ... starting from the initial phase[*] at n=0, the vector position

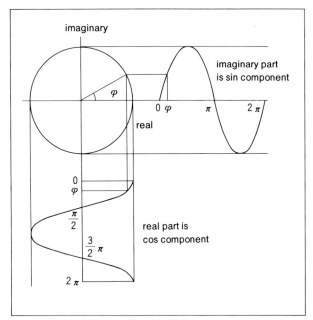

Fig. 2-5 Phase
Signal is a rotating vector of a circle. The radius is amplitude, rotating speed is frequency and the angle from the x-axis is phase.

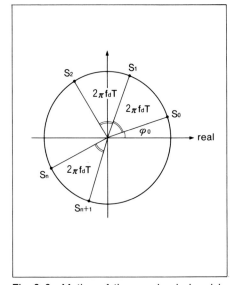

Fig. 2-6 Motion of the received signal in pulsed Doppler
The first received signal is S_0. The second signal reaches S_1 after rotating several times. The phase difference between S_0 and S_1 is the same as the one which is produced by Doppler effect.

[*] An actual received signal reaches position S_n after rotating several times as previously explained. In this case, the rotation is always in a counterclockwise direction. However, as only the final positions S_1, S_2, ... S_n are detected at pulse reception, the shift frequency of the blood flow receding from the transducer is indicated by a negative value and the detection signal rotation is clockwise.

changes to S_1, S_2, ... in sequence. The phase difference of the signal which is received is expressed by $2\pi f_d T$. If the phase of the received signal against that of the transmission signal is known at each pulse transmission, the Doppler frequency f_d can be estimated from Eq. 2-5.

When the value of phase differnce $2\pi f_d T$ exceeds π, it becomes ambiguous whether the rotation direction of the signal is counterclockwise (approaching blood flow) or clockwise (receding blood flow). Since the maximum detectable phase difference is π, the maximum detectable shift frequency is:

$$f_{d\ max} = \frac{1}{2T} = \frac{f_r}{2} \qquad\qquad 2\text{-}7$$

From the above formula, it is known that the maximum detectable frequency is half of the pulse repetition frequency f_r. If the Doppler frequency exceeds this value, the signal is recognized as if the signal vector is rotating in the reverse direction. This phenomenon is called "aliasing".

2-3 Basic Principle of Two-Dimensional Doppler

1. Differences compared with the conventional PW Doppler system

The main difference of 2-D Doppler from PW Doppler (generally, PW Doppler is a generic name for the pulsed Doppler system, but in this context it implies the conventional pulsed Doppler system which displays the frequency spectrum.) exists in the method of detecting frequency shift f_d. The 2-D Doppler method directly detects the phase difference $2\pi f_d T$ between two successively received echo signals as shown in Fig. 2-6. That is , if two echo signals S_n and S_{n+1} are known, the phase shift is measured. This was made possible by advances in digital technology.

On the one hand, in PW Doppler, the rotation speed f_d is estimated from about 100 points such as S_1, S_2 ... S_n which occur serially. To make this estimation, usually the FFT (Fast Fourier Transform) or the Chirp Z Transform are used. They enable display of a detailed distribution of the vector rotation, and they are called spectrum analysis. A vector rotation at constant speed results in a spectrum with a narrow frequency band, while that of variable speed results in a spectrum with a wide frequency band. Generally in frequency spectrum analysis, the longer the signal observation time the better is the resulting frequency resolution. This means that a better frequency resolution is achieved when the number of sample points S_1, S_2, ... S_n is increased. From clinical experiences, a measurement time of at least about 20 ms is required. Therefore this method is not practical for a 2-D Doppler, because about one second is needed to obtain one frame image. For this reason, PW Doppler is used only in the M-mode. In the M-mode, it is possible to obtain the velocity profile of depth direction from the spectrum analysis data providing many sample points, which is called the multi-channel method[5,6]. As the method requires analysis of frequency at each point in the depth direction to obtain the velocity profile, many analyzers with multiple channels must be prepared, and therefore the scale of electronic circuitry increases.

2. Two-dimensional Doppler method

The 2-D Doppler method directly detects the phase difference between consecutively received echo signals. This can be achieved by detecting the phase in Fig. 2-4, i.e., the time difference of the signals. However, the direct detection of phase is very difficult in practice, since the measurement must be made with a resolution of a few nano seconds ($1ns = 10^{-9}$ sec.). A typical alternative approach is the quadrature detection method in which the received signal is separated into the sine and cosine wave components as shown in Fig. 2-7. This is achieved by multiplying signals $\sin(2\pi f_0 t)$ and $\cos(2\pi f_0 t)$ with the received echo signal and by eliminating the high frequency component with a low-pass filter. This process is expressed by Eqs. 2-7 and 2-8 :

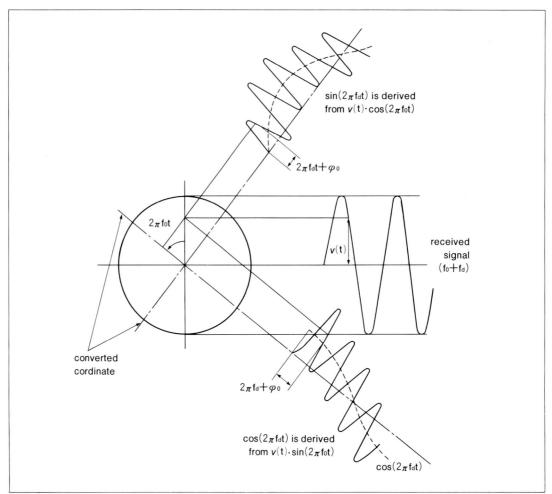

Fig. 2-7   Quadrature detection
The received signal is separated into the sine and cosine wave components.

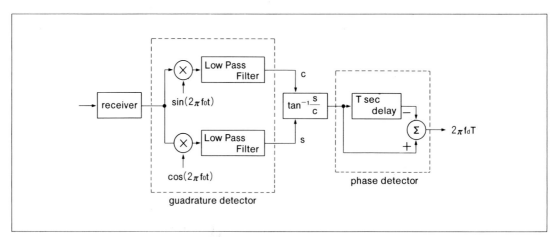

Fig. 2-8   Block diagram of the basic 2-D Doppler system

$$v_{in} \cdot \sin(2\pi f_0 t) = \sin(2\pi(f_0+f_d)t+\varphi_0) \cdot \sin(2\pi f_0 t)$$

$$= \frac{1}{2}\cos(2\pi f_d t+\varphi_0) - \frac{1}{2}\cos(2\pi 2f_0 t+\varphi_1) \qquad 2\text{-}7$$

$$v_{in} \cdot \cos(2\pi f_0 t) = \sin(2\pi(f_0+f_d)t+\varphi_0) \cdot \cos(2\pi f_0 t)$$

$$= \frac{1}{2}\sin(2\pi f_d t+\varphi_0) + \frac{1}{2}\sin(2\pi 2f_0 t+\varphi_1) \qquad 2\text{-}8$$

This operation converts the received signal to two quadrature Doppler signals with the sine wave and cosine wave components. This operation is called the quadrature detection method. The advantage of this method is that the hardware for following signal processing is less complex, since the converted Doppler signals are within the range of audio frequency.

After the separation of the received echo signal into the sine and cosine wave components, the phase of the signal is obtained by the following equation:

$$\varphi_n = \tan^{-1}\left(\frac{\sin(2\pi f_d nT + \varphi_0)}{\cos(2\pi f_d nT + \varphi_0)} \right)$$

$$= 2\pi f_d nT + \varphi_0 \qquad\qquad 2\text{-}9$$

Then if the phase difference between the two consecutive received signals is known, a value proportional to the velocity can be obtained by Eq. 2-10:

$$\varphi_{n+1} - \varphi_n = 2\pi f_d T \qquad\qquad 2\text{-}10$$

Fig. 2-8 shows a block diagram of the operation. In practice the signal is digital-converted after quadrature detection and the operation to obtain the value of $\tan^{-1}$ is performed digitally. In this manner, many channels and complex circuits which are required in the multi-channel method are not necessary to determine the velocity profile of the depth direction. In this method, signal processing can be achieved serially instead of parallel processing which is performed in the multi-channel method. In addition, as f_d can be estimated by two sound transmissions in principle, 2-D Doppler can be performed by high-speed scanning.

2-4 Implementation of Two-Dimensional Doppler System

As described in the previous section, a practical 2-D Doppler system can be made by using the principle shown in Fig. 2-8. Here in this section, an actual system that has been made available will be described[7].

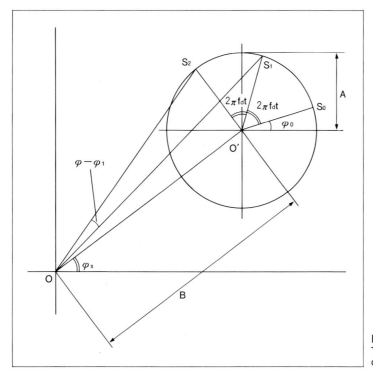

Fig. 2-9 Need for MTI filter
The distance B represents the clutter component of the received signal.

1. MTI filter

The MTI (Moving Target Indication) filter is also called the Delay Line Filter or Stationary Canceller. As it is used to eliminate signals caused by wall motion, it may also be called the Wall Motion Filter. As the name indicates, the MTI filter extracts only the signals from moving targets. As previously described, basic 2-D Doppler detects the phase difference $2\pi f_d T$ of consecutively receirved echo signals at each transmission. In this case, if the target is stationary, the MTI filter is not needed as $f_d=0$. However, when the 2-D Doppler system is applied to the human body, this kind of filter has an important role because the echo from blood is superimposed on a strong tissue echoe such as that from blood vessels and the heart wall. This aspect is shown in Fig. 2-9. The point O' which is the center of the blood signal vector is located at a distance B from the original coordinate O. This B represents the tissue echo signal such as a blood vessel. If the echo is from fixed tissue, the position of O' is stationary. However, when it is in motion, such as the heart wall, the point O' itself is rotating according to the moving velocity of the heart wall. The phase to be detected is expressed by Eq. 2-11:

$$\varphi_n = \tan^{-1} \frac{A \cdot \sin(2\pi f_d nT) + B \cdot \sin \varphi_s}{A \cdot \cos(2\pi f_d nT) + B \cdot \sin \varphi_s} \qquad 2\text{-}11$$

In this case, the detected phase difference between the received signals is $\varphi_{n+1} - \varphi_n$ but not $2\pi f_d T$. The stronger the fixed tissue echo over the blood echo, the larger is the value of B over A, and $\varphi_{n+1} - \varphi_n$ approaches zero. This means that blood flow information is not detected because it is buried in the fixed tissue echo. Unnecessary echos from blood vessels and the heart wall, i.e., the B components in Fig. 2-9 are generically called clutter.

The purpose of the MTI filter is to eliminate clutter. The simplest configuration of the MTI filter is shown in Fig. 2-10. Its operation is to subtract echo signals for consecutive sound receptions. It will be noted that when the signal processing shown in Fig. 2-10 is performed on the sine and cosine wave components, the tissue echo component B of Fig. 2-9 is eliminated. Fig. 2-11 (2) shows the characteristics of the filter where the sensitivity of f_d varies according to frequency. To improve this defect, various filters have been developed.

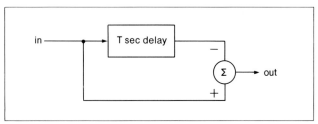

Fig. 2-10 Block diagram of the simplest MTI filter

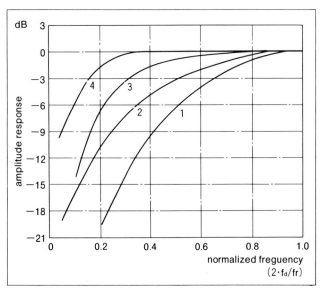

Fig. 2-11 Frequency characteristics of MTI filter

Frequency is normalized by $f_r/2$. (2) shows the characteristics of the filter shown in Fig. 2-10

Fig. 2-11 (1,3,4) shows some of them. When designing a filter not only the characteristics of frequency response, but also the time response must be considered carefully, but a detailed discussion of it is omitted[8,9].

2. Autocorrelation

In the present 2-D Doppler system, an autocorrelation technique is used, and Fig. 2-12 shows the operation principle. By the correlation operation, phase difference $\varphi = \varphi_2 - \varphi_1$ is directly obtained from signal S_2 with phase φ_2 and signal S_1 with phase φ_1. The operation is performed by Eq.2-12 :

$$
\begin{aligned}
\tan \varphi &= \frac{\sin \varphi}{\cos \varphi} = \frac{\sin(\varphi_2 - \varphi_1)}{\cos(\varphi_2 - \varphi_1)} \\
&= \frac{\sin \varphi_2 \cdot \cos \varphi_1 - \cos \varphi_2 \cdot \sin \varphi_1}{\cos \varphi_2 \cdot \cos \varphi_1 + \sin \varphi_2 \cdot \sin \varphi_1} \\
&= \frac{x_1 y_2 - x_2 y_1}{x_1 x_2 + y_1 y_2}
\end{aligned}
\qquad \text{2-12}
$$

Since x and y of Eq. 2-12 are the cosine and sine wave components of the Doppler signal obtained by the quadrature detector, the resultant signal in Eq. 2-12 is obtained by the system shown in Fig. 2-13. In the description in section 2-3, the phase of the received signal is detected first after which the phase difference between consecutive received signals is then obtained. In autocorrelation, the signals are first converted into a signal with the phase difference, and the phase of the converted signal is then detected. The entire system is shown in Fig. 2-14. The method used is different, but the same result as shown in Fig. 2-8 is achieved.

3. Restrictions on two-dimensional Doppler

A velocity profile in the depth direction is available by using a system shown in Fig. 2-8 or Fig. 2-14, without using parallel multi-channel operation. Since an MTI filter is used, the minimum number of sound transmissions in the same direction is three. However, in practice, an additional number of sound transmissions in the same direction is used to improve the flow image quality. This is because noise is reduced by averaging the flow information.

In 2-D Doppler, the frame rate or the view angle for one frame image is decreased compared with those for a black/white image, because a number of sound pulses must be transmitted in the same direction. Fig. 2-15 shows the relation between these, when 128 raster lines are scanned for a 90° view angle and the PRF is 4KHz. This condition corresponds to 18cm of diagnostic distance. The number of sound transmissions in a single

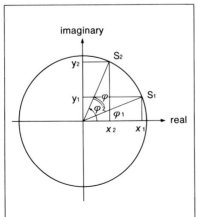

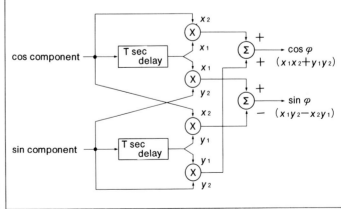

Fig. 2-12 Schematic understanding of autocorrelation.
Autocorrelation of S_1 and S_2 is the signal with the phase φ.

Fig. 2-13　Block diagram of correlator

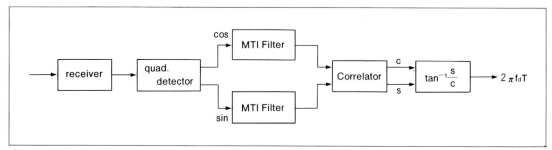

Fig. 2-14 Block diagram of available 2-D Doppler system

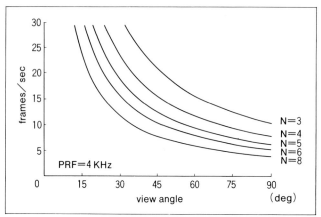

Fig. 2-15 Restriction of frame rate and view angle
Either the display view angle or frame rate must be reduced to improve the image quality of 2-D Doppler, that is to increase the number N.

direction is represented by value N, and when this value is larger a better image quality is obtained. As can be seen from Fig. 2-15, either the display view angle or the frame rate must be reduced to improve the output image quality. With a fixed value of N, the view angle must be reduced if the frame rate is increased. In this method, by increasing the PRF to 8KHz, the diagnostic distance is reduced to 9 cm. However, the restriction on the frame rate and the view angle is lightened because the value of N in Fig. 2-15 is doubled. Value N must be increased to reduce the noise level of the transmitter/receiver system and improve the S/N ratio.

4. Detection of variance information[10,11]

Variance of the Doppler signal indicates the degree of disturbance of blood flow. Qualitatively, narrow-band spectrum has a smaller variance and wide-band spectrum have a larger variance. A frequency spectrum displays a degree of variance from the spectrum span in addition to the velocity information. In 2-D Doppler the same kind of information can be obtained as follows.

Variance σ^2 in the statistical theory is expressed by the following equation:

$$\sigma^2 = \sum p(x_i)(x_i - \overline{x})^2 = \overline{x_i^2} - \overline{x}^2 \qquad \text{2-13}$$

In the formula, $p(x_i)$ is the probability that variable x takes value x_i; $\overline{x}$ is a mean value of x; and $\overline{x^2}$ is a mean value of x^2. Variance can be calculated by averaging the detected velocity. It is difficult to accurately estimate the variance, unless the averaging number N is larger than a certain value. For example, when N=3, a variance estimation according to Eq.2-13 is not possible, because there is only one velocity datum available.

For a discussion of variance, it is also important to know the time base of data dispersion. A displayed mean velocity is detected during transmission and reception for the same direction. Averaging time is about 2ms. Likewise, variance of velocity information is detected in almost the same time period.

5. Power display[12,13]

In some systems, attempts have been made to directly display the echo signal intensity of the blood flow, i.e., the power of the blood flow echo. Generally, the echo intensity is increased when the number of red blood cells, which are the echo source of the ultrasound wave, is increased. Therefore, the power display was originally used to determine the blood quantity. However, simply displaying the echo intensity is not significantly different from the normal black/white image display. As the echo from the blood flow has the same characteristics as random noise, it is impossible to distinguish blood flow signal from noise by simply amplifying the received signal. To selectively display the blood flow echo signal, movement information should be considered. As previously explained, the signal from a stationary object is eliminated by the MTI filter. In the power display, the output from the MTI filter is displayed according to its amplitude. In Fig. 2-6, a signal vector rotated on the circumference of a circle with radius 1, assuming that the vector amplitude was always constant. In actual cases however, the amplitude of the echo signal is changing all the time and hence the radius is also changing accordingly. While the velocity data are detected from the signal phase difference, power is detected from the amplitude information. If the same MTI filter is used, there is no difference concerning the flow display area between the power display and the 2-D Doppler.

At present, the power display is not fully used in clinical applications and several unknown factors still exist with respect to its usability and applications. However, the advantage of detecting the quantity of blood flow must be fully exploited in the future.

References

1) Grandchamp, P. A. : A novel pulsed directional Doppler velocimeter : The phase detection profilometer. Proc. Second European Cong. Ultrasoics Medicine Edited by E. Kanzer et al, 137 : 143, Excerpta Medica, Amsterdam, Oxford, 1975.

2) Brandestini, M. : Application of the phase detection principles in a transcutaneous velocity profile meter. Proc. Second European Cong. Ultrasonics Medicine Edited by E. Kanzer et al, 144 : 152, Excerpta Medica, Amsterdam, Oxford, 1975.

3) Angelsen, B. A. J. : On ultrasonic MTI measurement of velocity profiles in blood flow. IEEE, Vol.BME-26, No.12, Dec., 665 : 671, 1979.

4) White, D. N. : Johan Cristian Doppler and his effect - a brief history. Ultrasound in Med. and Biol., Vol.8, No.6, 583 : 519, 1982.

5) Fish, P. J. : Multichannel direction resolving Doppler Angiography. Proc. Second European Cong. Ultrasonics Medicine Edited by E. Kanzer et al, 153 : 159, Excerpta Medica, Amsterdam, Oxford, 1985.

6) Eyer, M. K., Brandestini, M. A. : Color digital echo/Doppler image presentation. Ultrasound in Med. and Biol., Vol.7, 21 : 31, 1981.

7) Namekawa, K., Kasai, C., Tsukamoto, M., Koyano, A. : Realtime bloodflow imaging system utilizing autocorrelation techniques. Ultrasound '82 Edited by R. Lerski and P. Morley, 203 : 208, Pergamon Press, London, 1983.

8) Shrader, W. W. : MTI rader. In Rader handbook. Edited by M. I. Skolnik, McGrow-Hill, 1970.

9) Harada, A., Kondo, Y., Namekawa, K., Kasai, C. : The studies on the effect of wall motion filters in real-time two-dimensional blood flow imaging system. Procedings of the 48th Meeting of the Japan Society of Ultrasonics in Medicine, 597, 1986.

10) Namekawa, K., Harada, A., Kasai, C. : Real time two-dimensional blood flow imaging-Variance display- . Proceedings of the 45th Meeting of the Japan Society of Ultrasonics in Medicine, 507, 1984.

11) Hongo, H., Shiki, E., Seo, Y., Iinuma, K. : 2-D color flow mapping system - Turbulent mode-. Proceedings of the 47th Meeting of the Japan Society Ultrasonics in Medicine, 481,1985.

12) Seo, Y. : Principle of Doppler method. In Clinical application of ultrasound Doppler method. Edited by J. Yoshikawa, 17 : 23, Medical Core, Tokyo, 1986.

13) Seo, Y., Shiki, E., Hongo, H., Iinuma, K. : 2-D color flow mapping system -Power mode-. Proceedings of the 47 th Meeting of the Japan Society of Ultrasonics in Medicine, 481, 1985.

Chapter 3　Equipment

3-1　Two-Dimensional Doppler Equipment

Fig. 3-1 shows an actual device which uses the principle described in the previous chapter. Today, the system most widely used for circulatory diagnosis is a phased array type.

The signal received by the probe of this system is detected by the quadrature detector. It is sent to the MTI filter after A/D conversion to eliminate various high harmonics components of PRF (Pulse Repetition Frequency) as well as frequency components induced by the motion of nearby walls. The output is applied to the autocorrelator to calculate the mean frequency and variance and the result is stored in the digital scan converter (DSC). In addition to the blood flow data, the tissue echo and PW Doppler data at a specific sample volume are also stored in the DSC after conversion into digital signals. The data in the DSC are digitally processed in the color signal processor and the results are converted to the three primary colors of red (R), green (G) and blue (B) of the analog signals to be displayed on a CRT. The output signals are also converted into the standard TV signals of NTSC or PAL via an encoder for connection with peripheral equipment such as a VCR.

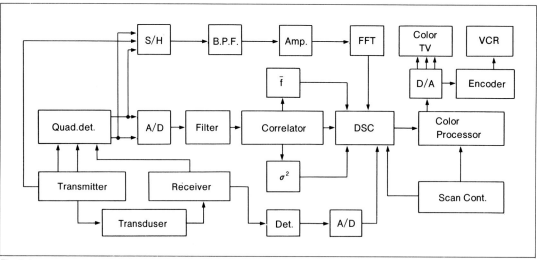

Fig. 3-1

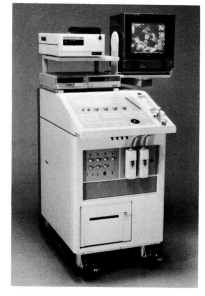

Fig. 3-2　2-D Doppler system.

Fig. 3-2 shows a view of a device which is commercially available as circulatory diagnostic equipment. The major diagnostic modes of the equipment are:

a) B-mode image
b) M-mode
c) PW Doppler
d) CW Doppler
e) 2-D Doppler
f) Flow mapping M-mode

It is important to selectively use the modes depending on diagnostic purpose. Various data displayed by the 2-D Doppler device are described below.

a) Display of Flow Direction

The blood flow approaching the probe is indicated by red, and the receding blood flow by blue.

b) Display of Flow Velocity

The blood flow velocity is indicated by the degree of brightness of the previous colors. That is, rapid blood flow in the direction of the probe is indicated by bright red and slow flow by dark red. There are 8 stages of brightness including the darkest (black).

In the 2-D Doppler system, aliasing occurs as in PW Doppler. Table 3-1 shows the brightness corresponding to the blood flow velocity. The vertical direction of the table shows the degrees of brightness of red and blue, and the lateral direction shows combinations of the PRF and ultrasound frequency. The PRF can be switched to 4 types, i.e., 4, 6, 8 and 12 KHz, and the ultrasound frequency to nominal 2.5, 3.5 and 5 MHz. As can be seen from the table, when a PRF of 12KHz is used, the highest detectable blood flow velocity is 96 cm/s with the ultrasound frequency of 5 MHz, and the blood flow of a normal infant can be diagnosed without aliasing. However, the maximum diagnostic distance is limited when the PRF is increased, and is 6 cm at a PRF of 12 KHz. As can be seen from the table, the color and brightness of the same blood flow velocity are different when the PRF is changed. Table 3-2 shows the relationship between color and brightness for 16 cm/s and 52 cm/s blood flow velocity with a 3.33 MHz ultrasound frequency. The 16 cm/s blood flow velocity is indicated by the 3 rd stages of brightness of red from the bottom when the PRF is 4 KHz. But, when the PRF is increased to 12 KHz, the same velocity is indicated by the 1 st stage of brightness of red which is darker than that of 4 KHz. On the one hand, a blood flow

Tab. 3-1

PRF (KHz)		4			6			8			12		
Freq of Probe (MHz)		2.5	3.33	5.0	2.5	3.33	5.0	2.5	3.33	5.0	2.5	3.33	5.0
Approaching Flow bright red	7	55~64	42~48	28~32	81~93	61~70	41~47	107~123	81~93	54~62	166~191	124~143	83~96
	6	47~55	35~42	23~28	68~81	51~61	34~41	90~107	68~81	45~54	140~166	105~124	70~83
	5	38~47	29~35	19~23	56~68	42~51	28~34	74~90	56~68	37~45	115~140	86~105	58~70
	4	30~38	22~29	15~19	43~56	33~42	22~28	57~74	43~56	29~37	89~115	67~86	45~58
	3	21~30	16~22	11~15	31~43	23~33	16~22	41~57	31~43	21~29	64~89	48~67	32~45
	2	13~21	10~16	6~11	19~31	14~23	9~16	25~41	19~31	12~21	38~64	29~48	19~32
dark red	1	4~13	3~10	2~6	6~19	5~14	3~9	8~25	6~19	4~12	13~38	10~29	6~19
	0	<4cm/s	<3cm/s	<2cm/s	<6cm/s	<5cm/s	<3cm/s	<8cm/s	<6cm/s	<4cm/s	<13cm/s	<10cm/s	<6cm/s
Receding Flow dark blue	1	4~13	3~10	2~6	6~19	5~14	3~9	8~25	6~19	4~12	13~38	10~29	6~19
	2	13~21	10~16	6~11	19~31	14~23	9~16	25~41	19~31	12~21	38~64	29~48	19~32
	3	21~30	16~22	11~15	31~43	23~33	16~22	41~57	31~43	21~29	64~89	48~67	32~45
	4	30~38	22~29	15~19	43~56	33~42	22~28	57~74	43~56	29~37	89~115	67~86	45~58
	5	38~47	29~35	19~23	56~68	42~51	28~34	74~90	56~68	37~45	115~140	86~105	58~70
	6	47~55	35~42	23~28	68~81	51~61	34~41	90~107	68~81	45~54	140~166	105~124	70~83
bright blue	7	55~64	42~48	28~32	81~93	61~70	41~47	107~123	81~93	54~62	166~191	124~143	83~96
View range		6, 9, 12, 18 cm			6, 9, 12 cm			6, 9 cm			6 cm		

Tab. 3-2

PRF \ velocity	16 cm/s	52 cm/s
4 KHz	red 3	blue 7
6 KHz	red 2	red 6
8 KHz	red 1	red 4
12 KHz	red 1	red 3

velocity of 52 cm/s in the direction of the probe has aliasing when the PRF is 4 KHz, and is indicated by the 7 th stage of blue which is the brightest color of receding flow. Along with increases of the PRF to 6, 8 and 12 KHz, aliasing is eliminated, and the velocity is indicated by the 6 th, 4 th and 3 rd stages of red brightness in darker order.

c) Variance Display

Variance is indicated by inclusion of green with red or blue. An approaching fast turbulent blood flow is indicated in yellow which is a mixture of red and green. On the other hand, a receding fast turbulent blood flow is indicated in cyan color which is a mixture of blue and green. The display condition is indicated by a color bar at the side of the screen as shown in "**Color Velocity Function**".

3—2 Flow Display Function

The instrument shown in Fig. 3-2 has six modes for display of the 2-D Doppler.

a) 28°

This mode has a small display angle but a high frame rate. When the PRF is 8 or 12 KHz, a single image can be drawn in 1/60 of a second.

b) 53°L

This mode has a display angle of 53° and a low frame rate. In this mode, the S/N ratio of color signals is improved.

c) 53°H

This mode has a display angle of 53° and a high frame rate and thus a shorter average time of signal processing.

d) 90°

This mode has a display angle of 90° and a lower frame rate than the other modes.

e) 46°/90°L

This mode enables display of a 46° 2-D Doppler in any direction in the 90° B-mode image. The frame rate is lower, but the S/N ratio is improved.

f) 46°/90°H

In this mode, the display is the same as item e) above, but the average signal processing time is shorter and the frame rate is high as in item c).

Table 3-3 shows the relationship between the display mode and frame rate. It is important to select the most appropriate display mode according to the purpose of application.

Tab. 3-3

Flow Display \ PRF	4 KHz	6 KHz	8 KHz	12 KHz
28°	30 F/S	30 F/S	60 F/S	60 F/S
53° L	10 F/S	15 F/S	20 F/S	30 F/S
53° H	15 F/S	20 F/S	30 F/S	30 F/S
90°	7.5 F/S	10 F/S	15 F/S	15 F/S
46°/90° L	10 F/S	15 F/S	20 F/S	30 F/S
46°/90° H	15 F/S	20 F/S	30 F/S	30 F/S

3—3 Flow Filter Function[1,2]

In a 2-D Doppler, the MTI filter is used to eliminate echoes from tissue which is

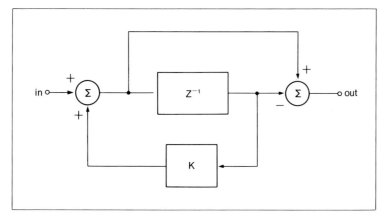

Fig. 3-3 First order MTI filter with feed back loop.

stationary or moving at low velocity. In order to make the filter characteristics variable, the feedback value applied to the MTI filter is changed as shown in Fig. 3-3. Fig. 3-4 shows the frequency characteristics of this filter, where K is the feedback value. As it is a high-pass filter, the low frequency components are suppressed and artifact due to the wall motion is reduced in diagnosis.

In the actual instrument, two stages of the MTI filter are connected, and the frequency characteristics can be switched-over depending on the purpose of application. It has four selectable ranges, LOW, MID 1, MID 2 and HIGH. In the LOW range, a color display is available even with very slow motion.

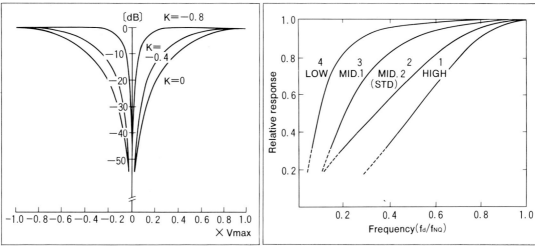

Fig. 3-4 Frequency characteristic of first order MTI filter.

Fig. 3-5 FLOW FILTER frequency-response.

3—4 Color Velocity Function[3]

This function allows switching to the display mode of the blood flow velocity in 2-D Doppler. There are four types of display modes as follows:

7-step display	: Displays approaching or receding flow in 7 stages of brightness.
1-step display	: Displays approaching or receding flow in the brightest color of red or blue regardless of flow velocity.
Approaching flow display	: Displays only approaching flow in red.
Receding flow display	: Displays only receding flow in blue.

○ P.49   "Color Velocity Function" shows examples of these modes.

3—5 Color Display Function[3]

◐ P.50

In the 2-D Doppler,the tissue echoes are shown in black/white and blood flow is shown in red or blue with green in proportion to the flow turbulence. The Color Display Function allows the blood flow data to be freely changed with respect to tissue echo, direction/ velocity and variance. When the variance function is turned off, only the data for direction and velocity of blood flow are displayed in pure red and blue with brightness change. When the echo function is turned off, the black/white B-mode image is erased, and only the blood flow data are displayed. Actual examples are shown in "**Color Display Function**".

3—6 Color Enhance Function[3]

◐ P.50

As shown in Table 3-2, when the PRF is increased, the brightness of color for the same blood flow velocity becomes darker. However, to diagnose fast heart beat rate such as that of an infant, the PRF must be increased to raise the frame rate as much as possible. To obtain a bright display even in such cases, the relationship between the velocity and the color brightness can be altered by the Color Enhance Function. Fig. 3-6 shows the relationship. When the Color Enhance Function is turned off, the color brightness is determined by the PRF and ultrasound wave frequency, and the intermediate color brightness is proportional to the flow velocity. In the LOW range, a flow velocity of more than 3/4 of the maximum is constantly displayed with the highest brightness. In the MID range when the velocity is more than 2/3 of the maximum, or in the HIGH range when the velocity is more than 1/2, the brightness is at the highest level. Differences on an actual display are shown in "**Color Enhance Function**".

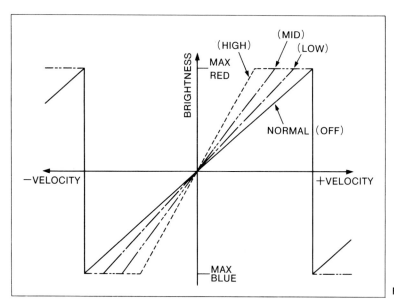

Fig. 3-6 Color Enhance.

3—7 Color Baseline Shift Function[3]

When aliasing occurs in 2-D Doppler, this function shifts the reference color level, so that correct observation is possible without color reversal up to double the maximum flow velocity (see Table 3-1). The principle is shown in Fig. 3-7. It is equivalent to the baseline shift functon seen in the conventional PW or CW Doppler system.

As can be seen from the principle, this function is used when the flow is uni-directional either approaching or receding, and the velocity is fast. When the shift value is set to the maximum, each of the 7 stages of brightness is assigned to double the normal flow velocity.

◐ P.51

Actual examples are shown in "**Color Baseline Function**".

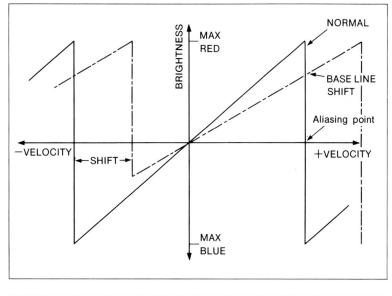

Fig. 3-7 Color Baseline shift.

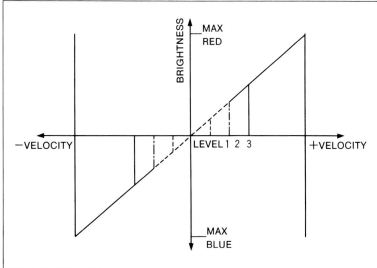

Fig. 3-8 Color Reject.

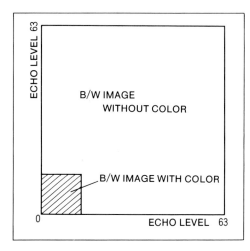

Fig. 3-9 Color Edge.

3—8 Color Reject Function[3]

When artifact due to wall motion occurs in 2-D Doppler, this function erases unnecessary colors from the artifact. Fig. 3-8 shows its operation. As can be seen from the figure, the color with low flow velocity can be suppressed by eliminating up to the lowest 4 of the 7 brightness stages. An actual example is shown in "**Color Reject Function**".

◯ P.51

3—9 Color Edge Function[3]

● P.51

When an echo of more than a certain level from a tissue is superimposed on 2-D Doppler data as shown in Fig. 3-9, the color of that portion is erased. As the echo from a tissue is larger than that of blood corpuscles, color on the black/white is eliminated by the use of this function. An example of this function is shown in "**Color Edge Function**".

3—10 PW Doppler Function

Existence/nonexistence of abnormal blood flow is easily diagnosed by the introduction of the 2-D Doppler system. In this system however, detailed data for flow velocity change in time at a specific location and the velocity distribution are not available. To obtain these data, the PW Doppler function used in the conventional instrument is attached to the present system. The specification of the pulsed Doppler function is shown below.

a) PRF : 4, 6, 8 and 12 KHz
b) Sample volume size : 2, 5 and 10 mm
c) Wall filter : 200, 400, 600 and 800 Hz
d) Baseline shift function
e) Display pattern : power spectrum display
f) Scanning mode : B/PW simultaneous mode and PW mode
g) Detectable velocity range : see Table 3-4

Tab 3-4 Detectable maximum velocity

Freq of probe \ PRF(Hz)	4 K	6 K	8 K	12 K
2.5 MHz	0.64	0.93	1.23	1.91
3.5 MHz	0.48	0.70	0.93	1.43
5.0 MHz	0.32	0.47	0.62	0.96

COS θ =1 (Dimension : m/s)

3—11 CW Doppler Function

As a pulsed ultrasound is used in either 2-D Doppler and PW Doppler method, aliasing occurs when the blood flow velocity exceeds a certain value. This means that a maximum limit exists in measurable blood flow velocity. On the other hand, it is possible to measure fast velocity without aliasing using the CW Doppler system. A variety of applications are possible with the CW Doppler system. A widely-used method is to approximate the pressure difference (Δp) between the stenotic valve from the maximum blood flow velocity passing through the valve. That is, the pressure difference can be determined using the simplified Bernulli's formula $\Delta p = 4 v^2$. The CW Doppler is important in measuring the intracardiac pressure.

In this method of measurement it has been assumed that the directions of the blood flow and ultrasound beam are identical. However, they are not in parallel in reality and error will occur as described later.

1. Probes for CW Doppler

The effectiveness is increased when CW Doppler and a 2-D Doppler are used in combination[4]. For this purpose, two types of duplex probe, as shown in Fig. 3-10, are available.

In one type, the direction of the CW Doppler beam is fixed for both transmission and reception. In the other type, the direction of the transmission beam is fixed, but that of the reception beam is variable with the phased array probe. With the first type of probe which is

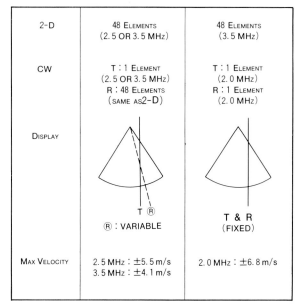

2-D	48 Elements (2.5 OR 3.5 MHz)	48 Elements (3.5 MHz)
CW	T : 1 Element (2.5 OR 3.5 MHz) R : 48 Elements (SAME AS 2-D)	T : 1 Element (2.0 MHz) R : 1 Element (2.0 MHz)
Display	T Ⓡ Ⓡ : VARIABLE	T & R (FIXED)
Max Velocity	2.5 MHz : ±5.5 m/s 3.5 MHz : ±4.1 m/s	2.0 MHz : ±6.8 m/s

Fig. 3-10 CW Doppler probes.

Tab. 3-5 Detectable maximum velocity CW Doppler

Probe freq	Range(Hz)	5.3 K	10.4 K	15.6 K	20.8 K	25 K	35.7 K
Indepent	2 MHz	±1.02	±1.99	±2.99	±3.98	±4.78	±6.83
	3 MHz	±0.68	±1.33	±1.99	±2.66	±3.19	±4.55
Duplex	2.5 MHz	±0.81	±1.59	±2.39	±3.19	±3.83	±5.46
	3.5 MHz	±0.61	±1.2	±1.79	±2.39	±2.87	±4.10

$\cos \theta = 1$ (Dimension : m/s)

fixed in the beam directions of both transmission and detection, the sound vibrator for the CW Doppler is independently provided beside a phased array probe, which means that the transmission frequency can be freely selected. However, a disadvantage is that operability declines as the probe size increases. In the other type with the variable direction of detection beam, a single transmission vibrator is provided beside the phased array. Therefore, the probe size is not much larger compared to the conventional phased array type. In addition, because of variable detection direction, it is possible to set the transmission and detection beams to intersect at a location with maximum blood flow velocity, so that the detection sensitivity can be increased. In this case however, the frequency for the CW Doppler is determined by the frequency of the phased array probe.

In addition to the above probes, an independent type of probe specific for CW Doppler is also available. This type of probe has wide frequency range, and the frequency can be switched between 2 MHz and 3 MHz.

Table 3-5 shows the highest flow velocities measurable by the different types of probes.

2. Error in flow velocity measurement

In detecting the highest flow velocity by CW Doppler, error is produced depending on the angle θ between the ultrasound beam direction and the blood flow direction. When the transmission and detection beams are in parallel, deviation is generally expressed by the following formula :

$$\alpha = (1 - \cos \theta) \cdot 100\%$$

However in an actual instument, the beams are not in parallel, and the equation can be modified as follows :

$$\alpha = (2 - \cos \theta_1 - \cos \theta_2) \cdot 50\%$$

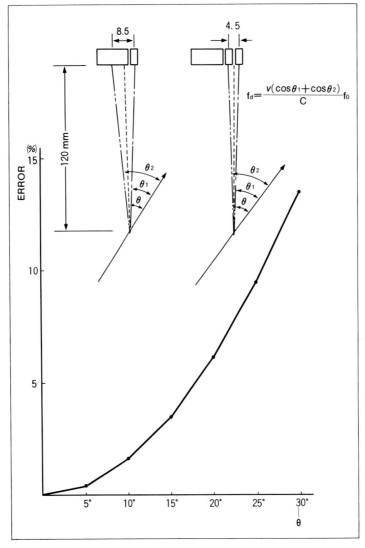

Fig. 3-11 Error in flow velocity measurement.

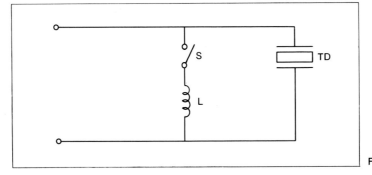

Fig. 3-12

where, θ_1 and θ_2 are the angles of the transmission and detection beams against the blood flow direction, respectively. As an example, let us calculate the errors for both a fixed transmission/detection beam method and a variable detection beam method. If the sound beams intersect with flow at the depth of 12 cm as shown in Fig.3-11, intersection angles become $\theta_1 = 19°$ and $\theta_2 = 21°$ for the fixed beam method, and $\theta_1 = 18°$ and $\theta_2 = 22°$ for the variable beam method. Substitution of these values in the above formula results in errors of 6.05 % and 6.09 %. These values are considered to be acceptable in actual clinical measurements. However, it is desirable to make the directions of blood flow and the ultrasound beam as parallel as possible to decrease the errors.

3—12 **Improvement of Image Quality**

In the clinical diagnosis , black/white image is important. To obtain a better result, the resolution and gray shades of the B-mode image must be improved. For this purpose, ultrasound wave transmission with a wide frequency band is required to make the receiving pulse width shorter. On the other hand, to increase the detection sensitivity of the 2-D Doppler and thereby improve the S/N ratio, it is better to transmit a large number of ultrasound waves with a narrow frequency band. Therefore, improvement in B-mode image quality is inconsistent with that in 2-D Doppler quality.

To satisfy both requirements a probe as shown in Fig. 3-12 has been developed, in which the switch S is turned off when transmitting short pulses in B-mode black/white operation, while it is turned on to an inductor L to make resonant oscillation with capacity C of the vibrator and a cable in 2-D Doppler operation.

In the previous 2-D Doppler, the inductor was always connected even in black/white operation, and hence the image quality was not adequate. By the development of the new probe, the problem of image quality has been overcome. Fig. 3-13 shows a comparison of the new and old probes.

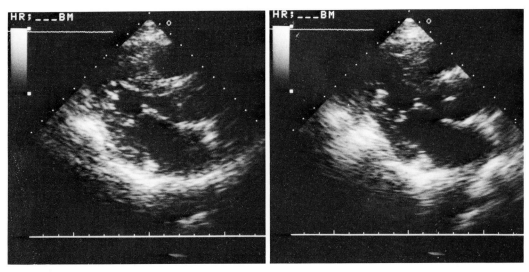

Fig. 3-13 Improvement of image quality.

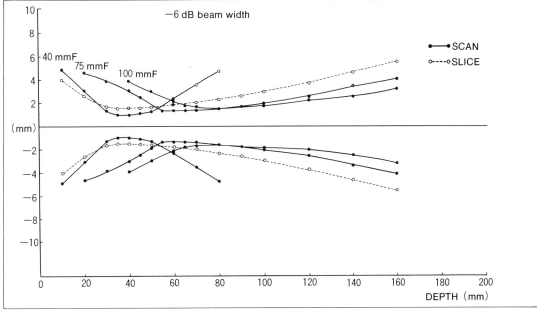

Fig. 3-14

28

3—13 Electronic Focusing

The present instrument uses an electronic focusing system for transmission and detection of sound waves to obtain a better image quality with improved resolution.

When the standard probe is used, the focus can be switched in three different ways : 40, 75 and 100mm. Fig. 3-14 shows the actual directivity pattern of ultrasound beams. The beam characteristics must be well understood for applications in clinical diagnosis.

References

1) Yoshikawa, Y. : 2-D Doppler equipment. In Medical Ultrasound Equipment Handbook. Edited by Y. Ohta et al., 173, Corona Publishing Co., Ltd. Tokyo, 1985.

2) Omoto, R., Kyo, S., Matsumura, M., Harada, A., Katabami, T., Namekawa, K., Proceedings of the 47 th Meeting of the Japan Society of Ultrasonics in Medicine., 477, 1985.

3) Miura, K., Kato, K., Hirosaka, L., Katabami, T., Yoshikawa, Y., Kyo, S., Matsumura, M., Omoto, R. : Proceedings of the 48th Meeting of the Japan Society of Ultrasonics in Medicine., 613, 1986.

4) Omoto, R., Yokote, Y., Takamoto, S., Kyo, S., Asano, H., Matsumura, M., Kasai, C., Namekawa, K., Miura, K., Kondo, Y., Koyano, A. : Clinical significance of combined use of color flow mapping and continuous wave Doppler in aquired valvular diseases. WFUBM '85. Edited by R. W. Gill and M. J. Dadd, 393, Pergamon Press, 1985.

Chapter 4 Cautions for Clinical Use of the Instrument

4—1 Basic Features

1. Angular dependency

As stated earlier in the Principles section, the Doppler frequency f_d is angle dependent and is given by:

$$f_d = \frac{2 v \cdot \cos \theta}{c} f_o \qquad 4\text{-}1$$

○ P.52

This has been verified by a model experiment. "**Transducer Position and Blood Flow Imaging**" shows the experimental setup. A latex tube with an internal diameter of 8 mm was placed horizontally in a water tank and water which contains sound reflection particles was pumped through the tube. The tube and sound beam were made to intersect at right angles in the center of the flow image. Therefore, the Doppler frequency or the flow color will be different depending on the positions of the tube.

The scanning sector angle of observation was $53°$ and the flow speed was set to the maximum detectable velocity at the edge of the tube inside the sector angle. The numbers (0 $\sim$7) given in the diagram indicate the color shades corresponding to the flow velocities. The area of non-detectable low velocity flow was within the range of $\pm 2°$ from the center of the sector image. From Eq. 4-1, the critical angle θ, where flow can be detected, is calculated to be $88°$. As the water is flowing through the tube from left to right, the flow direction is toward the transducer in the left portion of the tube and is away from the transducer in the right portion of the tube. Therefore the flow color is red in the left portion of the tube, and is blue in the right portion. Blood flow in the heart is three-dimensional. However, as is well known, only the flow component onto the sound beam of flow velocity is shown in the 2-D Doppler[1]. Therefore, it is essential to have a full understanding of this when interpreting the color images.

2. Time delay

In the analysis of pulsed Doppler signals by FFT (Fast Fourier Transform), there is an inevitable time delay resulting from data collection and processing[2]. On the one hand, in 2-D Doppler, data is displayed after it is integrated over the time period of 8 sound transmission intervals as shown in Fig. 4-1. As the output from the autocorrelator and B-mode image timing are synchronized, the maximum time delay between the B-mode image and the 2-D Doppler is 8 times that of the pulse transmission interval (8 T). For example, when the depth of diagnosis is 18cm and PRF (Pulse Repetition Frequency) is 4KHz, the delay time becomes 2.0ms, which does not cause any problem in actual clinical use. In the Flow mapping M-mode, the averaging time is lengthened to improve the S/N ratio.

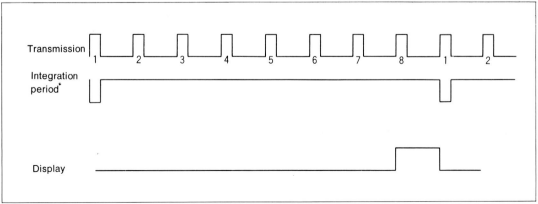

Fig. 4-1 Timing chart.

Tab. 4-1   Time Delay (Dimension : ms)

	2-D Doppler	Flow mapping M-mode	Pulsed doppler
①data collection time	2.0	16.0	25.0
②analysis time	0.005	0.005	8.0
③display time	−0.005	−0.005	8.0
$\frac{1}{2}×$①+②+③ mean delay time	1.0	8.0	28.5
	PRF＝4 KHz N＝8T	PRF＝4 KHz N＝64T	PRF＝4 KHz Number of data＝256

Table 4-1 shows the time delays for 2-D Doppler and FFT analysis. One must take into account that these time delays vary according to PRF, averaging and the devices used.

3. Frame rate and scanning directions

B-mode image is obtained by the scanning of sound beams. The time required for one scan, that is, the time required to obtain one frame image, is equal to the inverse value of the frame rate. For example, when a 30 frame per second image is displayed, the time needed for a single frame image is 33 ms. This means that the frame images are not real time in a strict sense. However, whether it is satisfactory to consider the image as real time or not, depends entirely on whether the time required to form the complete image is adequately short for imaging of the body's activities, such as heart movement.

◐ P.53 "Influence of Frame Rate" shows theoretical calculations for 2-D Doppler when the heart rate is changed. Frame rate is taken as 10 and heart rate is 60 in (**A**) and 120 in (**B**). In (**A**), one can recognize flow variation in three images, but in (**B**), virtually only one frame shows the flow and flow variation cannot be determined. Therefore, if the heart rate increases in relation the frame rate, an accurate evaluation of the flow becomes impossible. It is difficult to say in general, what value of frame rate is appropriate in relation to the heart rate, but in all cases, evaluation of flow on the basis of single frames taken randomly is a dangerous approach.

Sound beam scanning is conducted unidirectionally from right to left or from left to right. This scanning is commenced from the direction marked by the IMAGE DIRECTION in the device used. It is important to know that flow image will vary in accordance with the ◐ P.53 direction of scanning even if the frame rate is the same. "Influence of Scanning Direction" shows theoretical calculations which demonstrate this difference. The picture represents the image obtained with a frame rate of 10 and a heart rate of 120. Beam scanning is from right to left in (**A**) and is from left to right in (**B**). Since the flow is assumed to be flowing from left to right, the displayed flow area is larger when the scanning direction follows the flow as in (**B**), but it becomes smaller when the scanning direction is against the flow direction as in (**A**).

4. Variance and mosaic

In the 2-D Doppler instrument, the flow velocity is expressed by the brightness of red or blue colors, while variance is shown by a mixture of green with red or blue. That is, narrow band laminar flow is displayed by a pure red or pure blue color, while wide band turbulent ◐ P.54 flow is displayed by yellow or blue-green colors. "Expression of Variance" shows this phenomenon with the input of simulated electrical signals. (**A, C**) shows the input of a narrow band signal with the spectral display shown below and (**B, D**) shows when the input has a wide band spectrum. Colors in (**A, C**) are displayed in pure red and blue, while in (**B, D**) the colors are shown in yellow and blue-green.

If variance is further increased, and signals which have both positive and negative ◐ P.54 polarities are input, mosaic colors will develop as shown in "Display of Mosaic Pattern". That is, a mixed pattern which includes yellow and blue-green colors appear. In this case, the spectrum shows a wide frequency band. In an actual flow, a mosaic pattern appears when the flow velocity is very fast and the flow is disturbed.

4—2 Recording

The Doppler system is equipped with three devices for data recording. These are an instantaneous photo recorder, VCR and strip-chart recorder. Of these devices, the instantaneous photo recorder and VCR are used for color data recording, while the strip-chart recorder can only handle B-mode images.

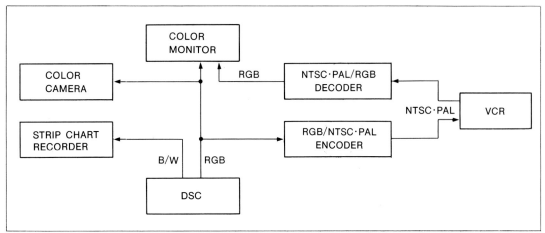

Fig. 4-2 Block diagram of the recording system.

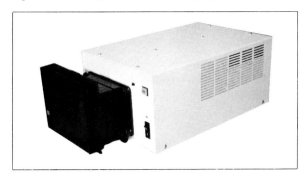

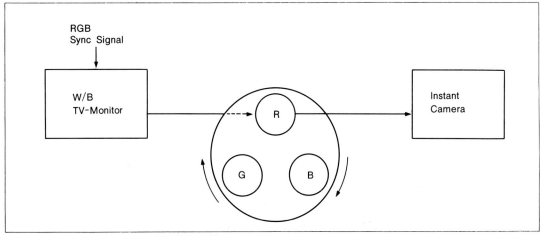

Fig. 4-3 Schematic diagram of the photo-taking system.

1. Recording by instantaneous photo recorder
The instantaneous photo recorder can record all of the images frozen on the observation monitor. Image freezing is accomplished at any desired time during the examination by pressing the freeze button. Image freezing is achieved instantaneously when the freeze

button is pressed in B-mode and M-mode when using scroll function. It also can be set by retarded times from electrocardiac R-wave in Pulse-synchronous-mode. After freezing an image, the camera button is pressed for photographic recording. It takes about 2～10 seconds for photographs to emerge. Fig. 4-3 shows the photorecording system, in which a flow image on a black/white monitor is recorded three times by changing filters of red, green and blue colors. By this operation, a highly resolved image is obtained, although a longer time is required.

Other methods for instantaneous photo recording have been developed. For example, (1) taking photo of color CRT display directly, (2) scanning a film on Optical Tube which has red, green and blue light emitter[3].

2. Recording by VCR

The recording of real-time images is conducted by a high capacity, low-price VCR[4]. Due care must be paid to this type of recording as the display format of the 2-D Doppler instrument differs from that of the VCR. In the 2-D Doppler instrument the RGB system, which is often employed in devices such as computers, is employed to display flow images. Though a highly resolved image is obtained with the RGB system, recording into a VCR is not possible. To do this, the RGB display format must be converted to the VCR format. NTSC is the format used in the U.S.A. and Japan for VCR recording. For this reason, a special signal convertor (ENCODER) has been built into the system to convert RGB format signals into NTSC format signals (PAL format in systems for Europe). This means that a TV monitor with either NTSC or RGB terminals can be connected to the main system. Recording can thus be accomplished by merely making a direct connection between the output terminals of the monitor and the input terminals of the VCR monitor. Doppler sound signal can also be obtained from the sound terminal.

In this video cassette recording however, the image may be slightly deteriorated due to the signal conversion.

As the 2-D Doppler system displays the flow data in colors, the colors displayed on the screen are extremely important. When a commercially available screen is used for play back, the image must be adjusted by the HUE and COLOR control knobs on the TV monitor. Use of the color test pattern displayed in the main monitor is recommended for this purpose.

A still image played back from a VCR generally displays only one field of data (two fields compose one frame image). This leads to a major reduction in image quality. It is therefore necessary to use a device to prevent image deterioration. Recently, VCR with inbuilt IC memory for single image holding have started to appear on the market, and they may provide significant improvement in the image quality.

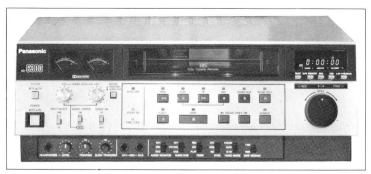

Fig. 4-4 Outlook of a commercially available VCR.

3. TV Syncronization and heart rate synchronization

In order to prevent the mixing of new and old image data in a single frame, 2-D Doppler image and TV image (1 frame or 1 field) are synchronized. This prevents the occurrence of a major time difference within the image. In this, the time difference between the right and left edges of a sector image is 1/7.5～1/60 seconds depending on the mode conditions. Fig. 4-5 shows an example when a TV image is not synchronized. As is seen from the figure, discontinuity of the image is produced. Normally when VCR replay images are frozen on

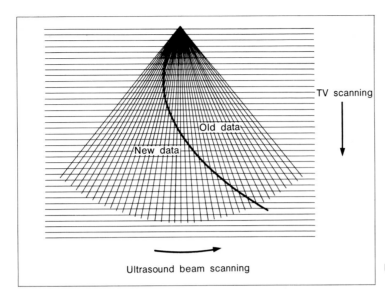

Ultrasound beam scanning

Fig. 4-5 The mixing of new and old image data on TV screen.

the monitor and observation of the image in the T period from the R-wave is desired, a time aberration of $1/7.5 \sim 1/60$ seconds may occur, thereby preventing appearance of the required image. However, if the heart rate synchronism function of the main unit is used, the recorded image will be synchronized with the T period and a time differnce will not occur. Therefore, heart rate synchronization is necessary when analysing a flow image.

4-3 Operation of the Instrument

As described in Chapter 3, various limitations exist when taking blood flow data. The 2-D Doppler system is optimally designed, but it is essential to have a full understanding of the device.

There are three interrelated items to be considered from the standpoint of using the device. These are:

(1) Selection of maximum flow velocity
(2) Selection of examination field of view
(3) Processing of color information

This relationship is shown in Fig. 4-6. Each of these operations consists of additional

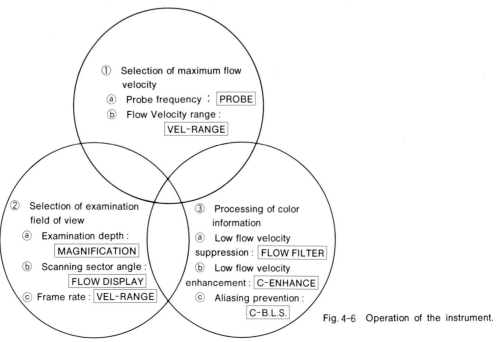

Fig. 4-6 Operation of the instrument.

complex functions and explanations of the switches provided for these operations are described below.

In addition, two further items are explained. These are:

(4) Optimal gain setting

(5) Selection of focal points

1. Selection of maximum detection flow velocity

Maximum detectable flow velocity is determined by the probe frequency and range of flow velocity.

(a) Probe frequency: PROBE switch

B-mode image quality is improved by increasing the probe frequency. However, as shown in Table 3-4, this causes a reduction in the detectable maximum flow velocity. For instance, the maximum detectable flow velocity for a probe frequency of 2.5 MHz is 0.64 m/s. By raising the frequency to 3.5 MHz the detectable velocity is decreased to 0.48 m/s (Doppler reference frequency is 3.33 MHz). When flow velocity exceeds this value, aliasing occurs. As for the color brightness, a higher probe frequency produces a brighter color as shown in

P.54 "**Selection of Maximum Detection Flow Velocity**"

(b) Flow velocity range: VEL-RANGE switch

The VEL-RANGE switch is used to change the maximum detection flow velocity. As shown in Table 3-4, the increase of PRF from 4 KHz to 6 KHz increases the detectable maximum flow velocity from 0.48 m/s to 0.70 m/s, thereby reducing the aliasing

P.55 phenomenon. "**Selection of Flow Velocity Range**" shows an example.

2. Selection of examination field of view

In 2-D Doppler, there exist various limitations between examination distance, scanning sector angle and frame rate. It is therefore necessary to understand their relationship when using the instrument.

(a) Examination depth: MAGNIFICATION switch

P.55 As shown in "**Selection of Examination Field of View**", when the MAGNIFICATION is 15 cm, and the VEL RANGE is changed from 4 KHz to 6 KHz, the magnification distance changes to 12 cm. The limitations on the examination depth caused by flow velocity range are shown in Table 3-1. When the examination depth and flow velocity range are large, it is necessary to select a low frequency probe.

(b) Scanning sector angle: FLOW DISPLAY switch

An effective way to expand a near range field of view is to widen the scanning sector

P.55 angle. "**Selection of Scanning Sector Angle**" shows the case where the scanning angle is changed from 53° to 90° with the FLOW DISPLAY switch. However, this alteration causes the frame rate to decrease from 15 f/s to 7.5 f/s when PRF is 4 KHz. When the PRF is doubled to 8KHz (90°) by the VEL-RANGE switch, a frame rate of 15 f/s and examination distance of 9 cm are achieved.

(c) Frame rate: FLOW DISPLAY switch

The inverse value of the frame rate is equal to the time required to make one frame image and it is therefore very important to analyze the cardiac cycle phase, particularly in infants

P.55 with a fast heart rate. "**Selection of Frame Rate**" shows the case where the frame rate is changed from 10 f/s to 30 f/s using the FLOW DISPLAY switch, while keeping the same scanning angle (B-mode: 90°, 2-D Doppler: 46°). This alteration however, decreases the averaging time which influences the S/N ratio. Other ways to increase the frame rate are either to increase the VEL-RANGE or to decrease the scanning sector angle.

3. Processing of color information

The data of the 2-D Doppler can be processed according to the various functions listed below. Please refer to sections 3-3, 3-6 and 3-7 where explanations of these functions are given.

(a) Low flow velocity suppression: FLOW FILTER switch

（b）Low flow velocity enhancement：COLOR ENHANCE switch
（c）Aliasing prevention：COLOR-B.L.S. switch

4. Optimal gain setting

In obtaining an accurate diagnosis, optimal gain setting is very important. If gain setting is not correct, it becomes difficult to take valid data and furthermore, an incorrect diagnosis can be made. Several important aspects of gain setting will be explained below：
（a）B-mode Gain

First, in order that the 2-D Doppler system is used properly, some basic understanding is required about the color display. All the colors displayed on a color TV screen consist of combinations of red（R）, green（G）and blue（B）. In the 2-D Doppler system, the brightness of red and blue colors on the TV screen is proportional to flow velocity in forward or reverse directions, while a mixture with green indicates the degree of flow disturbance. Therefore the color hue changes from red to yellow for the flow toward a transducer, while the color changes from blue to cyan（blue green）for the flow away from the transducer in accordance with the flow disturbance. Black/white tissue images are made by an equal mixture of the three primary colors, but with different intensities in proportion to the gray shades. Therefore, when the intensity or the contrast of the tissue image is changed, all three knobs of R, G, B must be adjusted in such a way that the tissue echoes are not colored. For instance, if the adjustment is not correct and a grey component overlays the blue color, the color becomes whitish,resulting in the loss of chroma. Correct adjustment of contrast also facilitates the valid evaluation of flow velocity. The following gain adjustments, **"Optimal Gain Setting"**（A）to（C）are examples where the settings of B-mode gain are changed in three ways.

⊙ P.56

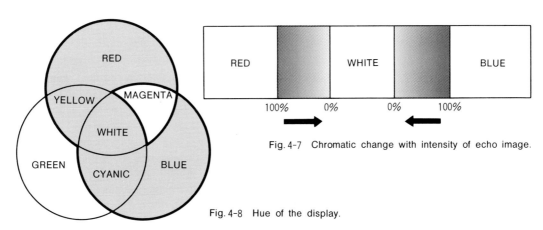

Fig. 4-7 Chromatic change with intensity of echo image.

Fig. 4-8 Hue of the display.

（**A**）: The B-mode gain is too weak. This prevents valid identification of tissue image.

（**B**）: The B-mode gain is too high. This also prevents clarity of color which readily leads to errors in evaluating the flow velocity and range.

（**C**）: This seems to be a correct setting of B-mode gain. It is important to produce an echo image that allows error-free evaluation of flow velocity data and easy identification of position.

（b）Flow Gain

Next, the gain setting for blood flow must be carried out carefully to obtain correct flow information. In particular, care must be paid to low flow velocity, since the signal gain for low Doppler frequency is smaller than for high frequency. This means that low flow velocity is displayed with a high flow gain. In **"Optimal Gain Setting"**（D）is the case when the flow gain is inadequate. However, it cannot be deduced from this photograph alone that the gain is too low. This is evaluated from increasing the gain slightly and expanding the display range on the basis of the condition before and after examination. Due care must be paid to avoid making gain settings that are too small in order to prevent underestimations of the clinical condition. On the other hand, when the gain setting is too large, the 2-D Doppler

⊙ P.56

image becomes noisy. (**E**) shows the case where yellow and blue-green noise appear over the entire screen. If the gain is further increased, a mosaic pattern of blood flow data indicating turbulence and noise arise, which may cause difficulties in making clinical evaluations and may lead to overestimations of the clinical condition. Therefore, the optimum gain setting may be that which is increased until only a slight amount of noise appears on the screen.

As explained in Section 3-5, the use of the COLOR DISPLAY function allows the display of only a black/white image or of a color flow image. This function is useful to determine the boundary of the endocardium.

5. Selection of focal points

In the present system, a focal point of the transducer is automatically varied according to the examination distance when the transducer frequency is 2.5 or 3.5 MHz. Table 4-2 shows the relation between the focal ranges and focal points. In addition, focussing at the region of interest independent of the examination distance can be made manually. By the use of this function, the sensitivity and resolution of the point is improved. Concrete examples are shown in "**Selection of Focal Points**".

○ P.56

Tab. 4-2 Focal range corresponding to selection of focal points

Focal point	Focal range	Examination depth (automatic setting)
40 mm	20 ~ 70 mm	6 cm
75 mm	20 ~ 120 mm	9, 12, 15, 18, 22 cm
100 mm	30 ~ 150 mm	

References

1) Fukaya, T., Yoshikawa, J., Yoshida, K., Yamakawa, M., Tomita, Y., Baba, K. : The problems in visualizing blood flow dynamics in real-time two-dimensional Doppler echocardiography. Proceedings of the 45 th Meeting of the Japan Society of Ultrasonics in Medicine., 175, 1984.

2) Kitabatake, A., Inoue, M. : Ultrasonic Doppler method in cardiology., 27, Marzen Co., Ltd. Tokyo, 1986.

3) Katabami, T., Yoshikawa, Y. : Development of the hard-copy unit with natural colors for the real-time imaging of two-dimensional Doppler flow. Proceedings of the 48th Meeting of the Japan Society of Ultrasonics in Medicine., 627, 1986.

4) Sano, A. : Video recorder. In Medical Ultrasonic Equipment Handbook. Edited by Y. Ohta, et al., 214, Corona Publishing Co., Ltd. Tokyo, 1985.

Chapter 5 Clinical Use of 2-D Doppler as the Third Generation of Technology in Echocardiography

5–1 Third Generation of Technology in Echocardiography

This chapter describes skillful clinical applications of the 2-D Doppler instrument in its role as the third generation of echocardiography technology. Other third-generation methods of echocardiography besides the 2-D Doppler, include M-mode echocardiography, two-dimensional echocardiography, pulsed-wave Doppler (PWD), and continuous-wave Doppler. The third-generation echocardigraphy modes are shown in a table (Tab. 5-1). Applications of continuous-wave Doppler (CWD), have been increasing and rank with

Tab. 5-1 Two-dimensional Doppler system, available modes and applications.

Modes	Applications (example)
M-mode	Measurement of dimensions
2-D Echo (B-mode)	Definition of anatomy and morphology, segmental wall motion analysis
2-D Doppler	Real-time imaging of blood flow, regurgitant and shunt flows
PW Doppler	Sample volume analysis, aortic, mitral and tricuspid flows
CW Doppler	Measurement of velocity and pressure gradients across valves and stenotic orifices

those of 2-D Doppler in importance among the third-generation echocardiography techniques. Applications of CWD are by no means new, but, since this technique has the advantage of providing accurate measurement of high velocity blood flow, it has been reappraised of late. Regardless of the particular technique used, whether it be conventional pulsed-wave Doppler recording or 2-D Doppler color flow imaging, in principle, the phenomenon of aliasing will occur beyond a certain level of flow velocity. This means that an upper limit exists on measurement of the maximal flow velocity. However, "aliasing" does not occur using continuous-wave Doppler recording and a flow velocity with no upper limit can be measured. Various applications of CWD exist, but the most clinically appropriate is that for the approximation of pressure gradient (ΔP) across a stenotic valve using the maximal flow velocity (V) through the stenotic valve[1,2]. In other words, by using the simplified Bernoulli's equation,

$$\Delta P = 4 V^2$$

an approximate value for the pressure gradient can be obtained. Applications of CWD are important for measuring the pressure gradient. However, in this case, the direction of the high velocity jet flow caused by the stenosis ("best jet") is assumed to be the same as that of the ultrasonic beam. In reality, the angle (θ) between the direction of blood flow and that of the ultrasonic beam is always problematic. Ideally, when θ is zero, cos $\theta = 1$, but in general θ is not limited to zero, which is a source of error in this technique. When θ is 20 degrees, there will be a 12% error in the estimation of the pressure gradient; when θ is 30 degrees, a 28% error. Consequently, it is essential to keep θ to a maximum of 20 degrees when measuring the maximal velocity of blood flow using a continuous-wave Doppler. In general, when calculating the maximal flow velocity of the left ventricular blood inflow or the left ventricular blood outflow, the most convenient approach is from the apex. As 2-D Doppler imaging can be used to make a clear image of the maximal flow velocity, a very effective method is to combine the use of 2-D Doppler and CWD. When the two are combined, the cursor line of CWD may be set in the optimum position, parallel to the direction of the "best jet". The 2-D Doppler can be used in almost the same way as conventional echocardiography (Fig. 5-1). Various types of transducers are currently available for a wide range of applications (Fig. 5-2). The transesophageal transducer is also useful for intraoperative use in cardiac surgery and for diagnosis of the dissecting aneurysm.

It is advisable to take full advantage of the features of 2-D Doppler in clinical

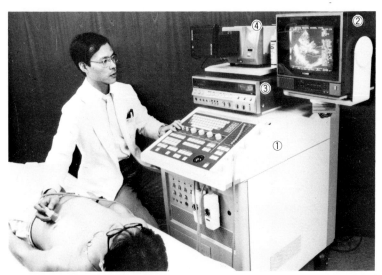

Fig. 5-1　Clinical examination of 2-D Doppler. (1) : 2-D Doppler system (Aloka-860), (2) : TV monitor, (3) : Video recorder, (4) : Instant photo camera.

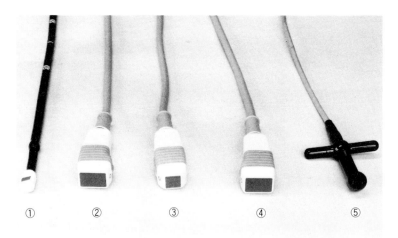

①　②　③　④　⑤

Fig. 5-2　Various types of probes. (1) : Transesophageal probe (3. 5 MHz, 11 mm), (2) : Probe for combined use with CWD (3. 5 MHz), (3) : 5 MHz, (4) : Probe for combined use with CWD (2. 5 MHz), (5) : Independent CWD probe.

applications. These features are outlined below :

1.　The display of the 2-D Doppler flow image is defined by the positional relationship between the direction of the ultrasound beam and the direction of the blood flow ○ P.57 **(Relationship between Direction of Beam Line and Blood Flow Imaging)**. Therefore, any change in the position of the transducer will result in reversal of the flow direction ○ P.57 display **(Transducer Position and Blood Flow Imaging)**. Selecting the most effective transducer position for flow imaging is also important in order to reduce the level of noise.

2.　To reconstruct a three-dimensional concept of intracardiac blood flow, 2-D Doppler images should be recorded from multiple planes. This kind of information cannot be ○ P.58 obtained by any other current invasive or non-invasive method **(Three-Dimensional Concept of Intracardiac Blood Flow (1))**. For example, mitral regurgitant turbulent flow is imaged as a single jet when recorded from the parasternal long-axis view and as two jets when taken from the apical four-chamber view. The simple combination of these two images provides a three-dimensional concept of intracardiac blood flow. In addition, the distribution of the left ventricular outflow blood, mitral inflow blood through the prosthesis and aortic regurgitant jet flow (AR-jet) can be imaged three-dimensionally from ○ P.59 long-axis and short-axis views **(Three-Dimensional Concept of Intracardiac Blood Flow (2))**.

3.　Skillful examination can be performed by selecting any of the five modes of third-generation echocardiography. Using continuous-wave Doppler, pressure gradients across stenotic valves and/or right ventricular systolic pressure can be estimated. The combination of these various modes can provide very useful information about a wide range of congenital and acquired heart diseases.

5-2 Clinical Examinations with 2-D Doppler

The technique of patient examination is similar to 2-D imaging except for the angle of the transducer and the variation in its position to optimize color flow data. As expected, the examination has some limitations resulting from the principles of the Doppler effect. First of all, the output of the Doppler effect is defined, in part, by the angle θ between the estimated intracardiac blood flow and the beam emitted from the transducer. Efforts should be made, therefore, to increase the Doppler output to a detectable level by making θ comparatively small. The S/N ratio when transmitting and receiving ultrasound is also important in detecting Doppler signals. The acoustic conditions which allow clear B-mode imaging with a favorable S/N ratio also produce desirable Doppler signals. Therefore, the following points should be taken into consideration: It is important to select the appropriate position for the transducer and an appropriate θ setting to facilitate both clear imaging of the B-mode and a display of the blood-flow image in the intended area of examination.

In the authors' institute, the following procedures are usually performed in routine 2-D Doppler examinations :

1） Start with B-mode echocardiography alone using the ASE standard views.

2） Superimpose color-coded 2-D Doppler images on B-mode echocardiograms, and change the position and/or the beam line direction of the transducer to obtain optimal blood-flow images.

3） Temporarily turn off the color mode, if necessary, to determine the anatomical structures using the wide angle B-mode.

4） Turn on the color mode and record 2-D Doppler images with VTR and/or instant color photos.

5） Routinely record data:

　　a） B-mode echocardiograms

　　b） 2-D Doppler images

　　c） flow-mapping M-mode

　　d） flow-mapping M-mode + pulsed-wave Doppler

　　e） continuous-wave Doppler (measurement of various parameters with a software program incorporated in the system)

As shown in the experimental data in Chapter 3, blood flow imaged at an angle θ only slightly off 90 degrees produces a sufficient Doppler output. Thus, using this system, sufficient Doppler output can be obtained even if the θ is near 90 degrees. Indeed, a number of clinical experiences have revealed that clear images of blood flow are obtainable in the left ventricular inflow and outflow tracts even in the standard parasternal view. These observations suggest that blood flow within the beating heart has such a complex flow that it produces a sufficient Doppler output even if the apparent angle between the blood flow and the beam line is near 90 degrees. Flow-mapping M-mode display has, in principle, a better S/N ratio and a lowered minimal detectable level of blood-flow velocity than 2-D Doppler alone, and the use of the flow-mapping M-mode is recommended.

Changes in the 2-D Doppler images according to the relative position of the transducer and the blood flow are demonstrated in the illustrations **"Relationship between Direction of Beam Line and Blood Flow Imaging"** and **"Transducer Position and Blood Flow Imaging"**. Another important point relating to the fundamental performance of this system is that the transducer should be placed at the most appropriate position on the chest wall for obtaining blood-flow images of optimal quality in the area of the cardiac chamber being imaged. The rationale for this is that "failure to image the blood flow in an area does not negate the existence of blood flow" but only indicates a "failure to detect blood flow for some reason". We should bear in mind, for example, that the best position for the transducer to obtain the blood-flow images in the left ventricular outflow tract is not necessarily the best position for the blood-flow imaging in the left ventricular inflow tract. For example, severe aortic regurgitant flow is not clearly observed using the transducer position where the blood flow from the left atrium to the left ventricle is best visualized. In such situations, the transducer should be angled appropriately.

References

1) Hatle, L.: Pulsed and continuous wave Doppler in diagnosis and assessment of various heart lesions. *In* Doppler Ultrasound in Cardiology, 2nd ed., Edited by L. Hatle and B. Angelsen, Philadelphia, Lea & Febiger, 1985.
2) Stamm, R. B., Martin, R. P.: Quantification of pressure gradients across stenotic valves by doppler ultrasound. J. Am. Coll. Cardiol., 2: 707-718, 1983.

Chapter 6   Pitfalls and Artifacts

Although Doppler echocardiography has been widely applied clinically, it is not without its problems of interpretation. These arise mainly from artifacts and pitfalls in reading due to the physical limitations of ultrasound itself and to the mechanical characteristics of the equipment. Since two-dimensional Doppler is no exception in this respect, particular care should be taken in reading.

6-1   Aliasing

Doppler shift frequency=f_d, is expressed as:

$$f_d = \frac{2v}{c} \cos \theta \cdot f_0$$

where: v=velocity of blood flow
c =velocity of ultrasound
where: θ=angle of incidence (between directions of blood flow and Doppler beam)
where: f_0=transmitted frequency
Maximal detectable Doppler shift frequency=f_{max}
is expressed as:

$$f_{max} = \frac{PRF}{2}$$

where: PRF=pulse repetition frequency

If $f_d > f_{max}$, this signal is displayed on the opposite side of the zero line in the spectral analysis, as shown in Fig. 6-1. Any 2-D Doppler signal where velocity is more than the maximal detectable velocity (or frequency) is displayed in the opposite color. This phenomenon is called aliasing. However, in 2-D Doppler, an aliased blood flow signal is usually surrounded by a lower velocity flow which is not aliased. In **Pitfall 1, A** the ○P.60 short-axis view of the aortic root shows aliased flow in the pulmonary artery that is displayed in yellow in the middle of a blue area when the frequency of the transducer is 4 KHz. With an 8 KHz transducer, this aliasing disappears. Aliasing is also seen in the flow-mapping M-mode, and the spectral analysis shows a "wrap-around" phenomenon

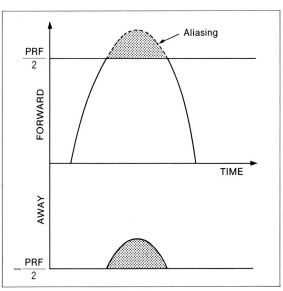

Fig. 6-1   Scheme of aliasing in the spectral analysis.

○ P.60 **(Pitfall 1, C).**

When it is very difficult to differentiate whether the signal is aliased or not, spectral analysis is an excellent method for differentiating, by means of the wrap-around signal. The other way to verify the presence of aliasing is to elevate the maximum detectable velocity by changing the transducer to a lower frequency, or to raise the pulse repetition frequency. If the area of yellow is reduced or disappears in such procedures, aliasing is confirmed. Tab. 6-1 shows that, the higher the pulse repetition frequency becomes, or, the lower the frequency of the transducer falls (or both), the greater the elevation of the maximal detectable velocity.

Tab. 6-1 Relationship between the maximal displayed velocity, frequency of the transducer and pulse repetition frequency.

Transducer	PRF			
	4 KHz	6 KHz	8 KHz	12 KHz
2.5 MHz	0.64	0.93	1.23	1.91
3.5 MHz	0.48	0.70	0.93	1.43
5.0 MHz	0.32	0.47	0.64	0.96

(m/s)

6-2 The Doppler Wall Motion Ghost Signal[1]

We found a certain pattern of Doppler signals in the spectral analysis when the pulsed-Doppler method was used in examinations of the intracardiac flow (Fig. 6-2).

The characteristics of the signal are described below:

(1) The direction of the signal is mainly towards the transducer in systole and away from the transducer in diastole.

(2) The frequency of the signal is low.

(3) The amplitude of the signal corresponds to the velocity of the cardiac wall motion which is in front of the sampling site.

(4) The signal is independent from definite signals of blood flow.

(5) The signal is demonstrated even at the sampling sites where there is definitely no blood flow.

We have found that this artifact signal arose from the cardiac wall motion as a result of reverberation, and was named the Doppler wall motion ghost signal[1,2,3]. This ghost signal is displayed not only in the pulsed-Doppler recording but also in the 2-D Doppler image[1,4].

The Doppler wall motion ghost signal in 2-D Doppler is shown widely and clearly in the

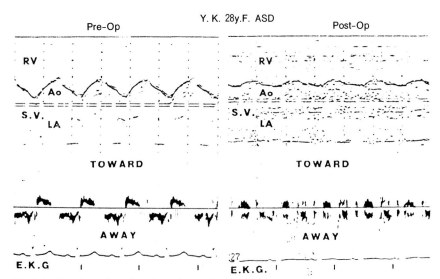

Fig. 6-2 Doppler wall motion ghost signal of an ASD patient before and after the operation. SV=sample volume ; RV= right ventricle ; LA=left atrium ; Ao=aorta.

B-mode image in patients whose wall motion is hyperdynamic. The Doppler wall motion ghost signal is displayed in red in systole and in blue in diastole and the area of this signal covers not only the intracardiac structure but also the extracardiac structure in the rear of the posterior wall of the left ventricle (**Pitfall 2, A, B**). In the M-mode display, the Doppler wall motion ghost signal is displayed as a slim red band in systole and as a slim blue band in diastole, both short in duration (**Pitfall 2, C**).

○ P.61

Spectral analysis data obtained in an ASD by scanning from the anterior wall of the right ventricle to the rear of the posterior wall of the left ventricle, are shown in **Pitfall 2, C**. These data show that the frequency of the Doppler wall motion ghost signal is low at the proximal sample volume, but higher at the distal sample volume. In the M-mode display the colors in the red and blue bands become brighter at the deeper site.

Experiment

An experiment was performed in order to determine the mechanism by which the Doppler wall motion ghost signal increases when the sample volume is deeper. A probe of 2-D Doppler was set just underneath the water surface, as shown in Fig. 6-3. An acrylic reverberation plate was placed at depth a as a model of the chest wall, and a plastic moving plate was moved up and down at a distance, b, deeper than the reverberation plate, as a model of the moving cardiac wall. The Doppler wall motion ghost signal was analyzed in B-mode, in M-mode and by spectral analysis.

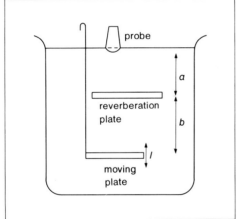

Fig. 6-3 Diagram of the experiment using a water bath.

○ P.61

○ P.62

In the B-mode, multiple oblique red bands are displayed when the moving plate came up, and multiple oblique blue bands were displayed when the motion plate went down (**Pitfall 2, D, E**). In the M-mode, multiple red or blue oblique bands appear simultaneously at various depths. The slope of the deeper bands is two or three times that of the uppermost band, and the color of the deeper bands is brighter (**Pitfall 3, G**). In spectral analysis the frequency of the Doppler wall motion ghost signal is low in the upper sample volume, but at the deeper sample volume, signals two and three times that of the original frequency appear simultaneously (**Pitfall 3, H, I, J, K**).

Fig. 6-4 illustrates the mechanism of generation of Doppler wall motion ghost signals according to the results of the experiment. The ultrasound waves that are reflected once at the moving plate and then rebound between the probe and the reverberation plate make multiple reverberations that apparently rebound from depths represented by b plus multiples of a, or $(na + b)$. The velocity of these reverberating echoes is the same as that of the wall motion (Fig. 6-4, A).

The waves that are reflected twice at the moving plate and then rebound between the probe and the reverberation plate make multiple reverberations apparently rebounding from depths represented by $2b$ plus multiples of a, or $(na + 2b)$. The velocity of these reverberating echoes is twice that of the wall motion (Fig. 6-4, B). Similarly, the waves reflected three times at the moving plate make multiple reverberations at depths $(na + 3b)$.

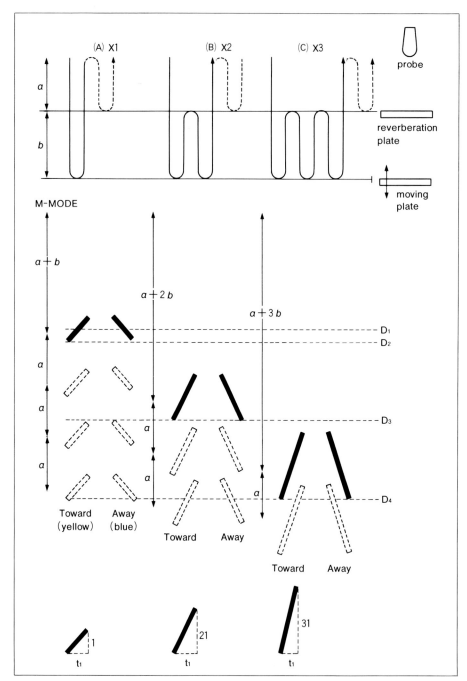

Fig. 6-4 Diagram of the mechanism of generation of the Doppler wall motion ghost signals. The signal with a velocity the same as that of the moving plate arises at the moving plate and is multiplied by reverberation between the probe and the reverberation plate. The signal whose velocity is twice that of the moving plate arises by double reflection at the moving plate and is multiplied by reverberation. Signals whose velocity is triple that of the moving plate arise by reflection three times at the moving plate.

The velocity of these echoes is three times that of the wall motions (Fig. 6-4, C). Thus, the multiple reflections at the moving plate determine the velocity of the Doppler wall motion ghost signal. These reverberating echoes are displayed simultaneously in a practical setting

◯ P.62 in **Pitfall 3, G**.

Theoretically, spectral recordings at the depth D_1 in Fig. 6-5 should represent the velocity of the reverberating echoes at that depth only. However, echoes reverberating more superficially than depth D_1 appear because reverberation occurs between the upper and lower surfaces of the reverberation plate. Therefore the solid line in Fig. 6-5 D_1 is displayed, but the dotted line is not. This fact is also represented in the spectrum in **Pitfall 3, H**. At depth D_1 in Fig. 6-5 the echo has the same velocity as the original signal, although only a part of the echo appears. At depth D_2, a complete echo, whose velocity is the same as that of

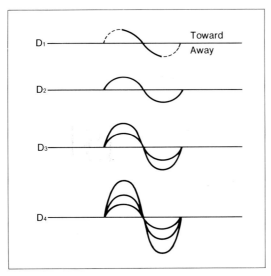

Fig. 6-5 Effect of depth (D_1-D_4) on the spectral display of theoretical Doppler wall motion ghost signal. At depth D_1 (Fig. 6-4) the spectral analysis displays only the center part where the signal is above depth D_1. At depth D_4 double-, and triple-velocity signals appear simultaneously.

the original, appears. At depth D_4 the echoes with velocities equal to and double and triple that of the original appear simultaneously (Fig. 6-5). Since the spectrum analysis shown in Fig. 6-5 theoretically displayed is almost the same as that in the experiment in **Pitfall 3, H, I, J, K**, this theory is confirmed.

○P.62

In a clinical setting, the Doppler wall motion ghost signal in the M-mode is shown as a longitudinal long band in **Pitfall 2, C**. It is thought that the reverberating echoes appeared continuously at all depths because multiple reverberation plates exist in the chest wall and the reverberation between these plates occurred in all combinations. Furthermore, in the case of clinical Doppler wall motion ghost signals, the attenuation of the sound at deeper sites, the wall motion of the posterior wall, and the valve motion may affect the image obtained. Cases in which the wall motion is vigorous demonstrate Doppler wall motion ghost signals clearly. Such cases include atrial septal defects, pericardial effusion and left atrial myxoma.

The following measures may be used to cope with Doppler wall motion ghost signals:

1) Using a flow filter that cuts off the low frequency level of the color signal.

○P.62

The effects of flow filters (1-4) on Doppler wall motion ghost signals are shown **(Pitfall 3, L, M, N, O)**. The cut-off level increases from Filter 1 to Filter 4. Note that the blue Doppler wall motion ghost signals have disappeared with Filter 4.

2) Elevating the level of the minimum detectable velocity by increasing the pulse repetition frequency.

3) Using the rejection function which cuts off the part of the signal below a certain level.

4) Employing the color edge function to eliminate color signals that overlap gray-scale signals from solid structures.

6–3 Artifacts Produced by the Valve

Since the velocity of the valve motion is much faster than that of the cardiac wall motion, and because reflection of the Doppler beam at the valve is very strong, the valve itself produces intense color signals. Even if Doppler penetration is weak, as in **Pitfall 4**, artifacts produced by the valve are well displayed. In the conventional long-axis view of the left ventricle, the anterior leaflet of the mitral valve, which moves anteriorly in early diastole, is shown in red, whereas it is displayed in blue in late diastole, when the valve closes with a

○ P.63

posterior motion **(Pitfall 4, B, D)**. The flow mapping M-mode shows the valve motion in color **(Pitfall 4, C)**. This artifact is frequently accompanied by a reverberation artifact, which is displayed just beneath the valve artifact **(Pitfall 4, B)**.

In 2-D Doppler, the reverberation from the prosthetic valve produced a strong artifact signal, which is seen extending down from just beneath the valve in 2-D Doppler **(Pitfall 4,**

E, G). Despite the strength of these artifact signals, they correspond well with the valve motion, which is very fast. Since these artifacts are of very short duration in comparison with the relatively long duration of the real blood flow signals (**Pitfall 4, F**), it is usually easy to distinguish between the two.

Care in differentiation is particularly required when the mitral flow signals are displayed simultaneously with artifact signals of the mitral valve. The valve artifacts may be suppressed by elimination by means of the color edge function, of the color signals that overlap the gray-scale signals from solid structures.

6—4 Artifacts Produced by Side Lobes

One characteristic of the phased-array system is the side lobe phenomenon, in which signals are displayed at locations different from those where they originate. Such artifact signals from solid structures are produced by the side lobes of the ultrasound beam, and are frequently encountered, but artifacts of blood flow signals caused by side lobes are seldom seen, because Doppler blood flow signals are about 40 dB weaker than those from solid tissues, and the signals from the side lobes are weaker than those from the main lobe. However, the artifact signals from a prosthetic valve that are due to the side lobes produce fairly strong screen images (**Pitfall 4, H**), but the main lobe artifact signals from the prosthetic valve are displayed more strongly (**Pitfall 4, G**), so that it is not difficult to identify the artifacts.

◐P.63

6—5 Mirror Image

Mirror images arise in 2-D Doppler when the Doppler beam is reflected once at a wall. Thus, with the precordial approach, the pericardium behind the posterior wall of the left ventricle is apt to act as a mirror. In **Pitfall 4, B,** the anterior leaflet of the mitral valve is displayed in red in early diastole, but its mirror image behind the left ventricle is seen as a blue artifact. When the anterior leaflet of the mitral valve appears blue in late diastole, its mirror image is red (**Pitfall 4, D**). In the flow mapping M-mode, the color signal of the anterior leaflet of the mitral valve was clearly seen to have a mirror image of the opposite color at a corresponding site on the other side of the pericardium (**Pitfall 4, C**).

Blood flow signals also produce mirror images under certain conditions. **Pitfall 5, A and B** show the left ventricular inflow through the mitral valve from the apical view. The 2-D echocardiogram reproduces the anterior and posterior leaflets of the mitral valve in the heart and their mirror images behind the left ventricle on the other side of the pericardium (**Pitfall 5, A**). The pericardium acts as a concave mirror. In 2-D Doppler, part of the real image of the blood flow through the mitral valve is represented in blue owing to aliasing due to its high velocity (**Pitfall 5, B**). However, its mirror image behind the concave pericardium is displayed in a weak yellowish color, because the velocity vector of this mirror image toward the transducer is small. Since Doppler flow signals in the more superficial regions of the body are generally strong, high blood flow rates may result in mirror images across the pericardium. Care should therefore be taken in relation to rapid flow near the transducer.

◑ P.64

6—6 Direction of Blood Flow in Sector Scanning

In sector scanning there are many beams radiating from the transducer. The color signals on each beam indicate the vector to the transducer, but not the true blood flow direction. In **Pitfall 5, D,** the flow in the tube running obliquely across the screen in the sector scanning B-mode is displayed in blue owing to aliasing in the deepest part, in a weaker red color at a

◐P.64

shallower site and by no color at all at the uppermost part of the tube. This is because the velocity vector of the flow in the oblique tube relative to the transducer varies from the deep to the shallow sites, not because the direction of the flow changes. In **Pitfall 5, E** a flow parallel to the transducer is also displayed in red, no color, and blue from the right to the left, owing to the change of the velocity vector to the transducer.

In linear scanning, on the other hand, flows with a certain direction and velocity have a fixed velocity vector to the transducer, and are displayed with a fixed color and brightness without change along the length of the tube **(Pitfall 5, F)**.

6—7　Frame Rate and Time Delay

The frame rate of the 2-D Doppler image related to the pulse repetition frequency, the display angle of the 2-D Doppler image, the frequency of the transmission of the Doppler sound on one beam and the maximum displayed depth (Fig. 6-6) (Tab. 6-2). The time taken to display a two-dimensional image with a broad display angle, and thus the time delay between the right and left edges of the image are determined by frame rate (Tab. 6-3) . If frame rate is low, this time delay is not negligible and the displayed image is a distortion of the real image. In infant cases with tachycardia, the high-velocity blood flow in the cardiac chamber cannot be properly evaluated at a low frame rate. If the frame rate is increased, 2-D images become more accurate representations of real-time images, but the maximum possible displayed depth becomes shallower (Tab. 6-2, 3). Accordingly, the optimal frame rate, pulse repetition frequency and displayed depth for the region under examination should be carefully selected.

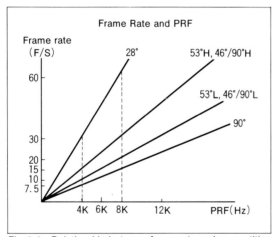

Fig. 6-6　Relationship between frame rate, pulse repetition frequency and display angle.

Tab. 6-2　Relationship between frame rate and the maximum displayed depth. (53°L)

	PRF			
	4 KHz	6 KHz	8 KHz	12 KHz
Frame rate　(p/s)	10	15	20	30
Maximum depth (cm)	18	12	9	6

Tab. 6-3　Frame rate and time delay between the right and the left edges.

Frame rate	Time delay
7.5 f/sec	128 msec
10　f/sec	96 msec
15　f/sec	65 msec
20　f/sec	48 msec
30　f/sec	32 msec

6—8　Significance of Non-Color Display

Although 2-D Doppler displays blood flow in color, areas of no color are frequently encountered. The possibility of the absence of any flow should first be considered; but it sometimes happens that flows of blood are not visualized in color and this might be misinterpreted as the absence of any flow. The principal conditions that may result in absence of color in areas of 2-D Doppler displays are listed below.

1) Absence of flow

Although no color display appears, a thrombus echo or a slight moving echo may be visualized in the gray scale if the resolution of the echo is good.

2) Excessively low setting of the color gain

This may be simply corrected by the operator. The optimal setting of the color gain is just below the level at which major areas of noise are eliminated.

3) Excessively low blood flow velocity

The minimal displayed velocity vector to the transducer in current sector scanning 2-D Doppler systems is 4-6 cm/sec. In the latest linear scanning 2-D Doppler equipment for peripheral vascular disease, which offer high-frequency transducers, and low pulse repetition frequencies, flow velocity vectors of about 2 cm/sec can be displayed in color.

4) Low flow velocity vector to the transducer

If the angle between a blood flow with sufficient velocity and the Doppler beam from the transducer is close to a right angle, the blood flow is not displayed in color. Accordingly, when color flow visualization is needed, the Doppler beam should be realigned closer to the axis of the flow.

5) Weak Doppler signal

Even if the color gain is adjusted properly, insufficient Doppler signal intensity will result in a failure to display in color. Doppler signals reflected from deep regions of the body or transmitted through a very thick body wall may be too weak to be displayed in color.

6) Excessively high setting of the flow filter

Various settings of the flow filter level may be tried in order to eliminate Doppler wall motion ghost signals. If the velocity vector of the blood flow is lower than this level, the blood flow will not be displayed in color, and so the flow filter level should be lowered. However, if this induces Doppler wall motion ghost signals, it becomes difficult to differentiate between these and real low velocity flow signals. This is the limitation of displays of low velocity flow, especially in the cardiac chamber, which tends to produce rather strong Doppler wall motion ghost signals.

7) Interference by artifacts in the gray scale

If a color display overlaps the echo of a structure, it may be eliminated by means of the Color Edge function. This function effectively eliminates Doppler wall motion ghost signals and valve artifacts, but mirror-image artifacts, side lobe artifacts and reverberations of gray-scale echoes may interfere with the real blood flow signals.

8) Display in the non-color zone

When the velocity vector of the blood flow is an even number multiple of the maximal displayed velocity, it is not displayed in color, because such blood flow velocities, which occur only during aliasing, are displayed at the zero level by spectral analysis, and occupy the non-color zone of a color flow display. However, since the blood flow is usually pulsatile even in the veins and since its velocity vector has some range of variance, it may nevertheless be intermittently displayed in color.

References

1) Takamoto, S.: Pitfalls in Reading, Artifacts Signals. *In* Color Atlas of Real-Time Two-Dimensional Doppler Echocardiography. 1st Ed. Edited by R. Omoto. Tokyo, Shindan-to-Chiryo Co., 1984.

2) Takamoto, S., Asano, H., Kondo, Y., Miura, K., Kubota, S., Omoto, R.: Clinical analysis of wall motion ghost signal in pulsed-Doppler echogram. Proceedings of the 43rd Meeting of the Japan Society of Ultrasonics in Medicine, 171, 1983.

3) Kondo, Y., Miura, K., Kubota, S., Takamoto, S., Asano, H., Omoto, R.: Some considerations for artifacts on an ultrasonic pulsed Doppler method. Proceedings of the 42nd Meeting of the Japan Society of Ultrasonics in Medicine, 299, 1983.

4) Takamoto, S., Asano, H., Kyo, S., Ueda, K., Omoto, R., Kondo, Y.: Experimental analysis of Doppler wall motion ghost signal by real-time two-dimensional Doppler echocardiography system. Proceedings of the 43rd Meeting of the Japan Society of Ultrasonics in Medicine, 435, 1983.

49

Color Velocity Function

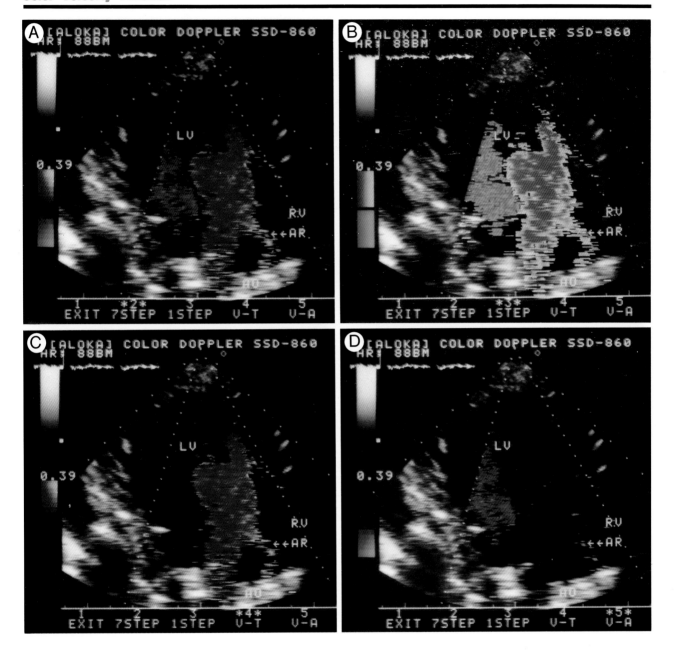

Ⓐ Ⓑ Ⓒ Ⓓ Color -bar in the left side of display shows color coding. Ⓐ 7-step display. Ⓑ 1-step display. Ⓒ Approaching flow display. Ⓓ Receding flow display.

Color Display Function

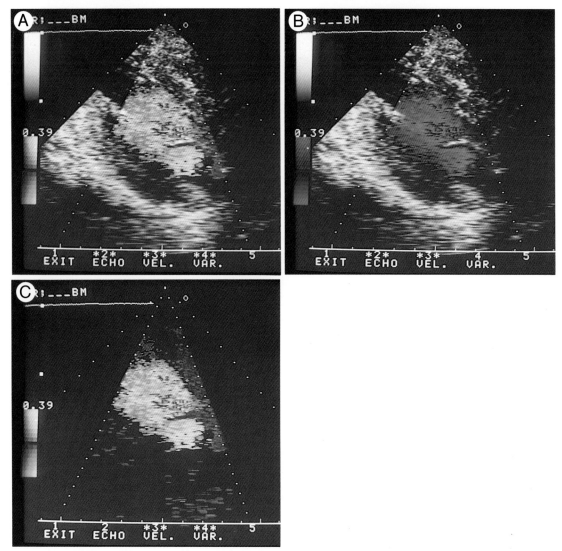

Ⓐ ECHO : ON, VEL : ON, VAR : ON, **Ⓑ** ECHO : ON, VEL : ON, VAR : OFF, **Ⓒ** ECHO : OFF, VEL : ON, VAR : ON.

Color Enhance Function

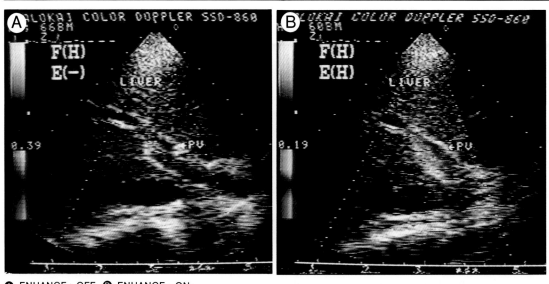

Ⓐ ENHANCE : OFF. **Ⓑ** ENHANCE : ON.

Color Baseline Shift Function

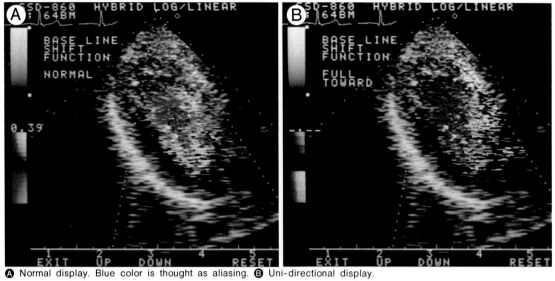

Ⓐ Normal display. Blue color is thought as aliasing. Ⓑ Uni-directional display.

Color Reject Function

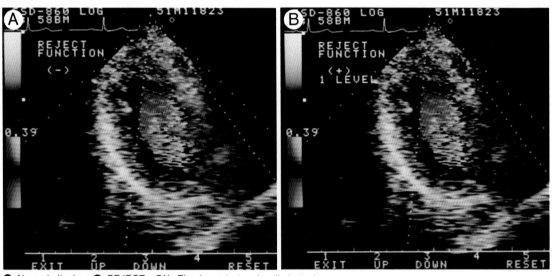

Ⓐ Normal display. Ⓑ REJECT : ON. The lowest step is eliminated.

Color Edge Function

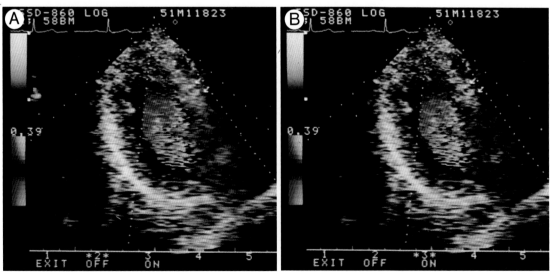

Ⓐ Normal display. Ⓑ COLOR EDGE : ON. Color is eliminated where black/white image is dominant.

Transducer Position and Blood Flow Imaging

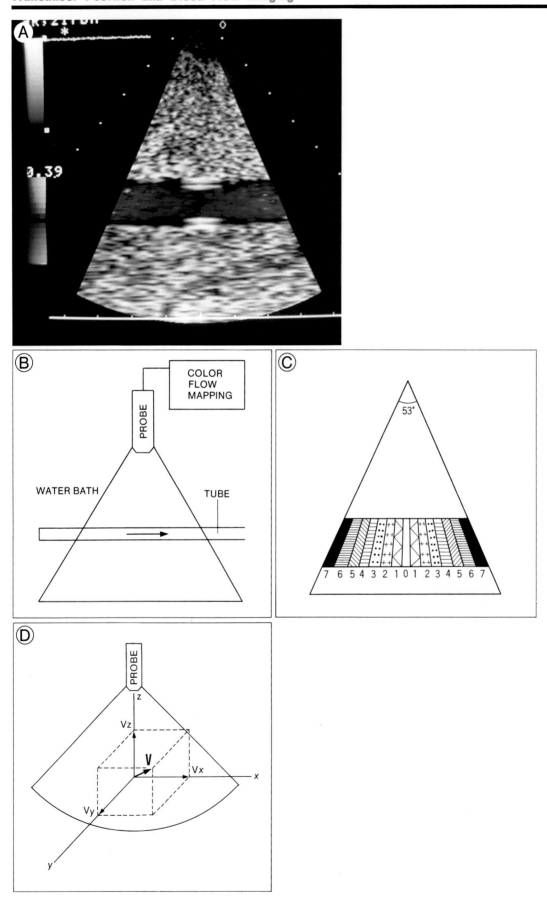

Ⓐ Detection of flow velocity in a latex tube placed in water. ⒷⒸ Simulation of flow detection. Output estimation in case of static flow. Ⓓ Flow velocity obtained as the velocity components of three-dimensional flow in the direction of the probe.

53

Influence of Frame Rate

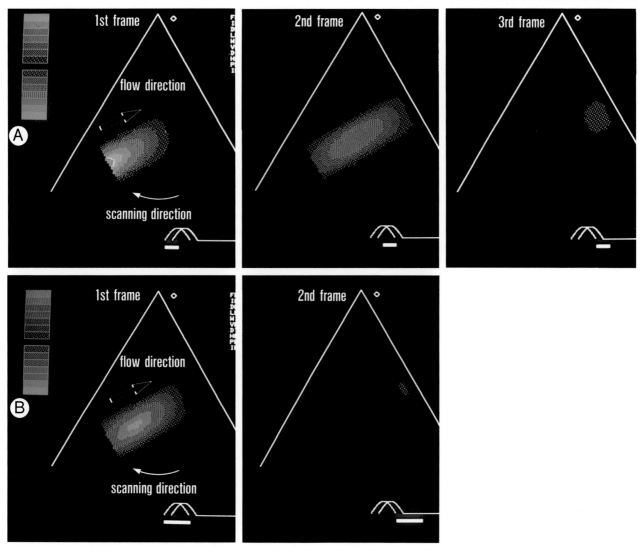

A Heart Rate : 60/min, Frame rate : 10 f/s. **B** Heart Rate : 120/min, Frame rate : 10 f/s.

Influence of Scanning Directions

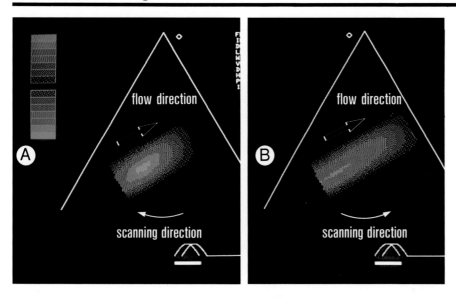

A Beam scanning is from right to left. **B** Beam scanning is from left to right.

Expression of Variance

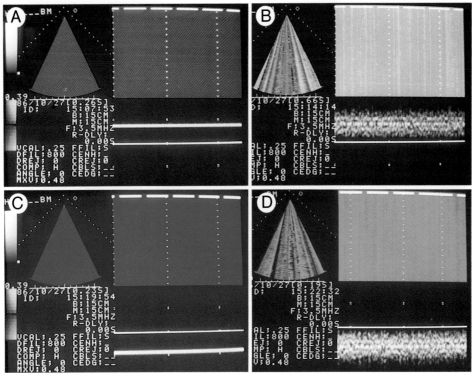

A● Diagrams showing pure red or blue colors with input of narrow frequency band electrical signals. **B**● Diagrams showing yellow and blue-green colors with wide frequency band electrical signals.

Display of Mosaic Pattern

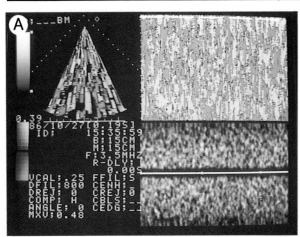

A A mosaic pattern is obtained when wide frequency band electrical signals are input.

Selection of Maximum Detection Flow Velocity

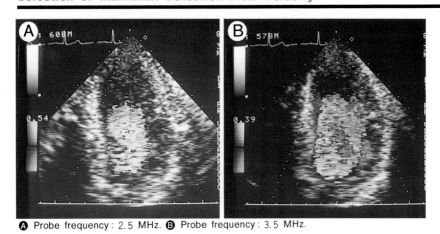

A Probe frequency : 2.5 MHz. **B** Probe frequency : 3.5 MHz.

Selection of Flow Velocity Range

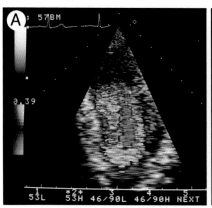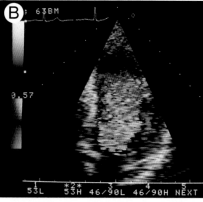

Ⓐ Flow velocity range : 4 KHz.
Ⓑ Flow velocity range : 6 KHz.

Selection of Examination Field of View

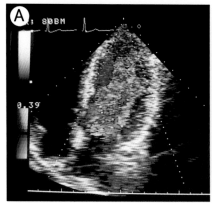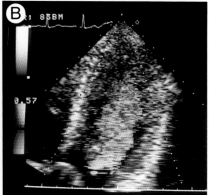

Ⓐ Examination depth : 15 cm (Flow velocity range : 4 KHz).
Ⓑ Examination depth : 12 cm (Flow velocity range : 6 KHz).

Selection of Scanning Sector Angle

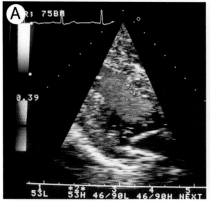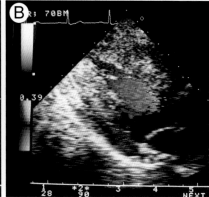

Ⓐ Scanning sector angle : 53°.
Ⓑ Scanning sector angle : 90°.

Selection of Frame Rate

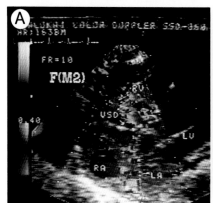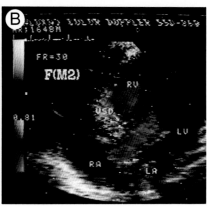

Ⓐ Frame rate : 10 f/s.
Ⓑ Frame rate : 30 f/s.

56

Optimal Gain Setting

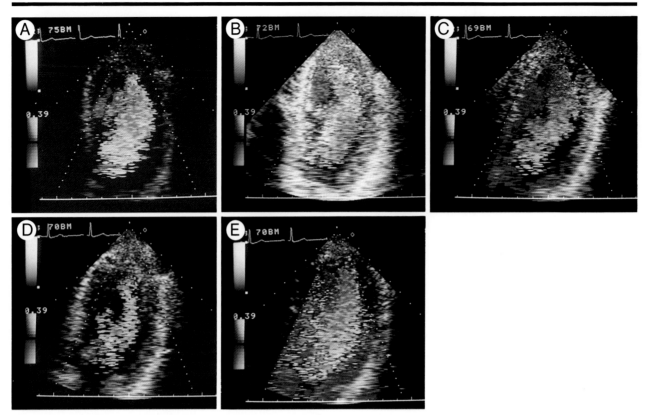

Ⓐ The B-mode gain is too weak. Ⓑ The B-mode gain is too high. Ⓒ The B-mode and flow gain is a correct setting. Ⓓ The flow gain is too weak. Ⓔ The flow gain is too high.

Selection of Focal Points

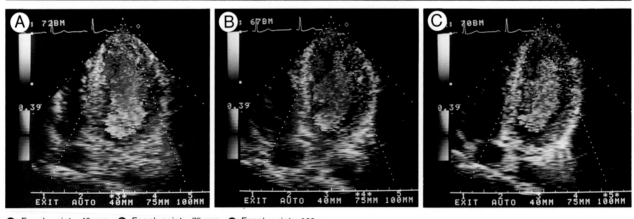

Ⓐ Focal point: 40 mm. Ⓑ Focal point: 75 mm. Ⓒ Focal point: 100 mm.

Relationship between Direction of Beam Line and Blood Flow Imaging

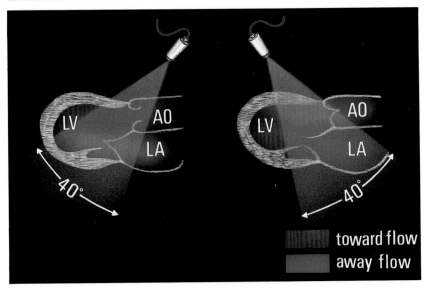

toward flow
away flow

Diagram showing the relationship between direction of beam line and blood flow imaging.
The colors in high parasternal view (left) and those in low parasternal view (right) are exactly reversed.

Transducer Position and Blood Flow Imaging **Normal heart** 6-year-old male

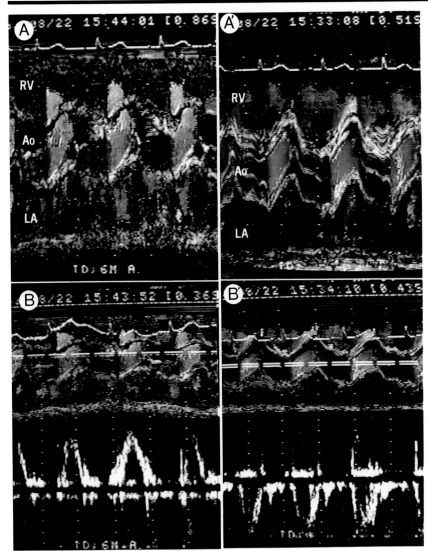

2-D Doppler images demonstrating the relation between transducer position and blood flow imaging.
ⒶⒷ Transducer position is located in the higher left sternal border. ⒶⒷ Transducer position is located in the lower left sternal border. ⒶⒶ Flow-mapping M-mode at the level of the aortic valve. ⒷⒷ Simultaneous display of flow-mapping M-mode and pulsed-wave Doppler.

Three-Dimensional Concept of Intracardiac Blood Flow (1) Mitral Stenosis and Regurgitation
48-year-old female

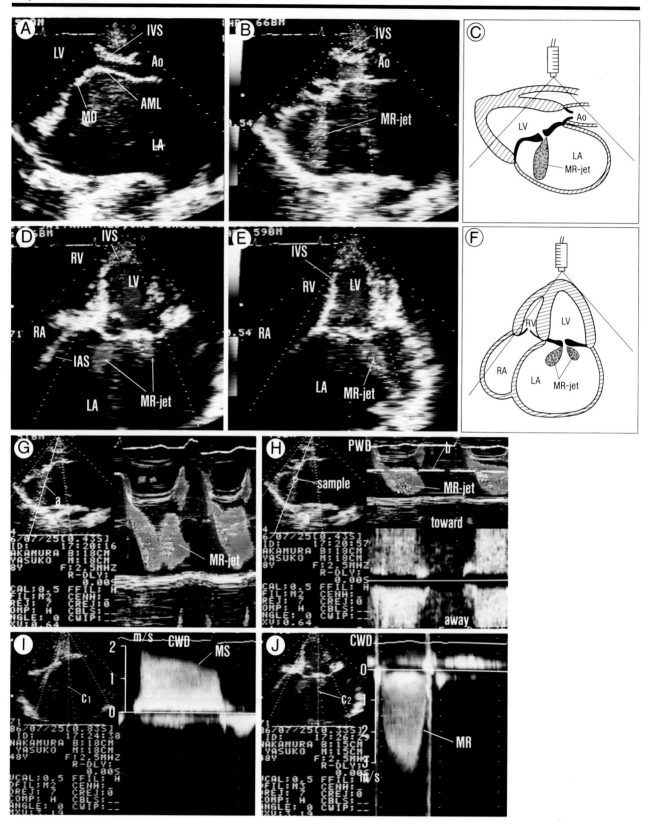

2-D Doppler images in a patient with mitral stenosis and regurgitation (MS·MR).
Ⓐ B-mode in long-axis view in diastole. Ⓑ 2-D Doppler same view, systole. One mitral regurgitant jet (MR-jet) is shown in parasternal long-axis view. Ⓒ Diagram of Ⓑ. Ⓓ 2-D Doppler in apical four-chamber view in systole. Two regurgitant jets are demonstrated in this view. Ⓔ 2-D Doppler in apical four-chamber view in systole. The cross-sectional plane of Ⓔ is slightly different from that of Ⓓ. Ⓕ Diagram of Ⓓ. Ⓖ Flow-mapping M-mode (beam line : a). Ⓗ Pulsed-wave Doppler (sample volume : b). Ⓘ Continuous-wave Doppler of mitral valve flow (beam line : c_1). Ⓙ Continuous-wave Doppler of mitral regurgitant flow (beam line : c_2). Maximal velocity of mitral regurgitant flow is 3.2 m/s.
[Evaluation of mitral stenosis]
max V=1.8 m/s, max ΔP=6 mmHg, P1/2T=0.20 sec, MVA=1.0 cm².

Three-Dimensional Concept of Intracardiac Blood Flow(2) Mitral Valve Prosthesis (St. Jude Valve) and Aortic Regurgitation (Sellers' grade 2)   43-year-old male

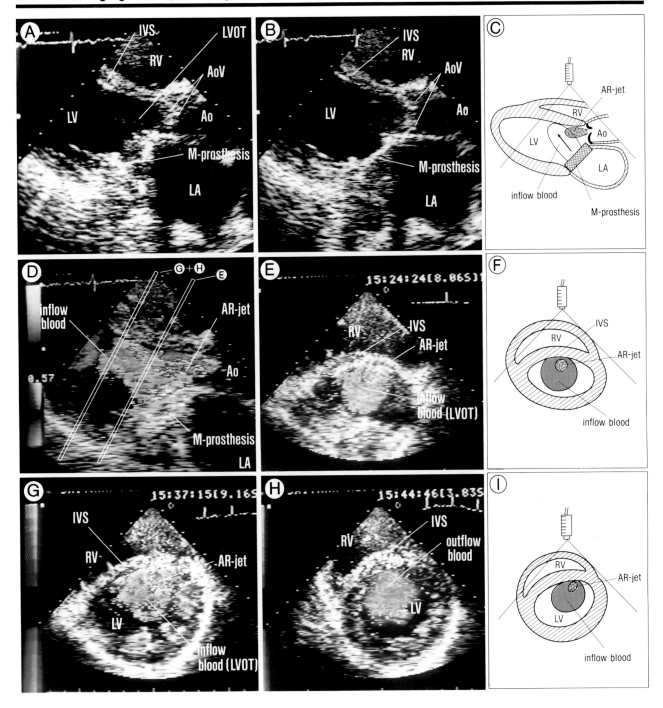

2-D Doppler images in a patient with mitral valve prosthesis and aortic regurgitation(MVR+AR).
A B-mode in long-axis view in diastole. **B** B-mode same view, systole. **C** Diagram of **D**. **D** 2-D Doppler in long-axis view in diastole. Mitral blood flow through prosthesis is displaced medially and strikes the interventricular septum, as it is crossed by aortic regurgitant flow having mosaic pattern toward the apex. **E** 2-D Doppler in short-axis view in diastole. The cross-sectional plane is indicated in **D** as Ⓔ. Aortic regurgitant flow shares the left ventricular outflow tract with mitral inflow blood. **F** Diagram of **E**. **G** 2-D Doppler in short-axis view in diastole. The cross-sectional plane is indicated in **D** as Ⓖ+Ⓗ. **H** 2-D Doppler same view, systole. Cross-sectional plane is indicated in **D** as Ⓖ+Ⓗ.

60

Pitfall 1 Aliasing

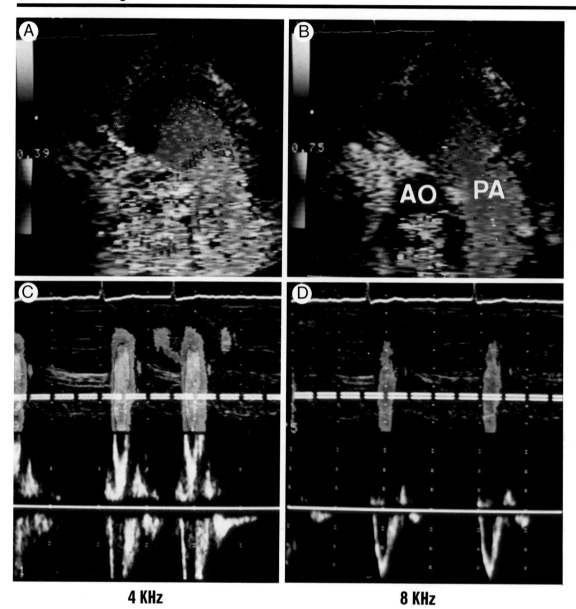

4 KHz　　　　　　　　　**8 KHz**

Effect of change of pulse repetition frequency on aliasing phenomenon.
AB 2-D Doppler images of short-axis view of the aortic root.
CD Flow mapping M-mode and spectral analysis of the pulmonary artery (PA) flow.
With 4 KHz of pulse repetition frequency (PRF) flow in the pulmonary artery is demonstrated by yellow due to aliasing in the middle of blue area.
With 8 KHz of PRF PA flow is demonstrated only by blue color.

Pitfall 2 Doppler Wall Motion Ghost Signal (1)

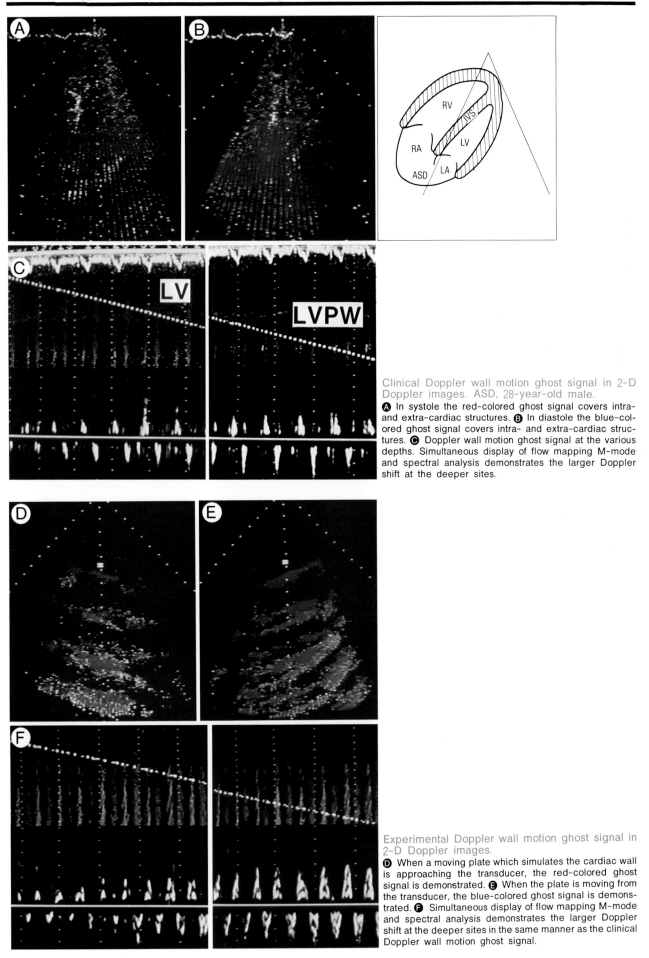

Clinical Doppler wall motion ghost signal in 2-D Doppler images. ASD, 28-year-old male.
A In systole the red-colored ghost signal covers intra- and extra-cardiac structures. **B** In diastole the blue-colored ghost signal covers intra- and extra-cardiac structures. **C** Doppler wall motion ghost signal at the various depths. Simultaneous display of flow mapping M-mode and spectral analysis demonstrates the larger Doppler shift at the deeper sites.

Experimental Doppler wall motion ghost signal in 2-D Doppler images.
D When a moving plate which simulates the cardiac wall is approaching the transducer, the red-colored ghost signal is demonstrated. **E** When the plate is moving from the transducer, the blue-colored ghost signal is demonstrated. **F** Simultaneous display of flow mapping M-mode and spectral analysis demonstrates the larger Doppler shift at the deeper sites in the same manner as the clinical Doppler wall motion ghost signal.

Pitfall 3 Doppler Wall Motion Ghost Signal (2)

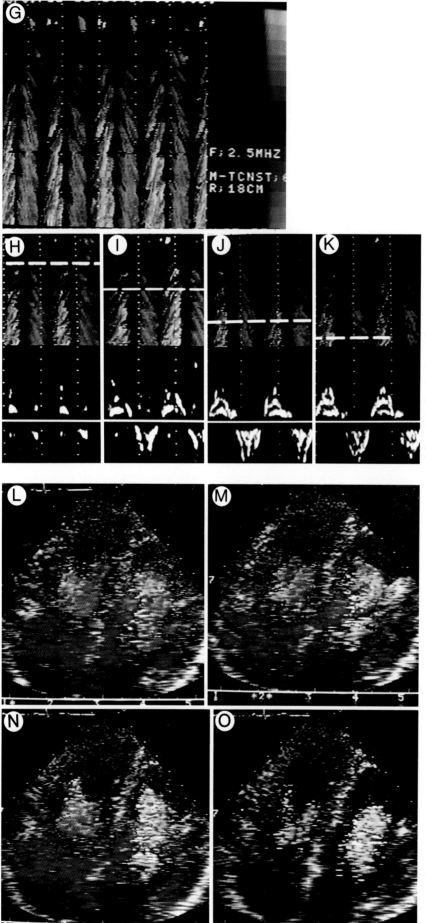

Experimental Doppler wall motion ghost signal in 2-D Doppler images (continued).

Ⓖ Experimental Doppler wall motion signal (color flow mapping M-mode). The slopes of the yellow or blue oblique bands which represent the velocity of the motion plates become steeper at the deeper sites. Each slope change represents multiple reflection of the Doppler wave at the moving plate. Ⓗ Ⓘ Ⓙ Ⓚ Experimental Doppler wall motion ghost signal at various depths (spectral analysis). At the deeper sites the signals of the original, double and triple velocities are displayed simultaneously.

Effects of the color filter on Doppler wall motion ghost signal (blue color).

Ⓛ Filter 1 Ⓜ Filter 2 Ⓝ Filter 3 Ⓞ Filter 4. The level of elimination of low frequency signals is increasing from Filter 1 to Filter 4. Doppler wall motion ghost signal is eliminated only by Filter 4 in this case.

Pitfall 4 Artifacts by Valves

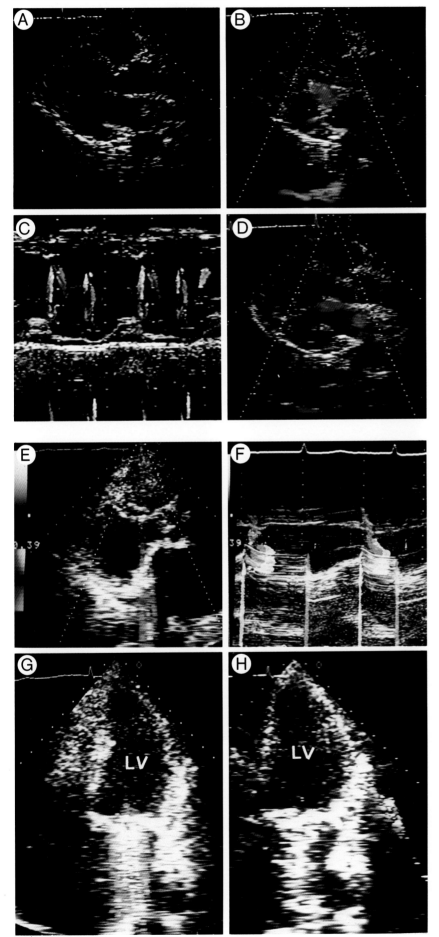

Artifacts by valves (A, B, C, D).
A Long-axis view of the left ventricle of 2 D echo. B 2-D Doppler demonstrates the red-colored artifact by the opening anterior leaflet of the mitral valve and its reverberation during early diastole. The mirror image of this artifact behind the pericardium is demonstrated in blue color. C Flow mapping M-mode demonstrates the artifacts and its mirror image of the mitral valve. D 2-D Doppler demonstrates the blue-colored artifact by the closing anterior leaflet of the mitral valve and the red-colored artifact by the posterior leaflet. The mirror images are demonstrated by the opposite colors.

Artifacts by the prosthetic valve (E, F, G, H).
E 2-D Doppler demonstrates the artifact of the prosthetic valve (SJM valve) due to reverberation at its rear side. F Flow mapping M-mode demonstrates the artifact of the prosthetic valve in very short duration. G 2-D Doppler demonstrates the artifact of the prosthetic valve at its rear side. H 2-D Doppler demonstrates the artifact of the prosthetic valve due to side lobe at the right posterior portion of the valve.

Pitfall 5 Mirror Image, Blood Flow Direction

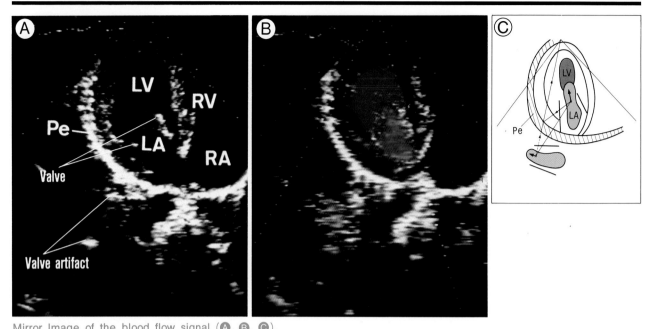

Mirror Image of the blood flow signal (Ⓐ, Ⓑ, Ⓒ).

Ⓐ 2-D echo demonstrates the mirror image of the mitral valve behind the heart, as if the pericardium works as the concave mirror. ⒷⒸ 2-D Doppler demonstrates the blood flow through the mitral valve in high velocity with aliasing and its mirror image at the rear side of the heart. The mirror image is displayed in yellow color of low brightness, since its velocity vector to the transducer is low. Pe=pericardium.

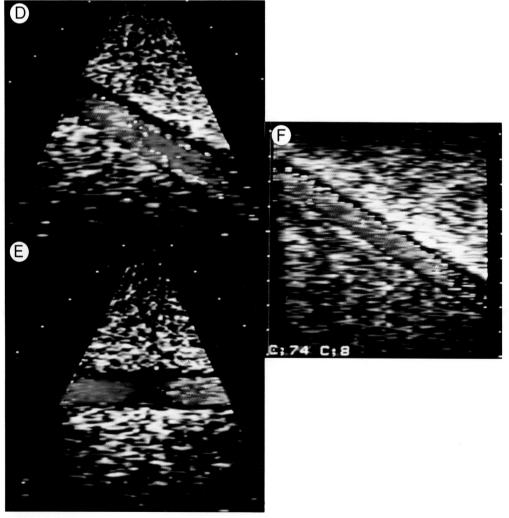

Display of the blood flow direction, Difference between Sector Scanning and Linear Scanning (Ⓓ, Ⓔ, Ⓕ).

By Sector Scanning (Ⓓ, Ⓔ) the flow with a certain direction and velocity is displayed with various colors and brightness, while by Linear Scanning (Ⓕ) that flow is displayed with a certain color and brightness.

Chapter 7   2-D Doppler Images in Normal Hearts

7—1   Adults

⊙P.81

Schematic representation and actual findings of the 2-D Doppler blood-flow images in a normal adult heart are shown in **Normal Heart (1)**. When the transducer is placed in the lower parasternal position with an ultrasound beam directed cranially, the blood-flow images of the inflow and outflow tracts of the left ventricle in the long-axis view are displayed in red in diastole, and in blue in systole. These findings in relation to the blood flow in the left ventricle are also demonstrated in the flow-mapping M-mode and in

⊙P.82

pulsed-wave Doppler recordings **(Normal Heart (2))**. In flow-mapping M-mode, the blood-flow images above the anterior mitral leaflet (AML) are clearly separated from the blood-flow images below the AML by the difference in color **(Normal Heart (2), A and B)**. The correlation between the findings by 2-D Doppler and conventional pulsed-wave Doppler recordings is demonstrated in **Normal Heart (2), C** and **D**.

⊙P.83

The 2-D Doppler findings in another normal adult heart in an apical long-axis view are shown in **Normal Heart (3)**. As shown in **Normal Heart (1), (2), and (3)**, the 2-D Doppler findings of the left ventricular blood-flow images in the parasternal view are similar to those in the apical view. However, in the angular relationship between the blood flow direction and the beam direction in the parasternal view, there is a significant difference from that in the apical view, since the beam direction is nearly parallel to the blood flow direction in the latter view. Thus, in observing the maximal velocities of the left ventricular inflow blood and/or outflow blood an approach from the apex is advantageous because the angle requires hardly any correction. Furthermore, when measuring the maximal blood flow velocity the use of a continuous-wave Doppler - one that is free from "aliasing" - is preferable. The analysis of the diastolic inflow blood pattern of the left ventricle is important in order to evaluate the left ventricular function, in particular its diastolic characteristic. In the left ventricular diastolic blood-flow pattern the height of the R wave corresponding to the rapid filling of the left ventricle, and the height of the A wave corresponding to the left atrial contraction are parameters of interest.

7—2   Child Cases

Children under ten years old usually have a good echo window, so that clear and distinct blood flow images can be readily obtained. Especially in infants, a parasternal or suprasternal approach yields clear blood flow images in the aortic arch and the descending aorta. The subcostal approach is another effective echo window for visualizing the blood flow in the right atrium through an atrial septal defect in children.

There are a number of reasons why clear blood flow images are easy to obtain in pediatric patients :

(1) The shallow scanning depth;

(2) The small echo attenuation through the subcutaneous tissue, the ribs, and the sternum;

(3) The ease of finding a good echo window avoiding the lung tissue, especially in the higher parasternal approach, and the presence of the thymus, which causes far less echo attenuation than lung tissue; and

(4) The good spatial resolution obtainable with a higher transducer transmitting frequency in infants and small children, who have high blood flow velocities and small hearts.

With the relatively shallow scanning depth required in pediatric cases, the higher echo attenuation that occurs at higher transmitting frequencies is negligible. However, the maximum velocity detectable without aliasing is relatively low in transducers with higher

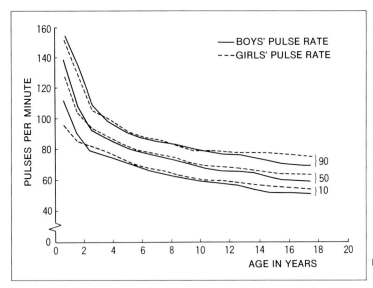

Fig. 7-1-a Pulse rates in infants and children.

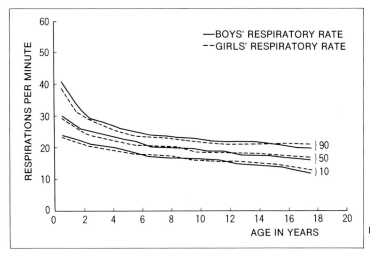

Fig. 7-1-b Respiratory rates in infants and children.

transmitting frequencies. This maximum detectable velocity can be expressed as follows :

$$V_{max} = \frac{C^2}{8 \times f_0 \times D \times \cos \theta} \quad \cdots\cdots\cdots\cdots\cdots\cdots\cdots\cdots\cdots\cdots\cdots\cdots\cdots\cdots\cdots\cdots \quad (1)$$

where: V_{max} = maximum detectable velocity
f_0 = transmitting frequency
D = scanning depth
C = velocity of sound
θ = angle of incidence

The scanning depth is

$$D = \frac{C}{2 \times PRF} \quad \cdots\cdots\cdots\cdots\cdots\cdots\cdots\cdots\cdots\cdots\cdots\cdots\cdots\cdots\cdots\cdots\cdots\cdots \quad (2)$$

where: PRF = pulse repetition frequency
Thus, equation (1) can be re-written as follows:

$$V_{max} = \frac{C \times PRF}{4 \times f_0 \times \cos \theta} \quad \cdots\cdots\cdots\cdots\cdots\cdots\cdots\cdots\cdots\cdots\cdots\cdots\cdots\cdots\cdots \quad (3)$$

When a transducer of higher frequency is employed, a relatively higher PRF should be selected for an appropriate range of V_{max}.

Tab. 7-1 Number of blood flow image frames in one cardiac cycle (diastolic/systolic time ratio=2).

A) Number of image frames in systole

FR \ HR	30	60	90	120	150	180	210
7.5	5	2.5	1.7	1.3	1	0.8	0.7
10	6.7	3.3	2.2	1.7	1.3	1.1	1.0
15	10	5	3.3	2.5	2	1.7	1.4
20	13.3	6.7	4.4	3.3	2.7	2.2	1.9
30	20	10	6.7	5	4	3.3	2.9

B) Number of image frames in diastole

FR \ HR	30	60	90	120	150	180	210
7.5	1.0	5	3.3	2.5	2	1.7	1.4
10	13.3	6.7	4.4	3.3	2.7	2.2	1.9
15	20	10	6.7	5	4	3.3	2.9
20	26.7	13.3	8.8	6.7	5.3	4.4	3.8
30	40	20	13.3	10	8	6.7	5.7

HR=heart rate, FR=frame rate

1. Images of older children

Normal Heart 4, 5: 8-year-old male (BW=27 kg, BH=127 cm)

Color images are almost the same for infants and children as for adults, but the heart rate is somewhat higher in children and markedly so in infants (Fig. 7-1). It is therefore important to select a transducer of the appropriate frequency, scanning depth, and pulse repetition frequency. Moreover, heart wall motion in an infant is very rapid, so that in 2-D Doppler examinations of infants, a cut-off filter of higher frequency should generally be selected in order to avoid the wall motion ghosts. Aliasing is often observed in 2-D Doppler images of intracardiac flows in normal infants and small children. For example, in **Normal Heart 4, B**, a part of the blood inflow into the left ventricle is depicted in red and in **Normal Heart 4, D**, the major part of the left ventricular ejection flow appears in red owing to aliasing. To differentiate between normal aliasing and abnormal turbulent flow, the range of V_{max} may be changed, thus avoiding the aliasing.

With the use of a 5 MHz transducer with a PRF of 4 KHz ($V_{max}=32$ cm/sec) the left ventricular ejection flow is depicted in red, owing to aliasing, as is shown in **Normal Heart 4, D**, but when a 3.5 MHz transducer with a PRF of 8 KHz is utilized, this flow is depicted in the normal blue color (**Normal Heart 5, B**). It is important for 2-D Doppler examinations in infants and small children to appropriately adjust the velocity range. In the long-axis view of the left ventricle the blood inflow into this ventricle during diastole is depicted in red (**Normal Heart 4, D ; 5, B ; 6, D ; 7, C ; and 8, C**). The left ventricular ejection flow in systole appears in blue (**Normal Heart 4, B ; 6, B ; 7,D ; and 8, B**).

The blood flow in the atria is clearly observed in the apical four-chamber view. The blood flows into the ventricles in diastole appear red (**Normal Heart 4, F ; and 8, F**) and the left ventricular ejection flow observed along the interventricular septum is represented in blue. The short-axis view at the aortic valve level is important for the observation of the right ventricular inflow and outflow tracts. The blood flows in the pulmonary trunk and the aortic root flow are shown in blue in systole (**Normal Heart 5, F ; 5, G ; and 8, H**).

Normal Heart 6: 9-year-old male (BW=32 kg, BH=139 cm)

As children grow, the velocities of the intracardiac blood flow approach the same levels as those of adults, so that aliasing does not occur so often in older children as in infants or small children. In **Normal Heart 6**, little aliasing can be seen in the parasternal long-axis view using a 3.5 MHz transducer. **Normal Heart 6, B** is a display in diastole at a PRF of 6 KHz ($V_{max}=70$ cm/sec) and **Normal Heart 6, D** is taken in systole at a PRF of 4 KHz ($V_{max}=48$ cm/sec. No aliasing can be seen in either figure.

2. Images of younger children and infants

Normal Heart 7: 3-year-old female (BW=14 kg, BH=95 cm)

Even in normal children, the heart rate is usually high in children under 3 years old, and

◐P.84
◐P.85
◐P.86
◐P.86

that of infants often exceeds 150/min (Fig. 7-1). Consequently, a skilled examiner is required in infant cases. The heart rate in **Normal Heart 7** is about 100/min, so that even at a frame rate of 15 frames/sec, only nine blood flow image frames are obtained from one cardiac cycle. When this heart was scanned at a lower frame rate, the visualized image was markedly distorted owing to the time lapse between the beginning and end of each scan. In the most advanced scanner currently available, the heart can be scanned at a frame rate of 30/sec (PRF=12 KHz) to a scanning depth of 6 cm, or at a frame rate of 20/sec (PRF=8 KHz) to a depth of 9 cm. It is also preferable in infants and small children to use higher PRF's, because the higher the PRF (and therefore the V_{max}), the less aliasing occurs in normal intracardiac blood flows, with the more appropriate V_{max} (Tab. 7-1).

Normal Heart 8: 4-month-old male (BW=8 kg, BH=65 cm)

○P.87

The heart rate of infants is higher than that of small children. In **Normal Heart 8** the heart rate is about 140/min. When the heart is scanned at a frame rate of 20/sec, only 8.5 blood flow image frames are produced in one cardiac cycle. The visualized images of intracardiac blood flow may still be markedly distorted when the frame rate is 20/sec as a result of the time taken to scan.

In infants the thymus gland occupies the area in front of the ascending aorta, so that it is usually easy to observe the ascending aorta, the aortic arch, and the thoracic descending aorta (**Normal Heart 8, I** and **8, J**) from the higher parasternal or suprasternal windows. These views are useful for diagnosing PDA in premature infants, interruptions of the aortic arch, and aorto-pulmonary fenestration.

Chapter 8   Acquired Valvular Disease

8－1   2-D Doppler Findings in Valvular Regurgitation

The first clinical application of 2-D Doppler was in acquired valvular diseases. "Valvular stenosis" can be adequately diagnosed by demonstrating organic changes using conventional echocardiography (2-D echo). However, 2-D echo is inadequate in diagnosing "valvular regurgitation". Contrast echocardiography is a technique that has been applied to compensate for this limitation. Therefore, evaluation of valvular regurgitation has become the first clinical application using the 2-D Doppler modality. Investigations using 2-D Doppler clinically have shown that it is very useful in the detection of aortic, mitral and tricuspid regurgitations, and that it offers a favorable correlation with angiography and/or with surgical findings in the semi-quantitative grading of the severity of valvular regurgitation. The 2-D Doppler findings in valvular regurgitation show the following two distinct characteristics of the Doppler signals: most regurgitant blood flows are characterized as (1) wide-band or broad-band patterns and (2) bi-directional flow patterns. To be more specific, in color-coded flow mapping, the regurgitant flow is inlaid with red-and-blue mosaic patterns which are further superimposed with green (indicating variance). The first characteristic "wide-band or broad-band" is common to all types of valvular regurgitation, but the second, "bi-directionality", does not always occur to the same degree. In some cases, Doppler signals of one direction corresponding to the direction of the regurgitating flow take predominance over signals from the reverse direction. A precise analysis of blood flow can also be achieved by simultaneous displays of the flow-mapping M-mode and pulsed-wave Doppler.

We compared the 2-D Doppler findings with the angiography or surgical findings, and set criteria for the semi-quantitative evaluation of valvular regurgitation[1]. Sellers' classification[2] is used as the criteria for evaluating aortic and mitral regurgitations by angiography. On the other hand, there are various criteria for the semi-quantitative evaluation of valvular regurgitations by 2-D Doppler. From the outset of our study the authors have used the maximum distance reached by the jet-form mosaic pattern (regurgitant jet pattern) exhibited by valvular regurgitation. The simplicity of this evaluation method — which uses the maximum distance attained by regurgitant jet flow — and the favorable correlation it has with angiographic and surgical findings, provide some practical advantages. However, the method has various weaknesses. If both narrow and wide regurgitant jets extend over the same distance, the severity of regurgitation is, clearly,

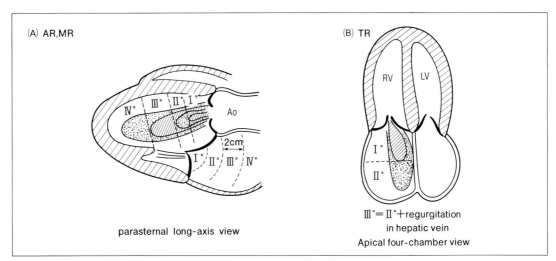

Fig. 8-1   Diagrams demonstrating how 2-D Dopper findings can be used to quantitate the severity of valvular regurgitation on a four-grade scale. Severity of valvular regurgitation by 2-D Doppler is mainly determined from the farthest distance reached by the regurgitant jets (see Tab. 8-1, 2, 3).

greater in the latter. For grading the severity of mitral regurgitation, a four-point scale classification based on 1.5 cm stepwise[3] increases in distance was reported, indicating fairly good correlation between the grading by 2-D Doppler and that by left ventriculography. In a recent report[4], an excellent angiographical correlation was achieved with the maximum area of the regurgitant jet signals expressed as a percentage of the left atrial area in all three planes, namely the apical four-chamber, parasternal long-axis, and right parasternal short-axis views. As for the 2-D Doppler assessment of aortic regurgitation, for example, the cross-sectional area of aortic regurgitant jets during diastole depicted at the level of the aortic annulus in the short-axis plane showed high correlation with the severity of aortic regurgitation[5]. As described above, the criteria used in the authors's studies were based on the farthest distance reached by the regurgitant jets. Although fairly good correlation was obtained with angiographical grading, as shown in Tabs. 8-1, 2, and 3, the authors are still now evaluating several criteria for grading of valvular regurgition by 2-D Doppler[6,7,8]. As for

Tab. 8-1 The correlation of 2-D Doppler and cineangiography in grading the degree of aortic regurgitation in 156 patients. Angio: cineangiographic grading (Sellers' classification), 2-D Doppler: Severity of aortic regurgitation (AR) determined by 2-D Doppler imaging on a four-grade scale.

Angio \ 2-D Doppler	0°	I°	II°	III°	IV°
0°					
I°	3	20	7		
II°		3	42	13	
III°			9	43	4
IV°				4	8

(May, 1986 Saitama)

The criteria for assessing the severity of AR by 2-D Doppler are based mainly on the maximal distance reached by regurgitant blood-flow images (RFIs) in the left ventricular outflow tract (in long-axis view):

(I°)	RFIs are localized between the region just inferior to the aortic valve and the middle of the level of the anterior mitral leaflet (AML).
(II°)	RFIs reach the level of the tip of AML.
(III°)	RFIs extend further to the level of the papillary muscle.
(IV°)	RFIs are visualized more deeply and extensively beyond the papillary muscles to the apex.

AML : anterior mitral leaflet.

Tab. 8-2 The correlation of 2-D Doppler and cineangiography in grading the degree of mitral regurgitation in 109 patients. Angio: cineangiographic grading (Sellers' classification), 2-D Doppler: Severity of mitral regurgitation (MR) by 2-D Doppler imaging on a four-grade scale.

Angio \ 2-D Doppler	0°	I°	II°	III°	IV°
0°					
I°	4	14	3		
II°		4	38	4	
III°			5	25	2
IV°				3	7

(May, 1986 Saitama)

The criteria for assessing the severity of MR by 2-D Doppler are based mainly on the maximal distance reached by regurgitant blood-flow images (RFIs) from the mitral orifice into the left atrium.

(I°)	RFIs are localized immediately posterior to the mitral valve in the left atrium not exceeding the middle level between the mitral orifice and the valve ring.
(II°)	RFIs reach almost to the level of the mitral valve ring.
(III°)	RFIs are present deeply within 2 cm from the level of the mitral valve ring.
(IV°)	Deeply RFIs are present beyond 2 cm from the level of the mitral valve ring, often visualized diffusely in the entire left atrium.

Tab. 8-3 The correlation of 2-D Doppler and operative findings in grading the degree of tricuspid regurgitation in 73 patients. Ope : grading from operative finding, 2-D Doppler : Severity of tricuspid regurgitation (TR) evaluated pre-operatively by 2-D Doppler on a three-grade scale.

Ope \ 2-D Doppler	0°	I°	II°	III°
0°		8	3	
I°		18	8	
II°			18	6
III°				12

(May, 1986 Saitama)

The criteria for assessing the severity of TR by 2-D Doppler are based mainly on the maximal distance reached by regurgitant blood-flow images (RFIs) from the tricuspid valve in the right atrium (in apical four-chamber view) and presence of significant regurgitant blood flow in the hepatic vein (in subcostal view).

(I°)	RFIs are present within one half of the right atrium above the tricuspid valve.
(II°)	RFIs are present diffusely within the entire right atrium.
(III°)	RFIs are present in the entire right atrium. At the same time, significant regurgitant blood flows are demonstrated in the hepatic vein in systole.

the evaluation of tricuspid regurgitation, established diagnosis is made using surgical findings[9], since right ventriculography is not routinely performed in the authors' institute. Prior to the cannulation for cardiopulmonary bypass, the regurgitant jet is examined by the surgeon inserting his forefinger into the right atrium so that it is 1 cm above the center of the tricuspid valve. The size of the regurgitant jet is compared with that of the finger and is graded as I (grade 1 : smaller than the width of the forefinger), II (grade 2 : almost the same) or III (grade 3 : larger). The criteria used for the semi-quantitative evaluation of valvular regurgitation with 2-D Doppler are described in Tab. 8-1 (aortic), Tab. 8-2 (mitral) and Tab. 8-3 (tricuspid). As shown in Tabs. 8-1, 2 and 3, 2-D Doppler has revealed its sensitive diagnostic capability in valvular regurgitation and correlated well with cardiac catheterization data and surgical findings. In tricuspid regurgitation, however, compared with the operative evaluation we tend to over-assess by about one grade when using 2-D Doppler. However, one must take into consideration the time lag between the 2-D Doppler examination and the operation. Continuing studies are being conducted, accounting for and correcting the time variance between the 2-D Doppler examination and surgery.

8—2 Doppler Findings in Valvular Stenosis

Anatomical changes in valvular stenosis have been diagnosed in detail with conventional 2-D echocardiography (B-mode). In other words, determining anatomical changes, such as the degree of calcification; size of valve opening; ventricular wall thickness; and diameter of cardiac lumen allow diagnosis of stenosis of the mitral valve and aortic valve to a certain extent. The defect in the evaluation of stenosis with conventional echocardiography is that it cannot reveal the pressure gradient in the stenotic region. Used together with CWD, 2-D Doppler has overcome such shortcomings. The approximation of the pressure gradient (ΔP) across a stenotic valve is obtained from a simplified Bernoulli's equation[10-14] using the maximal velocity (V) ($\Delta P = 4 V^2$). The mean pressure gradient (mean ΔP) is usually calculated by integrating the velocity profile every 0.04 second through diastole. A planiometered mean velocity does not provide an accurate mean pressure gradient due to the squared relation between velocity and pressure[15]. Usually, a mean pressure gradient is calculated by a software program already incorporated in the system. Hatle et al. have calculated the stenotic valve area from the mitral "pressure half-time[16] (P1/2T)", obtained by the CWD. This is, indeed, a unique concept and, at the same time, a practical method. Pressure half-time is the time required for the pressure differential to drop to half its peak value. Based on the equation $\Delta P = 4 V^2$, P at pressure half-time can be obtained by a simple graphic procedure from the record of the CWD (Fig. 8-2). When it is normal, the pressure half-time is below 60 ms and 100-400 ms in mitral valve stenosis[17]. The following practical formula applies:

$$MVA(cm^2) = \frac{220}{\text{pressure half-time}}$$

The most typical 2-D Doppler display of valvular stenosis is found in mitral stenosis. Using an apical four-chamber view, or low parasternal view, the inflow blood of the left ventricle is seen passing through the stenotic mitral orifice with increased velocity. The stenotic blood-flow image often appears as a flame. In the case of tricuspid stenosis, although its incidence is low, similar stenotic flow is noted clearly passing through the tricuspid valve orifice. In severe aortic stenosis, 2-D Doppler imaging from the apex or the left sternal border sometimes fails to produce a clear image of stenotic flow from the orifice. This could be due to the calcification around the valvular structure, which might decrease the Doppler signals. Similar phenomena are observed in cases with prosthetic valves, which may cause both increased attenuation of ultrasound and strong reverberation echoes. By contrast, turbulent stenotic flow is clearly visualized passing through the aortic orifice in mild aortic stenosis. In severe aortic stenosis, the best views may be obtained by a suprasternal or right sternal approach instead of a left parasternal or apical approach.

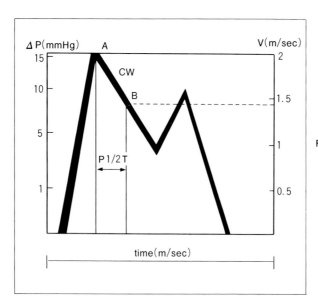

Fig. 8-2 Diagram illustrating method for calculation of mitral pressure half-time (P 1/2 T) from a continuous-wave Doppler velocity profile. The pressure half-time is the time required for the pressure gradient to drop to half its peak valve. Due to the squared relation between velocity and pressure gradient ($\Delta P = 4V^2$), the pressure half-time can be obtained from the velocity profile by dividing peak velocity by 1.4 (the square root of 2). Pressure half-time correlates with mitral valve area (MVA) [16,17]. An estimate of MVA is obtained by dividing 220 by the pressure half-time.

8-3 Approximation of the Right Ventricular Systolic Pressure

Tricuspid regurgitation (TR) may often be encountered in many valvular disorders. By applying the equation $\Delta P = 4 V^2$, through CWD, it is possible to approximate systolic pressure of the right ventricle[18,19,20]. The steps are as follows. Examine the tricuspid value by 2-D Doppler in the apical four-chamber view. On identifications of TR superimpose the CWD beam on the TR jet flow and measure, first of all, the maximum blood flow, max V. The pressure gradient (ΔP) across the tricuspid valve can be obtained in terms of mm Hg from this value. Add the mean right atrial pressure for an approximation of the right ventricular systolic pressure. The mean right atrial pressure may be obtained by using the measured value of the central venous pressure or, non-invasively, it may be estimated from the disappearance of the pulse wave of the jugular vein during elevation of the upper body[18]. In some cases, however, 10 mmHg[20] as a mean atrial pressure is added for the sake of simplicity. The right ventricular systolic pressure (RVP) thus obtained and the value obtained by cardiac catheter correspond well. For the sake of practicability, this approximate calculation of RVP by the continuous-wave Doppler technique is of definite clinical significance.

8—4 2-D Doppler Findings in Mitral Stenosis (MS)

○P.88
○P.89

As indicated in the previous section, in mitral stenosis turbulent blood flow through the stenotic orifice in diastole is seen as a flame[21),22)] in the long-axis view (**Cases 1** and **2**). The flow-mapping M-mode also shows rapid blood flow through the narrow slit-like mitral orifice. A 2-D Doppler image in the short-axis view in diastole is demonstrated in **Case 2, F**. Inflow blood through the fish-mouth shaped stenotic orifice in diastole is imaged in yellow.

○P.90

The concurrent use of 2-D Doppler and CWD in the evaluation of mitral valve stenosis provides data useful to the surgeon. Left atrial thrombus is often observed as a complication in mitral valve stenosis. A conventional 2-D echocardiogram is extremely useful in the diagnosis of left atrial thrombus (**Cases 3** and **4**).

8—5 2-D Doppler Findings in Mitral Regurgitation (MR)

○P.91

The imaging of mitral regurgitation by 2-D Doppler is particularly sensitive[4),23)-28)]. In this lesion, a regurgitant jet characterized by turbulent blood flow during systole is clearly observed in the left atrium. A case of mitral regurgitation (Sellers' grade 1) is shown in **Case 2, D**. In such a mild mitral regurgitation as Sellers' grade 1 or 2, the regurgitant blood-flow image is obtainable only in a limited direction and range within the left atrium. The detection may be rather difficult if the examination is carried out with the conventional pulsed-Doppler method. In **Case 5**, thorough scanning from multiple planes reveals the regurgitant image (Sellers' grade 2). As emphasized already in Chapter 5-1, the three-dimensional concept of intracardiac blood flow dynamics is essential in the 2-D Doppler examination. In angiography, the way in which the regurgitant jet runs varies according to the lesion of valvular structure causing mitral regurgitation. When mitral prolapse occurs at the anterior cusp, the regurgitant jet goes towards the posterior wall of the left atrium and conversely, when prolapse takes place in the posterior cusp, the

○P.92

regurgitant jet runs forward towards the aortic wall. In **Case 6**, the mitral regurgitation is due to rheumatic heart disease. The regurgitant jet flows from the anterior mitral cusp toward the posterior wall of the left atrium (Sellers' grade 3).

○P.93

Case 7 is also a mitral regurgitation (Sellers' grade 3). The anterior and posterior mitral cusps are destroyed by infective endocarditis, causing severe mitral regurgitation. Surgery revealed vegetations in the anterior and posterior mitral cusps.

○P.94

In **Case 8**, a severe mitral regurgitation is demonstrated. A mitral regurgitant jet (MR-jet) is diffused throughout the entire left atrium (Sellers' grade 4).

8—6 2-D Doppler Findings in Aortic Regurgitation (AR)

○P.95

2-D doppler findings in aortic regurgitation are displayed as characteristic turbulent flow occurring in the left ventricular outflow tract in diastole[29-33)]. In most cases, aortic regurgitant flow is also featured as wide-band and bi-directional in the pulse-wave Doppler. **Case 9** is a case of mild aortic regurgitation (Sellers' grade 1). In the 2-D Doppler image, regurgitant blood flow in diastole remains around the middle of the anterior mitral cusp level. **Case 10** is an aortic regurgitation (Sellers' grade 2), and 2-D Doppler images in aortic regurgitation

○P.96

○P.97

(Sellers' grade 3) are demonstrated in **Case 11**. The regurgitant flow is characterized by turbulence which runs along the anterior mitral leaflet toward the apex in the left ventricular outflow tract during diastole. The regurgitant flow extends almost to the level of the papillary muscles.

○P.98   In the case of Sellers' grade 4 aortic regurgitation (**Case 12**), the regurgitating jet flow, the AR-jet, is so wide as to completely occupy the left ventricular outflow tract and reaches as far as the apex. A case of aortic regurgitation of Sellers' grade 3 induced by infective

○P.99   endocarditis is shown in **Case 13**.

8-7 2-D Doppler Findings in Aortic Stenosis (AS)

    In the imaging of the jet-form mosaic flow pattern (AS-jet) caused by aortic stenosis, a position of the transducer must be selected such that the most intense Doppler signal can be obtained from the ascending aortic blood flow. Approaches from the apex, the upper part of the right sternal border[22] and the suprasternal notch must all be tried. Despite such a thorough approach there are cases with marked calcification causing a weak Doppler signal. Normally, CWD can be recorded without difficulty. The figures show the apical approach

○P.100
○P.101 (**Case 14**) and approach from the right sternal border (**Case 15**). If a 2-D Doppler image can be obtained, it will be extremely useful in determining the direction of the CWD beam axis[34].

8-8 2-D Doppler Findings in Tricuspid Regurgitation (TR)

○P.102   Tricuspid regurgitation is often secondary to the primary lesion, i. e., mitral and/or aortic valve lesions. **Case 16** is an example of tricuspid regurgitation, with associated mitral stenosis and regurgitation.

    In general, the apical four-chamber view is suitable for imaging tricuspid regurgitation[35,36]. Tricuspid regurgitation, even if it is mild, can be imaged by 2-D Doppler. Like other valvular regurgitation, blood flow is characteristically displayed as a mosaic pattern.

    As already mentioned, it is very common in marked tricuspid regurgitation (grade 3) for

○P.103 regurgitant flow to the hepatic vein to be observed in systole (**Case 17, F**). Flow-mapping M-mode findings and ECG timing confirm that flow into the hepatic vein (red) is indicative of significant tricuspid regurgitation (**Case 17, G**). This method is extremely sensitive to tricuspid regurgitation and can indicate even a small amount of regurgitant flow in the hepatic vein.

8-9 2-D Doppler Findings in Multivalvular Diseases

    Acquired valvular diseases often coexist with two or more valvular lesions. In addition, it is well known from previous clinical experience that 2-D Doppler is very advantageous in diagnosing multivalvular diseases. As emphasized earlier, the fundamental capability of 2-D Doppler is dependent upon the most appropriate positioning for investigating the respective valvular conditions. It is necessary, therefore, to select the most beneficial view for obtaining optimal blood-flow images.

○P.104   **Case 18** is of multivalvular disease, i.e., mitral stenosis associated with mitral regurgitation, aortic regurgitation, and tricuspid regurgitation. First of all, mitral regurgitation (Sellers' grade 2) is visualized in **Case 18, E**. In **Case 3, F**, the blood-flow image of the aortic regurgitation (Sellers' grade 2) is seen along with turbulent blood flow passing through the stenotic mitral valve during diastole (MS-jet). The tricuspid regurgitation (TR-jet) is demonstrated in the apical four-chamber view (**Case 18, J**). From the continuous-wave Doppler recordings, pressure gradients across mitral and tricuspid valves are calculated using a modified Bernoulli's equation ($\Delta P = 4V^2$).

○ P.105   Shown in **Case 19** is a multivalvular disease which exhibits aortic stenosis and regurgitation (Sellers' grade 2), mitral stenosis, and tricuspid regurgitation (grade 2).

Combined aortic regurgitation (AR-jet) and mitral stenosis (MS-jet) are simultaneously displayed as mosaic patterns with their respective characteristic turbulent flows (**Case 19, D**). In an apical five-chamber view, turbulent ejection flow at the aortic orifice (As-jet) is imaged. With the pressure gradient across the tricuspid valve calculated from the maximal velocity of tricuspid regurgitation, a non-invasive estimate of right ventricular systolic pressure can be obtained (**Case 18, K** and **Case 19, E, K**).

◯P.104
◯P.105

Of the combined valvular diseases, combined mitral stenosis and aortic regurgitation pose some problems which must be given special consideration in evaluating 2-D Doppler findings. The 2-D Doppler findings of aortic regurgitation are, as mentioned above, characterized by wide-band and bi-directional abnormal blood-flow signals elicited by regurgitation which are detected in the left ventricular outflow tract. On the other hand, it is also noted in mitral stenosis that the 2-D Doppler findings show similar characteristics of turbulent flow in the left ventricular inflow tract through the stenotic mitral orifice. Thus, both lesions are considered to generate analogous Doppler signals, although their detection sites are different. If mitral stenosis is associated with aortic regurgitation, a problem arises in evaluating the severity of aortic regurgitation by 2-D Doppler.

When turbulent blood flow due to either aortic regurgitation or to mitral stenosis is recognized as two independent jets, there is no difficulty in evaluating quantitatively the severity of aortic regurgitation. However, as is frequently experienced, turbulent blood flow due to aortic regurgitation (Sellers' grade 2) often appears along the anterior mitral cusp toward the left ventricular inflow tract. In this case the turbulent blood flow induced by aortic regurgitation might be visualized mixed with the turbulent blood flow elicited by the mitral inflow. There is also the possibility of misdiagnosis of severe aortic regurgitation, especially in the long-axis view, in which the turbulent blood flow due to aortic regurgitation appears to have joined the turbulent blood flow due to mitral stenosis in the form of a relay, this leads to the observation of turbulent diastolic blood flow in the apical direction. The distinction between these two flows is not clearly seen by pulsed-wave Doppler recordings. They both show analogous wide-band and bi-directional characteristics. Therefore, it is necessary to angle the transducer properly to delineate the abnormal flows in relationship to the separate anatomical structure. Using the parasternal short-axis view of the left ventricle is helpful in making this separation.

8—10 Valvular Regurgitation due to Infective Endocarditis (IE)

Cases of mitral regurgitation and aortic regurgitation induced by infective endocarditis have already been shown in **Cases 7** and **13**, respectively. In general, the diagnosis of infective endocarditis in its acute phase is often assessed by echocardiography alone[37-39]. Today, required surgery is usually indicated by the detection of valvular vegetations and evidence of valvular regurgitation obtained by 2-D echo and pulsed-wave Doppler. The advent of 2-D Doppler is thought to add comprehensive flow data for clinical and/or surgical management. In fact, 2-D Doppler can provide not only a direct observation of valvular regurgitation but also an evaluation of its severity. Another clinical application of this technique is in the defection of occult lesions of other valves.

8—11 Prosthetic Valves and 2-D Doppler Findings

There are special problems in 2-D Doppler findings of patients with prosthetic valves, particularly in the case of mechanical valves, where the two major problems are caused by the strong reflection by the metal stents of the prosthetic valve, and by acoustic attenuation.

Therefore, the direction of the beam should be carefully considered in examining a patient with a prosthetic valve by 2-D Doppler. It is necessary to direct the beam optimally to reduce disturbing reverberation due to the prosthetic valve structure.

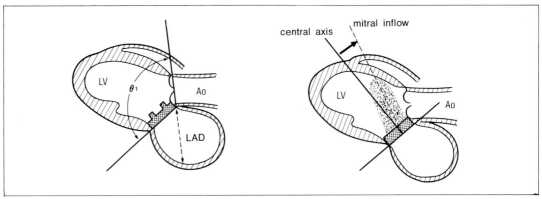

Fig. 8-3 Diagram illustrating altered mitral inflow after mitral valve replacement. The angle between the mitral and aortic annuli (θ_1) is narrowed and mitral inflow deviates medially from the central axis of the prosthesis regardless of model. With either a mechanical or bioprosthetic valve placed in the mitral position, ventricular diastolic flow patterns are reversed antero-posteriorly from normal. Diastolic inflow blood is directed toward the outflow tract and outflow blood, toward the inflow tract.

Tab. 8-4 Maximal transprosthetic mitral flow velocities from continuous-wave Doppler recordings and pressure gradients after the mitral valve replacement. Normally functioning prostheses have measurable gradients significantly different from normal native valves and maximal velocities <2 m/sec. The abnormally functioning prostheses, confirmed at the time of surgical replacement, all showed peak velocities of at least 2 m/sec and higher and obvious turbulence of inflow blood[47]. max V : maximal velocity, Δ P : pressure gradient.

	Control normal (n=10)	Normally functioning		Malfunctioning prosthesis (n=4)
		St. Jude valve(n=42)	Porcine valve(n=28)	
Measured maxV (m/s)	0.74±0.18	1.41+0.34	1.65±0.29	2.25±0.25
Calculated ΔP (mmHg)	2.19	9.95	10.1	20.3

Left ventricular blood flow in patients with prosthetic valves in the mitral position reveals a specific flow pattern[40]. In contrast to normal cases, diastolic blood flow through a prosthetic valve moves anteriorly and occupies the left ventricular outflow tract, appearing as if to strike the interventricular septum (Fig. 8-3, **Case 20, E**). In the left ventricular inflow tract the blood reverses and flows away from the transducer. An example of a Hancock valve is shown in **Case 20. Cases 20-22** have normally functioning valves.

Physiological leakage in prosthetic valves has been investigated in clinical as well as in experimental models. The slight leakage found in prosthetic valves remains a matter for further study.

There is another important point to be noted in the relationship between prosthetic valves and 2-D Doppler findings. It is desirable to use a noninvasive technique in the follow-up study of valve replacement patients. In particular, when the replacement of the native valve by a mechanical valve has been performed in the aortic position, left ventricular angiography is not usually conducted owing to the possible danger of damaging the leaflet of the mechanical valve. In this case 2-D Doppler provides information which cannot be obtained by any other noninvasive method.

The method is extremely effective in the post-operative follow-up[41] of patients who have undergone prosthetic valve replacement for the detection and evaluation of paravalvular leak and dysfunction of the prosthetic valve[42-46]. **Case 23** is an example of post-operative paravalvular leak in the replaced aortic valve. The authors' study[47] on the maximum mitral blood flow (max V) during post-operative follow-up after the mitral valve replacement is shown in Table 8-4. When the prosthetic valve is functioning normally the max V is below 2 m/s, be it a functional valve or an organic valve, and the 4 cases with malfunctioning prosthetic valve had max V above 2 m/s for both valve types. In the normally functioning prosthetic valve in the mitral position the mechanical valve tends to have a lower pressure gradient than the tissue valve. **Cases 24** and **25** are cases with dysfunction of the prosthetic valve in the mitral position. In either, the max V of mitral blood inflow is above 2 m/s and indicate mitral regurgitation caused by destruction of valvular tissue.

○ P.106
○ P.107
○ P.108

○ P.109

○ P.110
○ P.111

References

1) Omoto, R., Yokote, Y., Takamoto, S., Kyo, S., Ueda, K., Asano, H., Namekawa, K., Kasai, C., Kondo, Y., and Koyano, A.: The development of real-time two-dimensional doppler echocardiography and its clinical significance in acquired valvular disease with specific reference to the evaluation of valvular regurgitation. Jpn. Heart J., 25: 325-340, 1984.

2) Sellers, R. D., Levy, M. J., Amplatz, K., Lillehei, C. W.: Left retrograde cardioangiography in acquired cardiac disease: Technic, indication and interpretation in 700 cases. Am. J. Cardiol., 14: 437-447, 1964.

3) Miyatake, K., Izumi, S., Okamoto, M., Kinoshita, N., Asanuma, H., Nakagawa, H., Yamamoto, K., Takamiya, M., Sakakibara, H., and Nimura, Y.: Semiquantitative grading of severity of mitral regurgitation by real-time two-dimensional doppler flow imaging technique. J. Am. Coll. Cardiol., 7: 82-88, 1986.

4) Helmcke, F., Nanda, N., Hsiung, M. C., Sato, B., Adey, C. K., Goyal, R. G., and Gatewood, Jr., R. P.: Color Doppler assessment of mitral regurgitation with orthogonal planes. Circulation, 75: 175-183, 1987.

5) Kitabatake, A., Nakatani, S., Ito, H., Tanouchi, J., Ishihara, K., Fujii, K., Uematsu, M., Yoshida, Y., Tominaga, N., Inoue, M., and Kamada, T.: Cross sectional area of aortic regurgitant jet as an estimate of the severity of aortic regurgitation: A study with real-time two-dimensional doppler flow mapping technique. Proceedings of the 47th Meeting of the Japan Society of Ultrusonics in Medicine, 225-226, 1985. Abstract

6) Matsumura, M., Omoto, R., Kyo, S., Takamoto, S., and Yokote, Y.: Study on severity indexes of aortic regurgitation in real-time color flow mapping influenced by other factors. Jap. Circu. J., 50: 480, 1986. Abstract

7) Matsumura, M., Kyo, S., Takamoto, S., Yokote, Y., Morita, K., and Omoto, R.: Evaluation of severity of aortic regurgitation by real-time 2-D Doppler echocardiography. Comparison between parasternal and apical approaches. Proceedings of the 46th Meeting of the Japan Society of Ultrasonics in Medicine, 473-474, 1985. Abstract

8) Matsumura, M., Wong, M., Omoto, R., Yokote, Y., Takamoto, S., and Kyo, S.: The curvilinear relation between aortic regurgitant fraction and color flow jets: Intraoperative 2-dimensional doppler and electromagnetic flowmeter correlation. J. Am. Coll. Cardiol., 9(2): 66 A, 1987.

9) Kuwako, K., Tohda, E., Ino, T., Umeda, T., Furuta, S., Machii, K.: Echocardiographic evaluation of the tricuspid valve and ring: Diagnosis of tricuspid stenosis and regurgitation. J. Cardiography, 10: 947-966, 1980.

10) Holen, J., Aaslid, R., Landmark, K., and Simonsen, S.: Detemination of pressure gradient in mitral stenosis with a noninvasive ultrasound Doppler technique. Acta Med. Scand., 199: 455-460, 1976.

11) Hatle, L., Brubakk, A., Tromsdal, A., and Angelsen, B.: Noninvasive assessment of pressure drop in mitral stenosis by Doppler ultrasound. Br. Heart. J., 40: 131-140, 1978.

12) Hatle, L., Angelsen, B. A., Tromsdal, A.: Noninvasive assessment of aortic stenosis by Doppler ultrasound. Br. Heart. J., 43: 284- 292, 1980.

13) Hatle, L.: Noninvasive assessment and differentiation of left ventricular outflow obstruction with Doppler ultrasound. Circulation, 64: 381-407, 1981.

14) Berger, M., Berdoff, R., L., Gallerstein, P., E., and Goldberg, E.: Evaluation of aortic stenosis by continuous wave Doppler ultrasound. J. Am. Coll. Cardiol., 3: 150-156, 1984.

15) Stamm, R. B., Martin, R. P.: Quantification of pressure gradients across stenotic valves by doppler ultrasound. J. Am. Coll. Cardiol., 2: 707-718, 1983.

16) Hatle, L., Angelsen, B., and Tromsdal, A.: Noninvasive assessment of atrioventricular pressure halftime by Doppler ultrasound. Circulation, 60: 1096-1104, 1979.

17) Hatle, L.: Pulsed and continuous wave Doppler in diagnosis and assessment of various heart lesions. *In* Doppler Ultrasound in Cardiology, 2nd ed., Edited by L. Hatle and B. Angelsen, Philadelphia, Lea & Febiger, 1985.

18) Yock, P. G., Popp, R. L.: Noninvasive estimation of right ventricular systolic pressure by doppler ultrasound in patients with tricuspid regurgitation. Circulation, 70: 657-662, 1984.

19) Tei, C., Kisanuki, A., Arima, S., Arikawa, K., Otsuji, Y., and Tanaka, H.: Quantitative assessment of right ventricular pressure in patients with tricuspid regurgitation by continuous wave doppler echocardiogram. Proceeding of the 44th Meeting of the Japan Society of Ultrasonics in Medicine, 553-534, 1984. Abstract

20) Tei, C., Kisanuki, A., Arima, S., Arikawa, K., Otsuji, Y., Ri, S., Kashima, T., and Tanaka, H.: Non-invasive assessment of right ventricular pressure in patients with tricuspid regurgitation by

a continuous wave Doppler echocardiogram. Circulation, 70 : (Suppl. II), 116, 1984. Abstract

21) Yoshida, K., Yoshikawa, J., Kato, H., Yanagihara, K., Okumachi, F., Koizumi, K., Shiratori, K., Asaka, T., Shibuya, U., Sugita, I., Shono, H., and Akasaka, T.: Double inflow jets in mitral stenosis : A real-time two dimensional doppler echocardiographic study. Proceedings of the 45th Meeting of the Japan Society of Ultrasonics in Medicine, 417-418, 1984. Abstract

22) Morris, A. M., Roitman, D. I., Nanda, N. C., and Shah, M. R.: Color doppler assessment of stenotic valve area. Circulation, 72 : (Suppl. III), 100, 1985. Abstract

23) Switzer, D. F. and Nanda, N. C.: Color Doppler evaluation of valvar regurgitation. Echocardiography, 2 : 553-543, 1985.

24) Inaba, T., Ishimitsu, T., Noguchi, Y., Hiranuma, Y., Takano, S., Sugishita, Y., and Ito, I.: Cross sectional distribution of mitral regurgitant jet as an estimate of the severity and the cause of mitral regurgitation : A study with doppler color flow mapping. Proceedings of the 49th Meeting of the Japan Society of Ultrasonics in Medicine, 167-168, 1986. Abstract

25) Asaka, T., Yoshikawa, J., Yoshida, K., Koizumi, K., Okumachi, F., Yanagihara, K., Kato, H., and Shiratori, K.: Sensitivity and specificity of real-time two-dimensional doppler flow imaging systems in the detection of valvular regurgitation. Circulation, 70: (Suppl. II), 38, 1984. Abstract

26) Bommer, W. J., Rebeck, K. F., Laviola, S., Lafranchise, L., Jackson, T., and Keown, M.: Real-time two-dimensional flow imaging : Detection and semiquantification of valvular and congenital heart disease. Circulation, 70 : (Suppl. II), 38, 1984. Abstract

27) Mohr-Kahaly, S., Erbel, R., Esser, M., Drexler, M., and Zenker, G.: Different patterns of mitral regurgitation related to etiology analysed by color doppler. Circulation, 74 : (Suppl. II), 131, 1986. Abstract

28) Chandraratna, P. A. N., Minagoe, S., Wade, M., and Rose, J. S.: Demonstration of regurgitant stream shape and direction in mitral and tricuspid regurgitation by two-dimensional doppler color flow mapping. J. Am. Coll. Cardiol., 5 : 454, 1985. Abstract

29) Bouchard, A., Yock, P. G., Schiller, N. B., Newlands, J. S., Massie, B. M., Botvinick, E. H., Greenberg, B., and Cheitlin, M. D.: Quantitation of chronic aortic insufficiency using color doppler flow mapping. Circulation, 72 : (Suppl. III), 100, 1985. Abstract

30) Kitabatake, K., Ito, H., Tanouchi, J., Ishihara, K., Fujii, K., Yoshida, Y., Nakatani, S., and Kamada, T.: A new approach to quantitate aortic regurgitation by real time two-dimensional doppler echocardiography. Circulation, 72 : (Suppl. III), 306, 1985. Abstract

31) Perry, G. J., Helmcke, F., and Nanda, N. C.: Color doppler assessment of aortic insufficiency in tow orthogonal planes. J. Am. Coll. Cardiol., 7 : 101, 1986. Abstract

32) Pearlman, A. S., Otto, C. M., Janko, C. L., and Reamer, R. P.: Direction and width of aortic regurgitant jets : Assessment by doppler color flow mapping. J. Am. Coll. Cardiol. 7 : 100, 1986. Abstract

33) Diebold, B., Raffoul, H., Amiel, F., Guglielmi, J., Degroote, C., Ourbak, P., and Peronneau, P.: Quantification of aortic insufficiency using color Doppler flow imaging. J. Am. Coll. Cardiol., 9 (2), 66 A, 1987.

34) Helmcke, F., Perry, G. J., and Nanda, N. C.: Combined color doppler and continuous wave doppler in the evaluation of aortic stenosis. J. Am. Coll. Cardiol., 7 : 101, 1986. Abstract

35) Misawa, T., Miyatake, K., Izumi, S., Yamamoto, K., Nakagawa, H., Tomita, M., Kinosita, N., Sakakibara, H., and Nimura, Y.: Assessment of tricuspid regurgitation by real-time two-dimensional doppler flow imaging. Proceedings of the 46th Meeting of the Japan Society of Ultrasonics in Medicine, 463-464, 1985. Abstract

36) Suzuki, Y., Kambara, H., Kadota, K., Tamaki, S., Yamazato, A., Nohara, R., Osakade, G., and Kawai, C.: Detection and evaluation of tricuspid regurgitation using a real-time, two-dimensional, color coded, Doppler flow imaging system : Comparison with contrast two-dimensional echocardiography and right ventriculography. Am. J. Cardiol., 57 : 811-815, 1986.

37) Chandraratna, P. A. N., Robinson, J. J., Byrd, C., and Pitha, J. V.: Significance of abnormal echoes in left ventricular outflow tract. Br. Heart J., 39 : 381, 1977.

38) Ramirez, J., Guardiola, J., and Flowers, N. C.: Echocardiographic diagnosis of ruptured aortic valve leaflet in bacterial endocarditis. Circulation, 57 : 634, 1978.

39) Kleiner, J. P., Brundage, B. H., Ports, T. A., and Thomas, H. M.: Echocardiographic manifestation of flail right and noncoronary aortic valve leaflets : Studies in patients with bacterial endocarditis. Chest, 74 : 301, 1978.

40) Omoto, R., Asano, H., Yokote, Y., Takamoto, S., Kyo, S., and Matsumura, M.: Noninvasive analysis of left ventricular three-dimensional blood-flow dynamics in mitral valve replacement

by doppler color flow mapping. Circulation, 72: (Suppl. III), 206, 1985. Abstract

41) Asano, H., Yokote, Y., Morita, K., Kyo, S., Takamoto, S., and Omoto, R.: Study on blood flow through prosthetic mitral valves using real-time two-dimensional doppler echocardiography. Proceedings of the 45th Meeting of the Japan Society of Ultrasonics in Medicine, 141-142, 1984. Abstract

42) Akasaka, T., Yoshikawa, J., Yoshida, K., Kato, H., Okumachi, F., Koizumi, K., Shiratori, K., Takao, S., Asaka, T., Shakudo, M., and Shono, H.: Diagnostic value and limitations of two-dimensional doppler color flow mapping in the evaluation of bio-prosthetic valve dysfunction. Japanese Circulation J., 50: 749, 1986. Abstract

43) Yoshida, K., Yoshikawa, J., Kato, H., Okumachi, F., Koizumi, K., Shiratori, K., Asaka, T., Akasaka, T., Sugita, I., Shono, H., Maenishi, F., and Yagi, T.: Differential diagnosis of a paravalvular leakage from a transvalvular leakage by doppler color flow mapping. Proceedings of the 46th Meeting of the Japan Society of Ultrasonics in Medicine, 481-482, 1985. Abstract

44) Okumachi, F., Yoshikawa, J., Yoshida, K., Asaka, T., Takao, S., and Shiratori, K.: Diagnostic value and limitations of two-dimensional doppler color flow mapping in the evaluation of prosthetic valve dysfunction. Circulation, 72: (Suppl. III), 101, 1985. Abstract

45) Grube, E., Kuhnen, R., and Becher, H.: Combined use of 2D-color flow mapping (CFM) and continuous doppler echocardiography (CWD) to determine flow parameters in prosthetic valves. Circulation, 74: (Suppl. II), 389, 1986. Abstract

46) Yamagishi, M., Miyatake, K., Izumi, S., Nagata, S., Park, Y., Sakakibara, H., and Nimura, Y.: Bioprosthetic valve dysfunction studied by two dimensional color doppler flow imaging: Efficacies and pitfalls. Circulation, 74: (Suppl. II), 389, 1986. Abstract

47) Omoto, R., Matsumura, M., Asano, H., Kyo, S., Takamoto, S., Yokote, Y., and Wong, M.: Doppler ultrasound examination of prosthetic function and ventricular blood flow after mitral valve replacement. Herz, 11: 346-350, 1986.

Chapter 9　Intraoperative Use of 2-D Doppler

The use of color Doppler flow mapping, 2-D Doppler, during surgery is a new application of the technique. There have already been reports from several cardiac centers[1,2] on the usefulness of this application and we can expect substantial development in this field in the future. The 2-D Doppler technique has been employed during cardiac surgery at the author's institute since 1984. There are two approaches to using it in surgery. One is to place a probe in direct contact with the surgical field and to take an echogram from the surface of the heart (epicardial approach). The other approach uses a transesophageal probe (transesophageal approach[3], transesophageal echocardiography ; TEE). Both methods are necessary, but transesophageal echocardiography is likely to develop into the slightly more effective approach.

○ P.112

The main objectives of using this technique during surgery are outlined below:

1. Confirmation of Preoperative Diagnosis: Particularly in cases of congenital cardiac disease, the technique is useful immediately prior to cardiotomy to confirm the preoperative diagnosis made by cardiac catheter examination and angiography. The echo taken during surgery is especially significant in cases where preoperative examinations were not satisfactory or were inadequate. Moreover, Doppler color flow mapping used during surgery can detect complicating malformations not detected in preoperative examination.

2. Evaluation of the Effectiveness of Cardiac Surgery Prior to Chest Closure : Color Doppler assessment can be used before chest closure to check whether the patch closure of the intracardiac defect is completely repaired and to evaluate the effect of repairing the valve. Although it may rarely occur, the findings may indicate the need for additional surgery. The immediate evaluation of a repaired valve prior to chest closure may allow the cardiac surgeon to be more aggressive in salvaging a native valve. When mitral commissurotomy is performed, but significant mitral regurgitation occurs, valve replacement is usually performed, and in these cases intraoperative 2-D Doppler is also useful.

3. Evaluation of Cardiac Function: The 2-D Doppler can be used for pre- and post-operative monitoring of abnormalities of wall motion.

4. Evaluation During Surgery of an Untouched Lesion: The intraoperative 2-D Doppler examination is suitable where relatively slight aortic regurgitation is left untreated after performing mitral valve replacement.

5. Imaging of the Coronary Artery[4,1] : Even in cases where the stenotic site is clearly defined by selective preoperative coronary angiography, selection of the optimal area for bypass is not always easy. However, performing intraoperative imaging of the coronary artery during surgery allows confirmation of the precise site of anastomosis.

In conclusion, intraoperative 2-D Doppler can be a valuable new tool for providing information that may significantly improve surgical management in cardiovascular surgery.

References

1) Takamoto, S., Kyo, S., Adachi, H., Matsumura, M., Yokote, Y., and Omoto, R. : Intraoperative color flow mapping by real-time two-dimensional doppler echocardiography for evaluation of valvular and congenital heart disease and vascular disease. J. Thorac Cardiovasc. Surg., 90 : 802-812, 1985.

2) Maurer, G., Czer, L., De Robertis, M., et al : Intraoprative doppler color flow mapping in valvular and congenital heart disease. Circulation, 72 : (Suppl. III), 206, 1985. Abstract

3) Goldman, M. E., Thys, D., Ritter, S., Hillel, Z., and Kaplan, J. : Trans-esophageal real time doppler flow imaging : A new method for intraoperative cardiac evaluation. J. Am. Coll. Cardiol., 7 : 1, 1986. Abstract

4) Suzuki, S., Sasaki, T., Miyazawa, S., Morita, K., Horiguti, T., Mizuno, A., Takayasu, H., and Arai, T. : Observation of coronary artery by newly-developed 2-D echo equipment for operation. Proceedings of the 44th Meeting of the Japan Society of Ultrasonics in Medicine, 97-98, 1984. Abstract

Normal Heart (1) Adult 31-year-old male

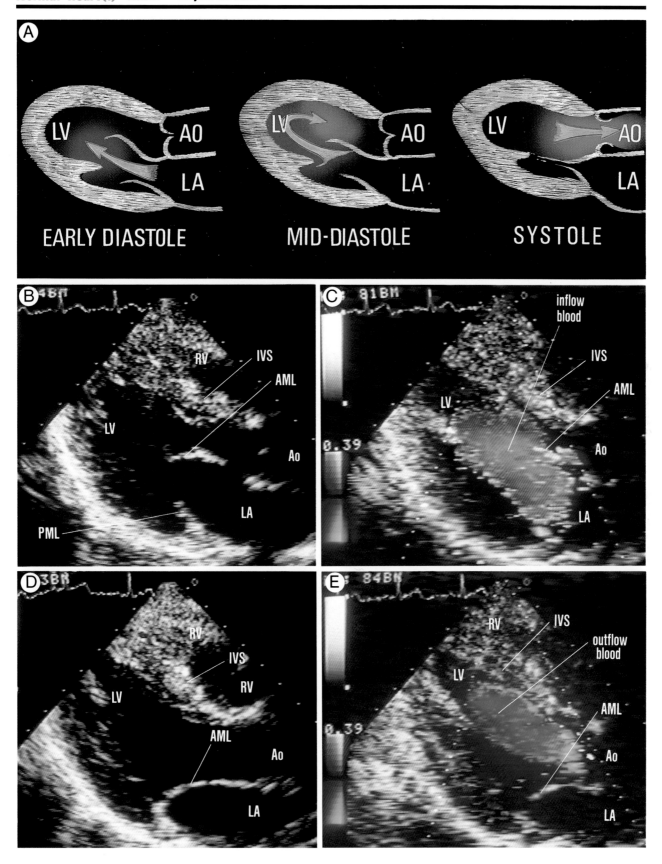

2-D Doppler images in a normal heart.
A Diagrams demonstrating diastolic flow (red) through the mitral orifice into the left ventricle and systolic flow from the left ventricle into the aorta (blue) with the transducer in the left parasternal position. **B** B-mode in long-axis view in diastole. **C** 2-D Doppler same vieiw, diastole. **D** B-mode same view, systole. **E** 2-D Doppler same view, systole.

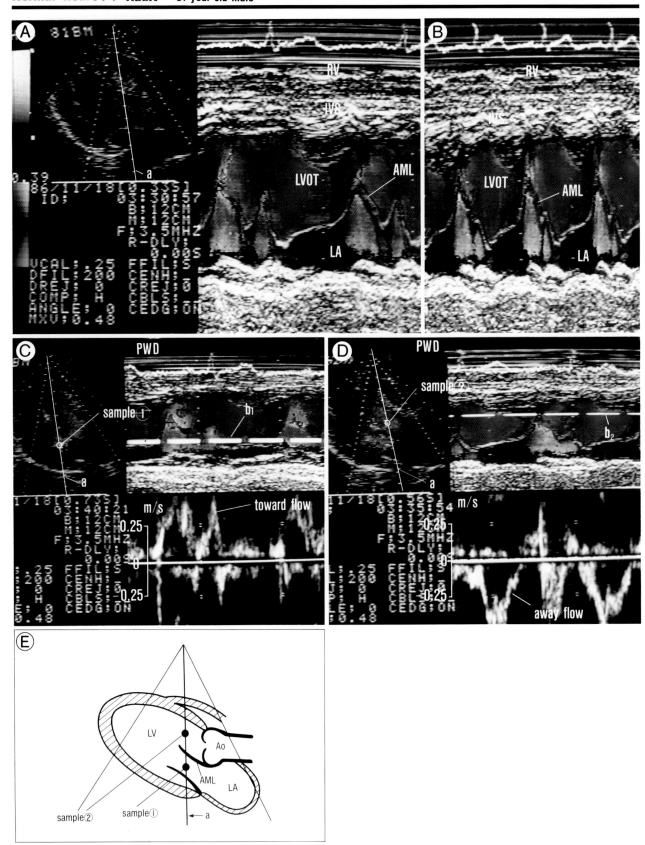

Flow-mapping M-mode and pulsed-wave Doppler in a normal heart.
Ⓐ Flow-mapping M-mode (beam line : a). Ⓑ Ditto. Ⓒ Simultaneous display of flow-mapping M-mode and pulsed-wave Doppler (sample volume : sample ① (b₁)). Ⓓ Ditto (sample volume : sample ② (b₂)) Ⓔ Diagram showing the transducer position, beam line, and sample sites.

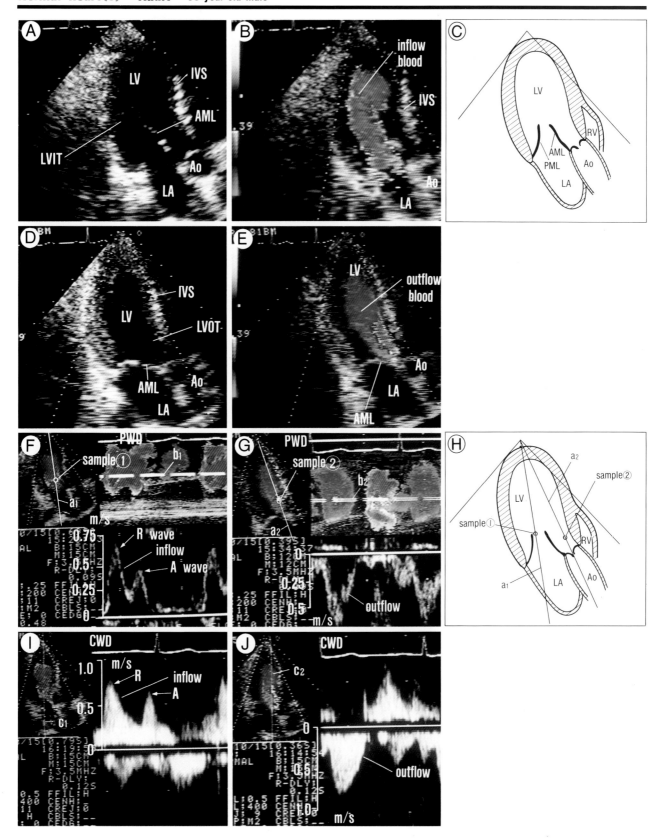

2-D Doppler, flow-mapping M-mode, pulsed-wave Doppler, and continuous-wave Doppler in a nomal heart.
A B-mode in apical long-axis view in diastole. **B** 2-D Doppler same view, diastole. **C** Diagram of **A**, **B**, **D**, and **E**. **D** B-mode in apical long-axis view in systole. **E** 2-D Doppler same view, systole. **F** Simultaneous display of flow-mapping M-mode and pulsed-wave Doppler (beam line : a₁, sample volume : sample ① (b₁)). R wave=62 cm/s, A wave=40 cm/s. **G** Ditto. (beam line : a₂, sample volume : sample ② (b₂)). **H** Diagram of **F** and **G**. **I** Continuous-wave Doppler (beam line : c₁). R wave=72 cm/s, A wave=56 cm/s. By switching from pulsed-wave Doppler (**F**) to continuous-wave Doppler, the maximal velocity is obtained. **J** Continuous-wave Doppler (beam line : c₂). max V=75 cm/s. Normally, mitral diastolic velocity spectra consist of R and A waves with the R wave predominant. R wave : early diastolic velocity, A wave : late velocity following atrial contraction.

Normal Heart (4) Child (BW=27kg, BH=127cm) 8-year-old male

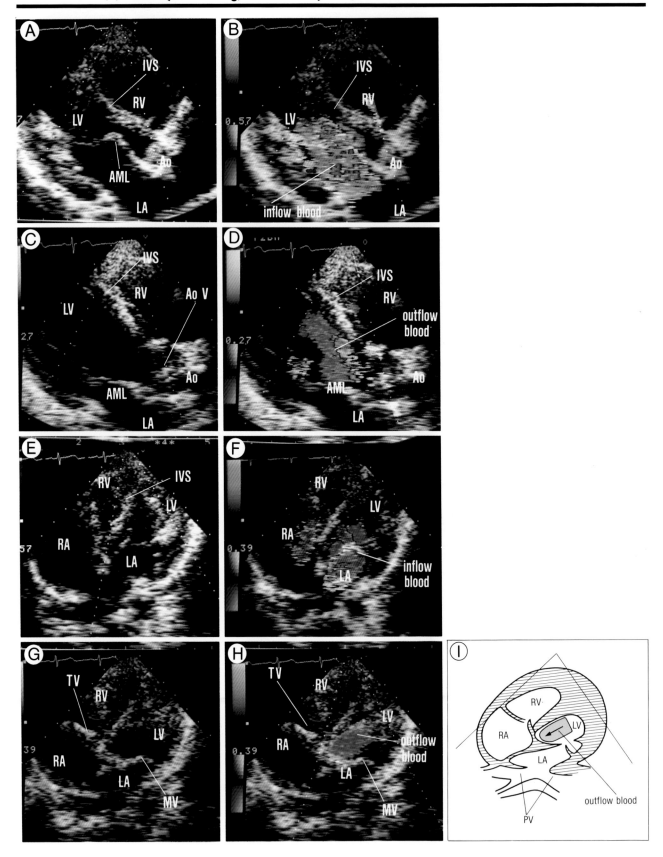

2-D Doppler images in long-axis view of the left ventricle.
Ⓐ Ⓑ The blood flow into the left ventricle in diastole is depicted with a red color as a flow towards the transducer . **Ⓒ Ⓓ** The left ventricular ejection flow in systole is depicted with a blue color as a flow away from the transducer in left ventricular outflow tract, but it changes into red color at the aortic valve due to aliasing in this scan (transducer=5 MHz, PRF=4 KHz).
2-D Doppler images in apical four-chamber view.
Ⓔ Ⓕ The blood flows into ventricles in diastole is depicted with red colors as a flow towards the transducer. **Ⓖ Ⓗ Ⓘ** The left ventricular ejection flow in systole is depicted with blue color as a flow away from the transducer along the interventricular septum in the left ventricle. In this view the right ventricular ejection flow cannot usually be seen. **Ⓘ** Schematic diagram.

Normal Heart (5) Child (BW＝27kg, BH＝127cm) 8-year-old male

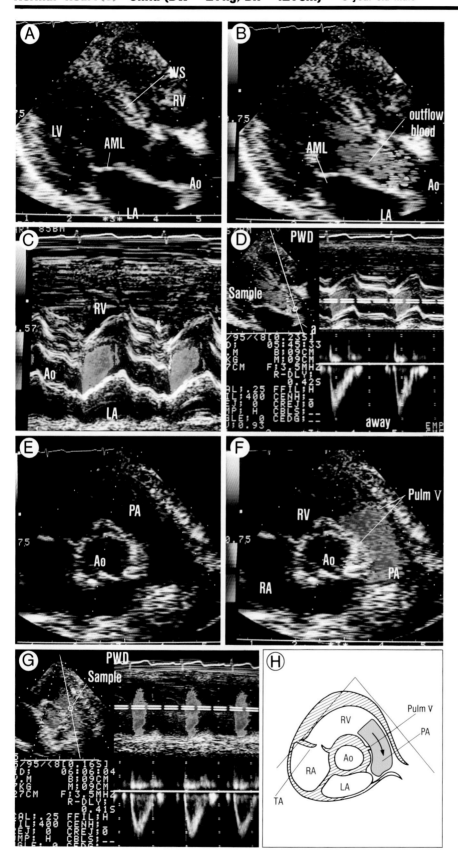

2-D Doppler images in long-axis view of the ventricle.

AB The left ventricular ejection flow in systole is depicted with a blue color as a flow away from the transducer in the left ventricular outflow tract, no aliasing is seen in this scan (transducer＝3.5 MHz, PRF＝8 KHz).

CD Flow mapping M-mode C and simultaneous display of M-mode and spectral analysis at the aortic valve level D demonstrate a parallelogram of the left ventricular ejection flow with a blue color and the laminar aortic ejection flow in systole.

Short-axis view at the aortic valve level.

EF The main pulmonary arterial flow in systole is depicted with a blue color. **G** Simultaneous display of flow mapping M-mode and spectral analysis demonstrates the laminar flow pattern of the normal pulmonary arterial flow with blue color as a flow away from the transducer. **H** Schematic diagram.

Normal Heart (6) Child (BW＝32kg, BH＝139cm) 9-year-old male

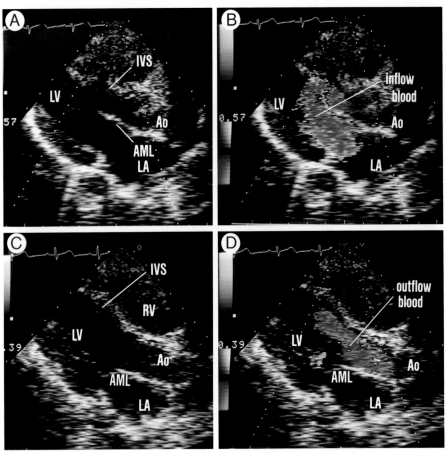

2-D Doppler images in long-axis view of the left ventricle.
A B The blood flow into the left ventricle in diastole is depicted with a red color as a flow towards the transducer.
C D The left ventricular ejection flow in systole is depicted with a blue color as a flow away from the transducer in the left ventricular outflow tract.

Normal Heart (7) Child (BW＝14kg, BH＝95cm) 3-year-old female

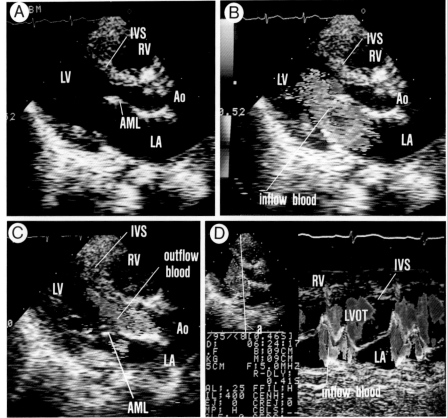

2-D Doppler images in long-axis view of the left ventricle.
A B The blood flow into the left ventricle in diastole is depicted with a red color as a flow towards the transducer.
C The left ventricular ejection flow in systole is depicted with a blue color as a flow away from the transducer in the left ventricular outflow tract. **D** Flow mapping M-mode at the mitral valve level (beam direction＝cursor line of ⓐ).

Normal Heart (8) Infant (BW＝8kg, BH＝65cm) 4-month-old male

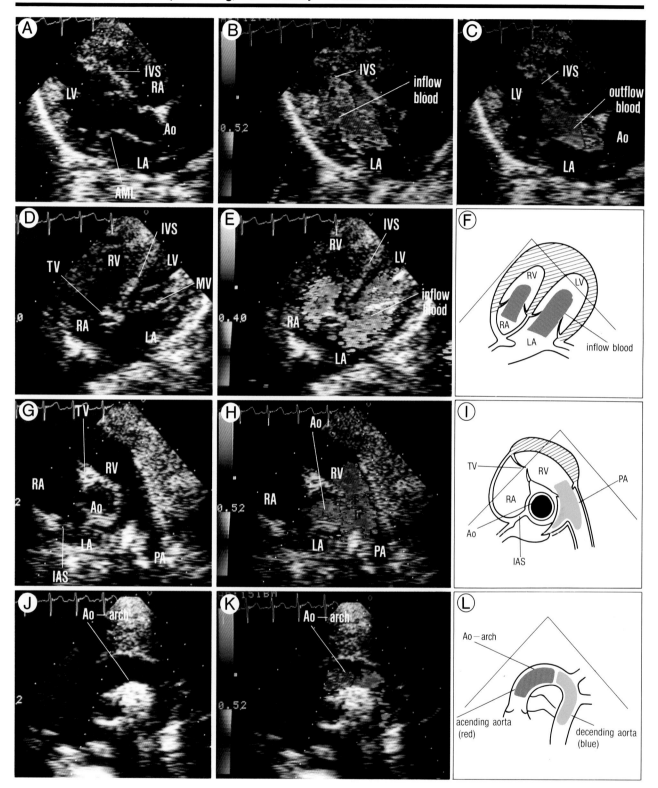

ⒶⒷⒸ Long-axis view of the left ventricle. The diastolic flow into the left ventricle is depicted with blue color Ⓑ as a flow away from the transducer and the left ventricular systolic flow is depicted with a blue color in systole as a flow towards the transducer.
ⒹⒺⒻ Apical four-chamber view. The diastolic blood inflow into the ventricles is depicted with red color as a flow towards the transducer Ⓔ.
Ⓕ Schematic diagram.
ⒼⒽⒾ Short-axis view at the aortic valve level. 2-D Doppler image in the right ventricular outflow tract is depicted with a blue color as a flow away from the transducer. Ⓘ Schematic diagram.
ⒿⓀⓁ Aortic arch view from the supra-sternum. The ascending aortic flow is depicted with a red color as a flow towards the transducer and the descending aortic flow with a blue color as a flow away from the transducer. Ⓛ Schematic diagram.

Case 1 **Mitral Stenosis** 36-year-old male

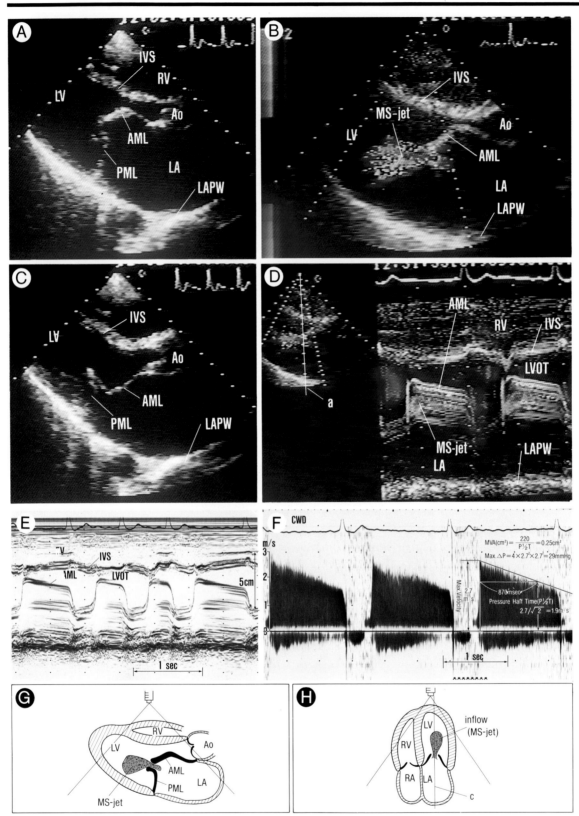

2-D Doppler images in a patient with mitral stenosis (MS).
Ⓐ B-mode in long-axis view in diastole. Ⓑ 2-D Doppler same view, diastole. Flame-shaped jet of inflow blood with mosaic pattern passes through the stenotic mitral valve into the left ventricle (MS-jet). Ⓒ B-mode in long-axis view in systole. Ⓓ Flow-mapping M-mode (beam line : a). Ⓔ Mitral valve echocardiogram. Ⓕ Continuous-wave Doppler of mitral valve flow (beam line : c in Ⓗ). Ⓖ Diagram of Ⓐ and Ⓑ. Ⓗ Diagram of continous-wave Doppler recording of mitral valve flow in Ⓕ.
[Evaluation of mitral stenosis]
  max V=2.7 m/s, mean V=2.1 m/s, max △P=29 mmHg, meam △P=16 mmHg, P 1/2 T=0.087 sec, MVA=0.35 cm².
The pressure gradient from cardiac catheterization (PAW-LVEDP) was 17 mmHg. PAW : pulmonay arterial wedge pressure, LVEDP : left ventricular end-diastolic pressure.

Case 2 Mitral Stenosis and Regurgitation (Sellers' grade 1) 66-year-old female

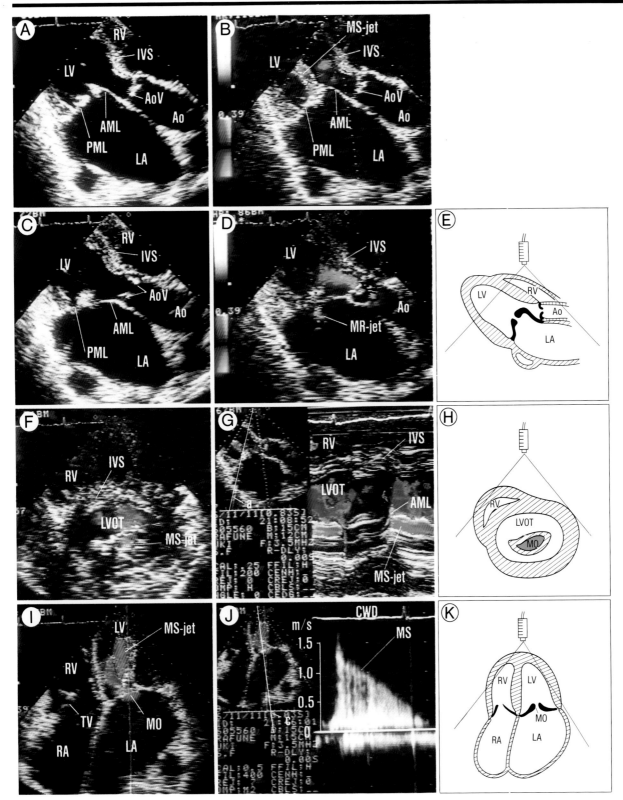

2-D Doppler images in a patient with mitral stenosis and regurgitation (MS·MR).

A B-mode in long-axis view in diastole. **B** 2-D Doppler same view, diastole. **C** B-mode same view, systole. **D** 2-D Doppler same view, systole. Mild mitral regurgitant jet (MR-jet) is shown. **E** Diagram of **D**. **F** 2-D Doppler in short-axis view in diastole. Stenotic mitral orifice is occupied by MS-jet. **G** Flow-mapping M-mode (beam line : a). **H** Diagram of **F**. **I** 2-D Doppler in apical four-chamber view in diastole. **J** Continuous-wave Doppler of mitral valve flow (beam line : c). **K** Diagram of **I** and **J**.

[Evaluation of mitral stenosis]

max V : 1.7 m/s, mean V : 1.2 m/s, mean ΔP : 5 mmHg, P 1/2 T : 0.18 sec, MVA : 1.2 cm².

The pressure gradient from cardiac catheterization (PAW-LVEDP) was 5 mmHg. PAW : pulmonay arterial wedge pressure, LVEDP : left ventricular end-diastolic pressure.

Case 3　Mitral Stenosis＋Left Atrial Thrombus　61-year-old female

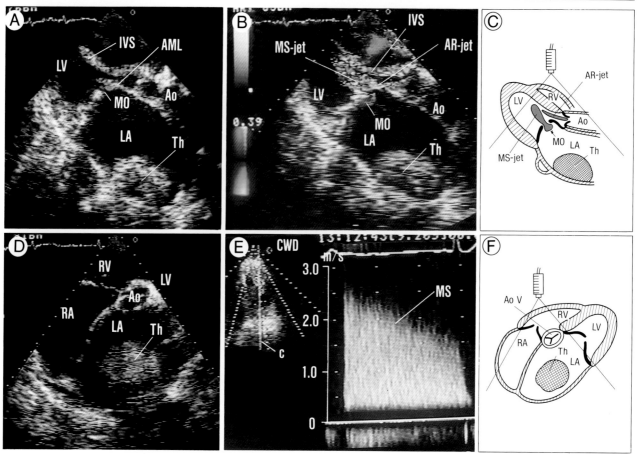

2-D Dopper images in a patient with mitral stenosis and left atrial thrombus.
A B-mode in long-axis view in diastole. A large clot (Th) is shown in the left atrium. **B** 2-D Doppler same view, diastole. Aortic regurgitant jet (AR-jet) as well as MS-jet is shown. **C** Diagram of **B**. **D** B-mode in apical four-chamber view in systole. **E** Continuous-wave Doppler of mitral valve flow (beam line : c). **F** Diagram of **D**.
[Evaluation of mitral stenosis]
　max V : 2.6 m/s, mean, ΔP : 13 mmHg, P 1/2 T : 0.38 sec, MVA : 0.58 cm^2.

Case 4　Mitral Stenosis and Regurgitation (Sellers' grade 3) ＋Left Atrial Thrombus　65-year-old female

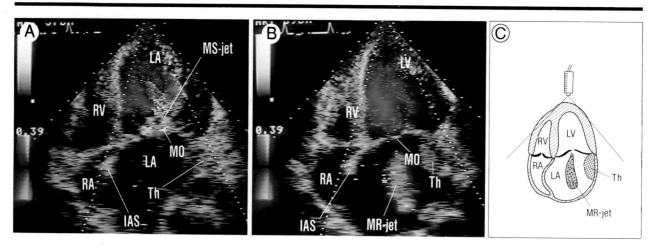

2-D Doppler images in a patient with combined mitral stenosis and regurgitation and left atrial thrombus.
A 2-D Doppler in apical four-chamber view in diastole. A large clot (Th) is demonstrated in the left atrium near the mitral valve. **B** 2-D Doppler same view, systole. **C** Diagram of **B**.

Case 5 Mitral Stenosis and Regurgitation (Sellers' grade 2) 66-year-old female

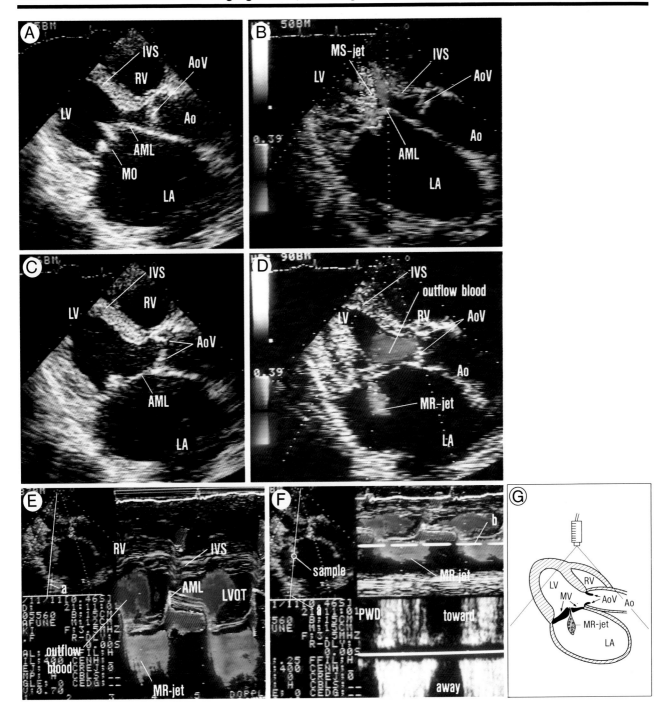

2-D Doppler images in a patient with mitral stenosis and regurgitation (MS·MR).

A B-mode in long-axis view in diastole. **B** 2-D Doppler same view, diastole. **C** B-mode same view, systole. **D** 2-D Doppler same view, systole. Mitral regurgitant jet (MR-jet, Sellers' grade 2) is shown in the left atrium. **E** Flow-mapping M-mode (beam line : a). **F** Simultaneous display of flow-mapping M-mode and pulsed-wave Doppler (beam line : a, sample volume : sample (b)). Regurgitant blood flows are characterized as wide-band (or broad-band) and bi-directional flow patterns in pulsed-wave Doppler recording. **G** Diagram of **D**.

92

Case 6 Mitral Stenosis and Regurgitation (Sellers' grade 3) 32-year-old female

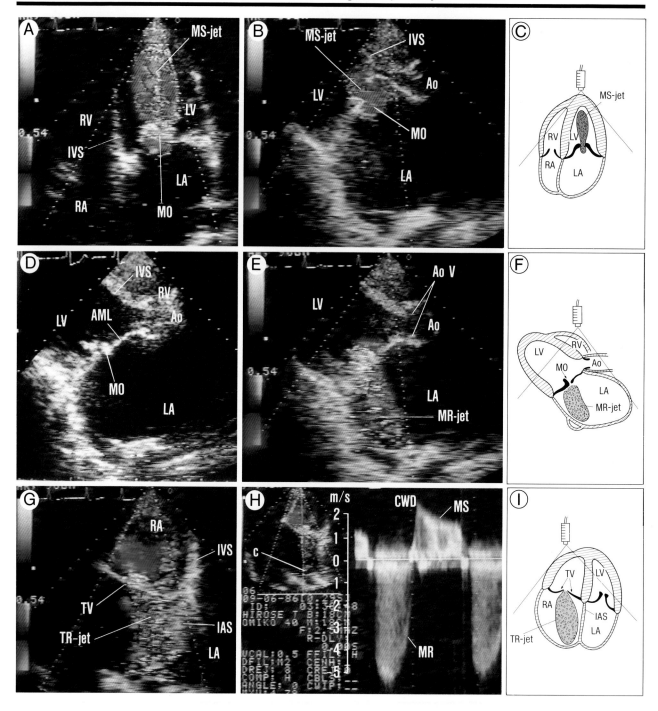

2-D Doppler images in a patient with mitral stenosis and regurgitation (MS·MR).
Ⓐ 2-D Doppler in apical four-chamber view in diastole. **Ⓑ** 2-D Doppler in long-axis view in diastole. **Ⓒ** Diagram of **Ⓐ**. **Ⓓ** B-mode in long-axis view in systole. **Ⓔ** 2-D Doppler same view, systole. Severe mitral regurgitation (Sellers' grade 3) is demonstrated. **Ⓕ** Diagram of **Ⓔ**. **Ⓖ** 2-D Doppler in apical four-chamber view in systole. Tricuspid regurgitant jet (TR-jet) is seen in the right atrium. **Ⓗ** Continuous-wave Doppler of mitral valve flow (beam line : c). With continuous-wave Doppler from the apex, high velocities are recorded both away from the transducer in systole (mitral regurgitation) and toward the transducer in diastole (mitral stenosis). **Ⓘ** Diagram of **Ⓖ**.
[Evaluation of mitral stenosis]
max V=2.4 m/s, mean V=1.4 m/s, mean ΔP=8 mmHg, P 1/2 T=0.21 sec, MVA=1.1 cm².

Case 7　Mitral Regurgitation (Sellers' grade 3) due to Infective Endocarditis　39-year-old female

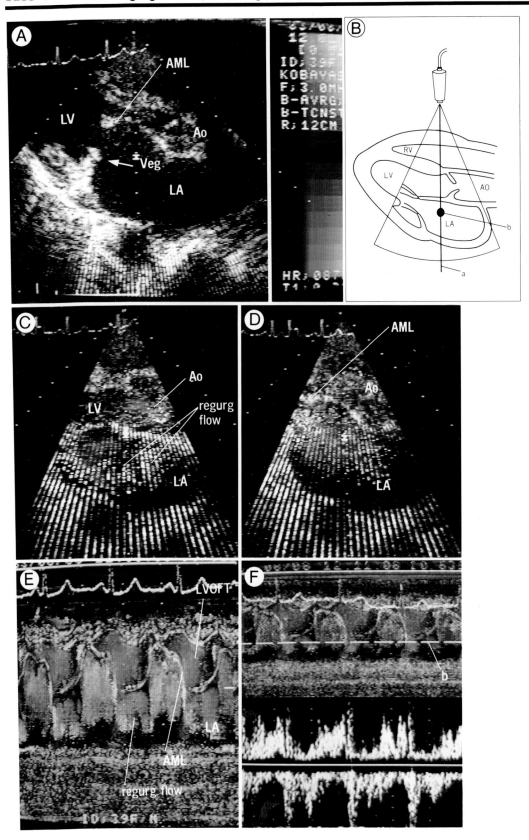

2-D Doppler images in a patient with mitral regurgitation due to infective endocarditis.
Ⓐ B-mode in long-axis view in diastole. Vegetation (Veg) is shown on the posterior mitral leaflet. Ⓑ Diagram of the transducer position, beam line, and sample site. Ⓒ 2-D Doppler in long-axis view in systole. Severe mitral regurgitation (Sellers' grade 3) is shown. Ⓓ 2-D Doppler same view, diastole. Ⓔ Flow-mapping M-mode (beam line : a in Ⓑ). Ⓕ Simultaneous display of flow-mapping M-mode and pulsed-wave Doppler (sample volume : b in Ⓑ and Ⓕ).

Case 8   Mitral Stenosis and Regurgitation (Sellers' grade 4)   49-year-old male

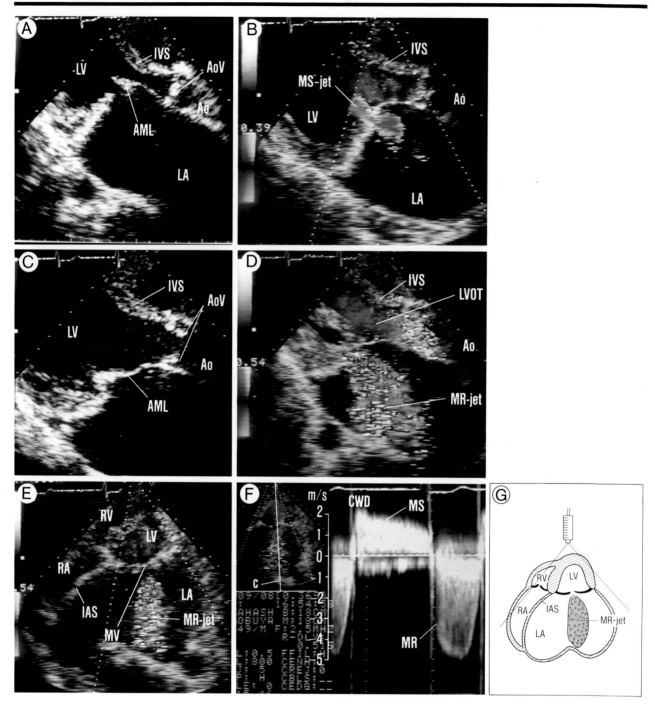

2-D Doppler images in a patient with mitral stenosis and severe mitral regurgitation (MS·MR).
A B-mode in long-axis view in diastole. **B** 2-D Doppler same view, diastole. **C** B-mode same view, systole. **D** 2-D Doppler same view, systole. Severe mitral regurgitantion (Sellers' grade 4) is demonstrated. **E** 2-D Doppler in apical four-chamber view in systole. **F** Continuous-wave Doppler of mitral valve flow (beam line: c).
[Evaluation of mitral stenosis]
  max V=2.3 m/s, mean ΔP=10 mmHg, P 1/2 T=0.21 sec, MVA=1.0 cm².

Case 9　Aortic Regurgitation (Sellers' grade 1)+ Mitral Stenosis　66-year-old female

2-D Doppler images in a patient with combined aortic regurgitation and mitral stenosis (AR + MS).
Ⓐ B-mode in long-axis view in diastole. **Ⓑ** 2-D Doppler same view, diastole. Mild aortic regurgitant jet (AR-jet) is demonstrated in mosaic patterns. **Ⓒ** 2-D Doppler in long-axis view in systole. Blood flow passes through aortic valve in mosaic patterns indicating mild aortic stenosis. **Ⓓ** Diagram of **Ⓑ**. **Ⓔ** Flow-mapping M-mode (beam line: a) **Ⓕ** Simultaneous display of flow-mapping M-mode and pulsed-wave Doppler (beam line: a, sample volume: sample (b)). Regurgitant jet is characterized as broad-band and bi-directional signals in pulsed-wave Doppler recording.

Case 10　Aortic Regurgitation (Sellers' grade 2)　29-year-old female

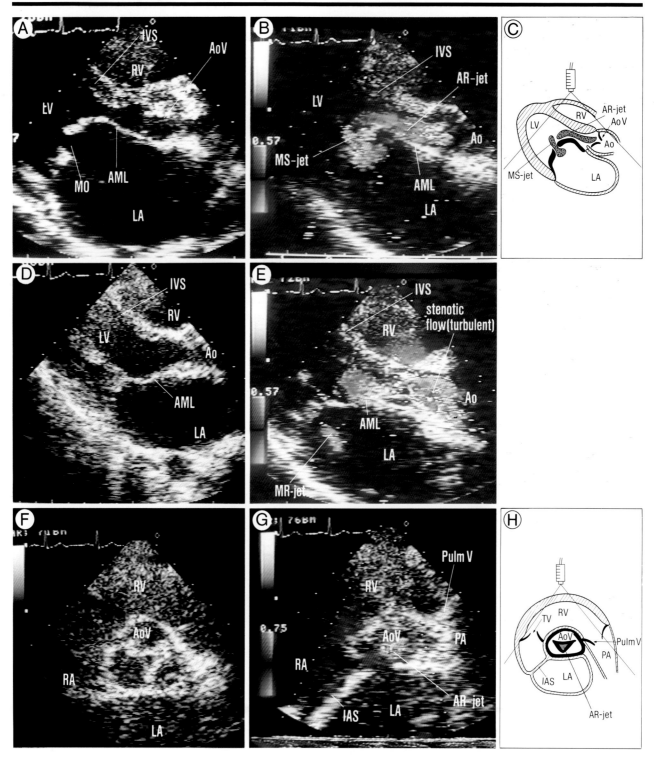

2-D Doppler images in a patient with combined mild aortic regurgitation and mitral stenosis and regurgitation（AR＋MS・MR）.
Ⓐ B-mode in long-axis view in diastole. **Ⓑ** 2-D Doppler same view, diastole. AR-jet reaches the level of the tip of the anterior mitral leaflet. MS-jet as well as AR-jet is seen in diaslole. **Ⓒ** Diagram of **Ⓑ**. **Ⓓ** B-mode in long-axis view in systole. **Ⓔ** 2-D Doppler same view, systole. Turbulent blood flow passes through aortic valve indicating mild aortic stenosis. **Ⓕ** B-mode in short-axis view at the level of the aortic valve in diastole. **Ⓖ** 2-D Doppler same view, diastole. AR-jet is seen in the incompetent aortic valve. **Ⓗ** Diagram of **Ⓕ** and **Ⓖ**.

Case 11 Aortic Regurgitation (Sellers' grade 3) 48-year-old female

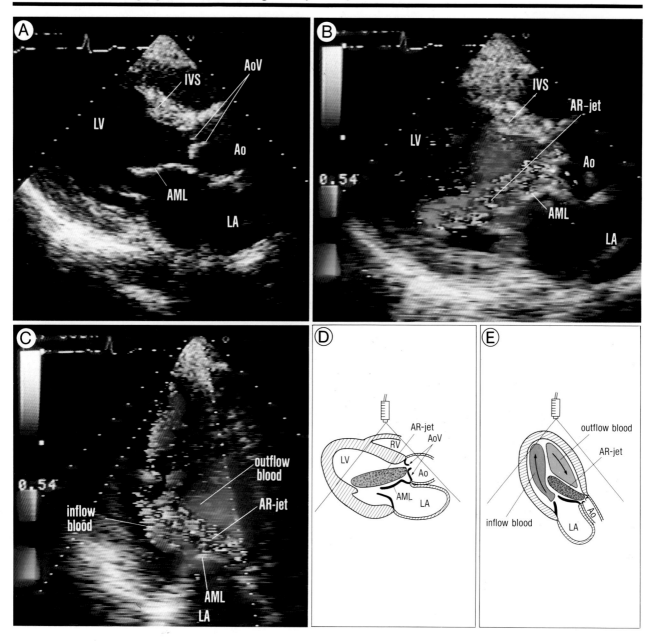

2-D Doppler images in a patient with severe aortic regurgitation (AR).
Ⓐ B-mode in long-axis view in diastole. Ⓑ 2-D Doppler same view, diastole. Ⓒ 2-D Doppler in apical four-chamber view in diastole. In this image, one can see sandwich-like three-layered blood flow image in diastole ; mitral valve flow (red), AR-jet (mosaic pattern), and outflow blood in the left ventricular outflow tract (blue). Ⓓ Diagram of Ⓑ. Ⓔ Diagram of Ⓒ.

98

Case 12　Aortic Regurgitation (Sellers' grade 4)　44-year-old female

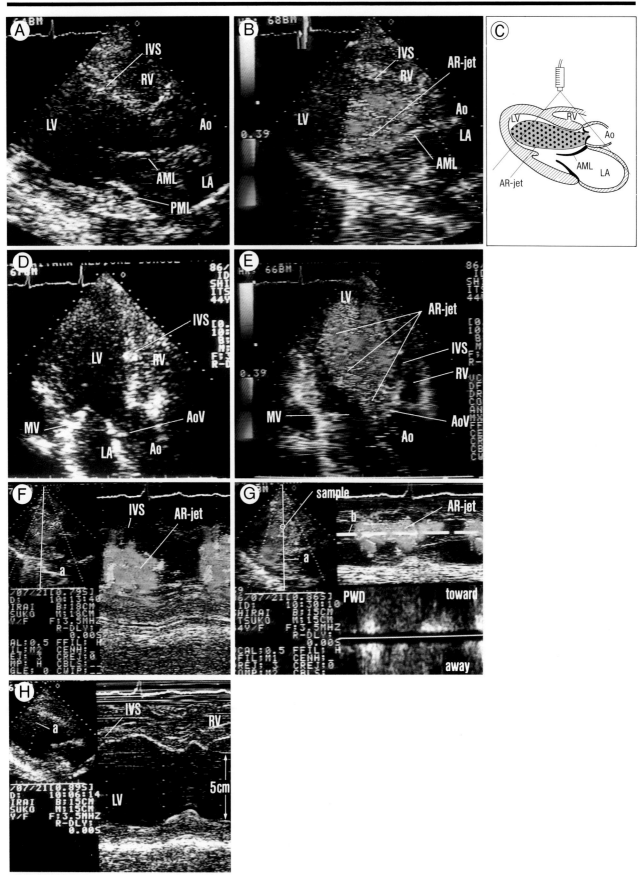

2-D Doppler images in a patient with severe aortic regurgitation (AR).
Ⓐ B-mode in long-axis view in diastole. Ⓑ 2-D Doppler same view, diastole. AR-jet occupies the entire left ventricular outflow tract.
Ⓒ Diagram of Ⓑ. Ⓓ B-mode in apical long-axis view in diastole. Ⓔ 2-D Doppler same view, diastole. AR-jet is shown deeper beyond the papillary muscles to the apex (Sellers' grage 4). Ⓕ Flow-mapping M-mode (beam line: a). Ⓖ Simultaneous display of flow-mapping M-mode and pulsed-wave Doppler (beam line: a, sample volume: sample (b)). Ⓗ M-mode echocardiogram (beam line: a). The left ventricle is remarkably dilated.

Case 13 Aortic Regurgitation (Sellers' grade 3) due to Infective Endocarditis 54-year-old male

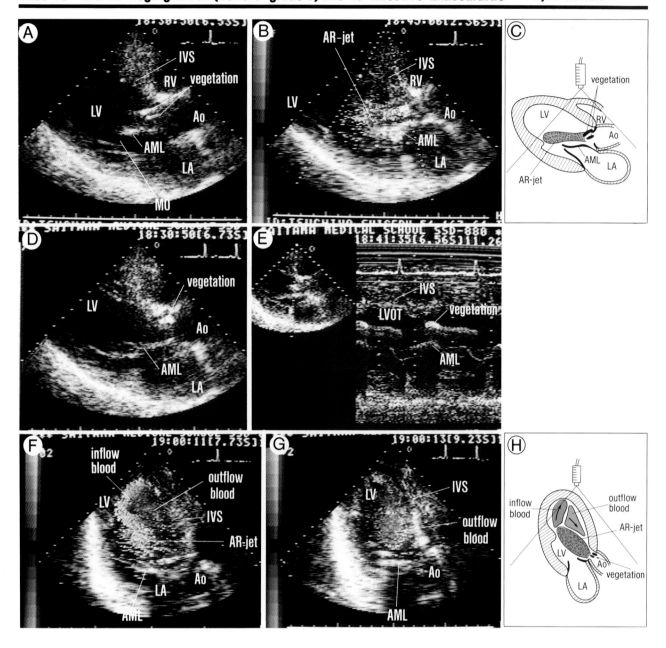

2-D Doppler images in a patient with aortic regurgitation due to infective endocarditis.
A B-mode in long-axis view in diastole. In diastole, vegetations on the aortic valve extend into the left ventricular outflow tract above the mitral valve. **B** 2-D Doppler same view, diastole. AR-jet corresponding to Sellers' grade 3 is demonstrated. **C** Diagram of **B**. **D** B-mode same view, systole. Vegetations on the aortic valve are shown. **E** Mitral valve echocardiogram. During diastole, echoes from the vegetations are recorded above the anterior mitral leaflet. **F** 2-D Doppler in apical long-axis view in diastole. Note the distribution of the three diastolic blood flow patterns in the left ventricle ; inflow blood, AR-jet, and outfow blood. **G** 2-D Doppler same view, systole. **H** Diagram of **F**.

Case 14 Aortic Stenosis 58-year-old female

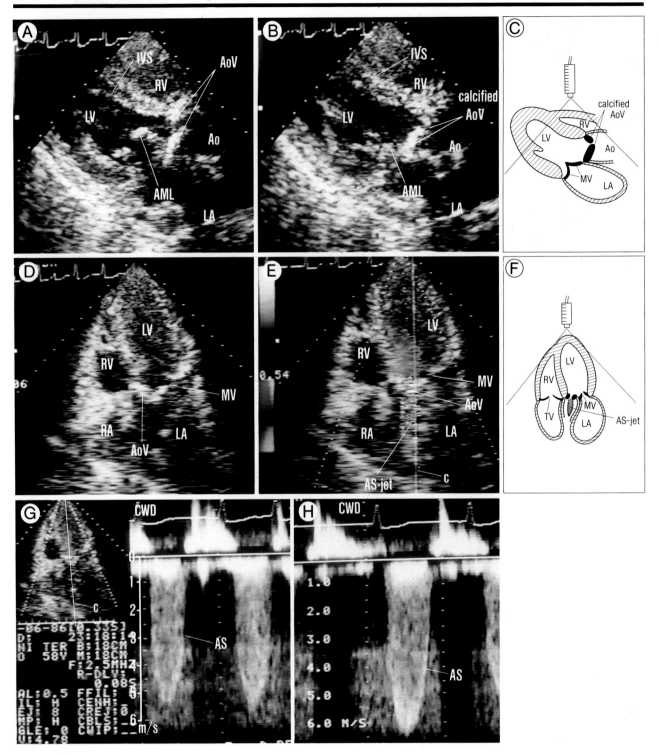

2-D Doppler images in a patient with severe aortic stenosis (AS).
Ⓐ B-mode in long-axis view in diastole. Ⓑ B-mode same view, systole. Calcific aortic cusps are shown. Ⓒ Diagram of Ⓑ. Ⓓ B-mode in apical five-chamber view in diastole. Ⓔ 2-D Doppler same view, in systole. Blood flow passes through stenotic aortic orifice into the ascending aorta in mosaic patterns (AS-jet) indicating significant aortic stenosis. Ⓕ Diagram of Ⓔ. Ⓖ Continuous-wave Doppler of aortic valve flow (beam line : c). Ⓗ Ditto.
[Evaluation of aortic stenosis]
　max V : 6.5 m/s, max △P : 165 mmHg.
Peak-to-peak pressure gradient from cardiac catheterization (LVP-AoP) was 152 mmHg. LVP : left ventricular systolic pressure, AoP : systolic pressure of the aorta.

Case 15 Aortic Stenosis 48-year-old male

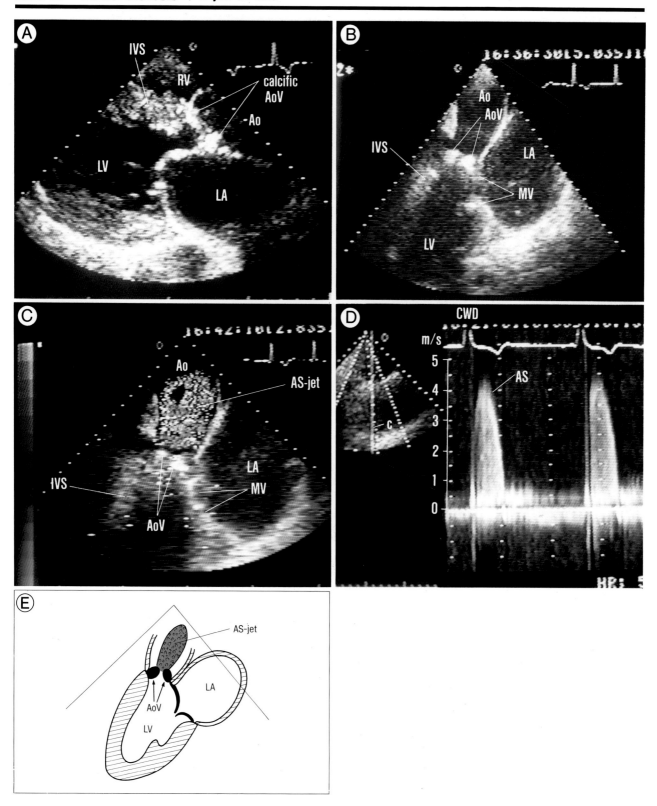

2-D Doppler images in a patient with mild aortic stenosis (AS).
Ⓐ B-mode in long-axis view in diastole. Calcific aortic valve is shown. Ⓑ B-mode in long-axis view from the higher right sternal border in systole. For obtainig the better flow signals from the ascending aorta the transducer was located in the higher right sternal border. Ⓒ 2-D Doppler same view, systole. AS-jet is clearly demonstrated. Ⓓ Continuous-wave Doppler of aortic valve flow (beam line: c).
[Evaluation of aortic stenosis]
 max V=4.7 m/s, max △P=88 mmHg.
Peak-to-peak pressure gradient from cardiac catheterization (LVP-AoP): 30 mmHg. LVP: left ventricular systolic pressure, AoP: systolic pressure of the aorta.

Case 16   Tricuspid Regurgitation (Grade 2) associated with MS·MR   66-year-old female

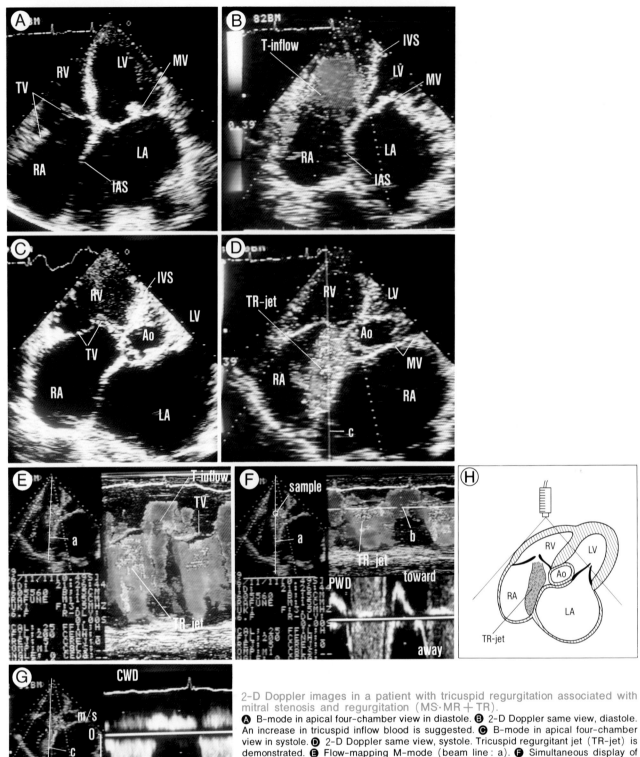

2-D Doppler images in a patient with tricuspid regurgitation associated with mitral stenosis and regurgitation (MS·MR + TR).
Ⓐ B-mode in apical four-chamber view in diastole. **Ⓑ** 2-D Doppler same view, diastole. An increase in tricuspid inflow blood is suggested. **Ⓒ** B-mode in apical four-chamber view in systole. **Ⓓ** 2-D Doppler same view, systole. Tricuspid regurgitant jet (TR-jet) is demonstrated. **Ⓔ** Flow-mapping M-mode (beam line : a). **Ⓕ** Simultaneous display of flow-mapping M-mode and pulsed-wave Doppler (beam line : a, sample volume : sample (b)). TR-jet is characterized as broad-band and bi-directional signals in pulsed-wave Doppler recording. **Ⓖ** Continuous-wave Doppler of tricuspid regurgitant flow (beam line : c). With the pressure gradient across the tricuspid valve, a noninvasive estimate of right ventricular systolic pressure can be obtained. **Ⓗ** Diagram of **Ⓓ**, **Ⓔ**, **Ⓕ**, and **Ⓖ**.
[Estimate of right ventricular systolic pressure (RVP)]
    max V=2.3 m/s, max ΔP=21 mmHg, RVP=21+10=31 mmHg (assuming that right atrial pressure is 10 mmHg).

Case 17 Tricuspid Regurgitation (Grade 3) associated with MS·MR 55-year-old female

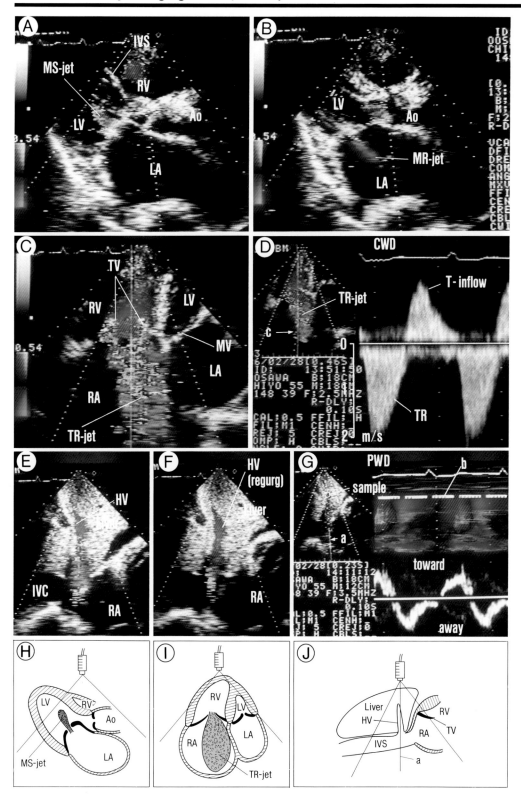

2-D Doppler images in a patient with tricuspid regurgitation associated with mitral stenosis and regurgitation (MS·MR + TR). **A** 2-D Doppler in long-axis view in diastole. MS-jet is shown. **B** 2-D Doppler same view, systole. Note the mild mitral regurgitation. **C** 2-D Doppler in apical four-chamber view in systole. Tricuspid regurgitant jet is present in the entire right atrium. **D** Continuous-wave Doppler of tricuspid regurgitant flow (beam line: c). **E** 2-D Doppler in subcostal view in diastole. **F** 2-D Doppler same view, systole. In systole, regurgitant flow to the hepatic vein (HV) can be observed in red color. **G** Simultaneous display of flow-mapping M-mode and pulsed-wave Doppler (beam line: a, sample volume: sample (b)). **H** Diagram of **A**. **I** Diagram of **C** and **D**. **J** Diagram of **E**, **F**, and **G**. [Estimate of right ventricular systolic pressure (RVP)]

max V=2.0 m/s, max ΔP=16 mmHg, RVP=16+10=26 mmHg (assuming that right atrial pressure is 10 mmHg).

104

Case 18　Multivalvular Disease (1): AR (Sellers' grade 2) + MS·MR (Sellers' grade 2) + TR (Grade 2)
29-year-old female

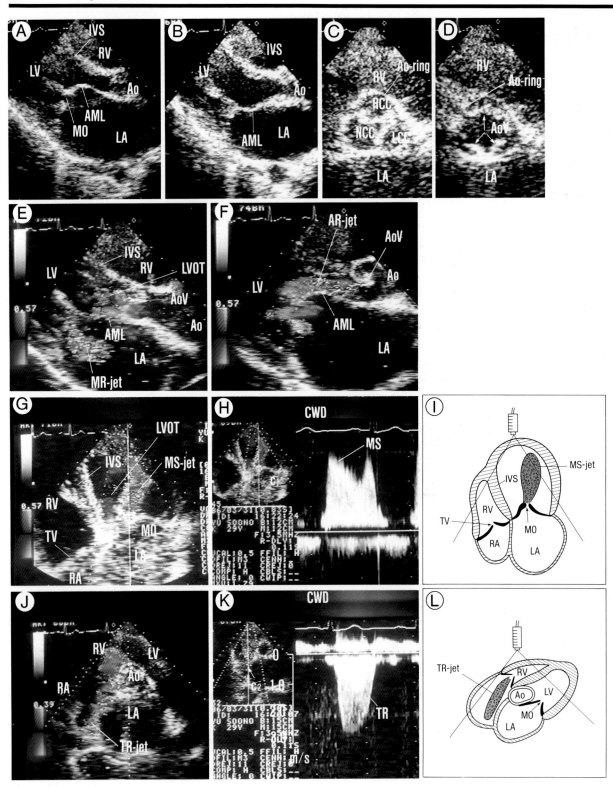

2-D Doppler images in a patient with multivalvular disease (AR + MS·MR + TR).
Ⓐ B-mode in long-axis view in diastole. Ⓑ B-mode same view, systole. Ⓒ B-mode in short-axis view at the level of the aortic valve in diastole.
Ⓓ B-mode same view, systole. Ⓔ 2-D Doppler in long-axis view in systole. MR-jet (Sellers' grade 2) is shown. Ⓕ 2-D Doppler same view, diastole. AR-jet (sellers' grade 2) is demonstrated. Ⓖ 2-D Doppler in apical four-chamber view in diastole. MS-jet is seen clearly in this plane.
Ⓗ Continuous-wave Doppler of mitral valve flow (beam line : c). Ⓘ Diagram of Ⓖ and Ⓗ. Ⓙ 2-D Doppler in apical four-chamber view in systole. TR-jet (grade 2) is seen along the interatrial septum in the right atrium. Ⓚ Continuous-wave Doppler of tricuspid regurgitant flow (beam line : c).
[Evaluation of mitral stenosis]
　max V=1.3 m/s, mean ΔP=4 mmHg, P1/2 T=0.20 sec, MVA=1.1 cm^2.
[Estimate of right ventricular systolic pressure (RVP)]
　max V=2.9 m/s, max ΔP=34 mmHg, RVP=34+10=44 mmHg (assuming that right atrial pressure is 10 mmHg).

Case 19　Multivalvular Disease(2):AS·AR (Sellers' grade 2)+MS+TR (grade 2)　54-year-old female

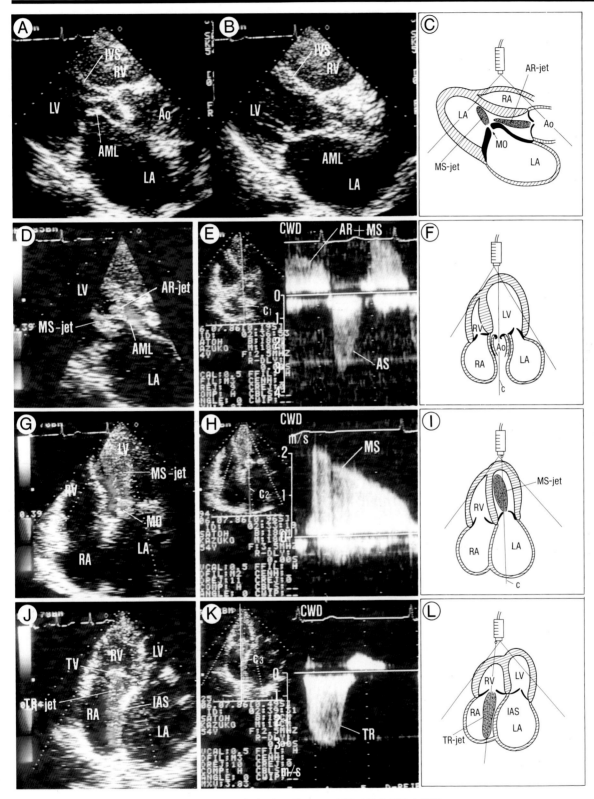

2-D Doppler images in a patient with multivalvular disease (AS·AR + MS + TR).
Ⓐ B-mode in long-axis view in diastole. Ⓑ B-mode same view, systole. Ⓒ Diagram of Ⓓ. Ⓓ 2-D Doppler in long-axis view in diastole. Both AR-jet (Sellers' grade 2) and MS-jet are demonstrated in this plane. Ⓔ Continuous-wave Doppler of aortic valve flow in apical five-chamber view (beam line : c_1). Doppler signals by aortic regurgitation and mitral stenosis are overlapping in diastole in this recording. Ⓕ Diagram of Ⓔ. Ⓖ 2-D Doppler in apical four-chamber view in diastole. MS-jet is clearly shown. Ⓗ Continuous-wave Doppler of mitral valve flow in apical four-chamber view (beam line : c_2). Ⓘ Diagram of Ⓖ and Ⓗ. Ⓙ 2-D Doppler in apical four-chamber view in systole. TR-jet is demonstrated. Ⓚ Continuous-wave Doppler of tricuspid regurgitant flow in apical four-chamber view (beam line : c_3).
[Evaluation of aortic stenosis]
　max V=3.0 m/s, max ΔP=36 mmHg.
[Evaluation of mitral stenosis]
　max V=2.0 m/s, mean V=1.6 m/s, mean ΔP=10 mmHg, P1/2 T=0.24 sec, MVA=0.9 cm^2.
[Estimate of right ventricular systolic pressure (RVP)]
　max V=2.7 m/s, max ΔP=29 mmHg, RVP=29+10=39 mmHg (assumng that right atrial pressure is 10 mmHg).

Case 20 Prosthetic Valve (1):Mitral Position (Hancock) 62-year-old female

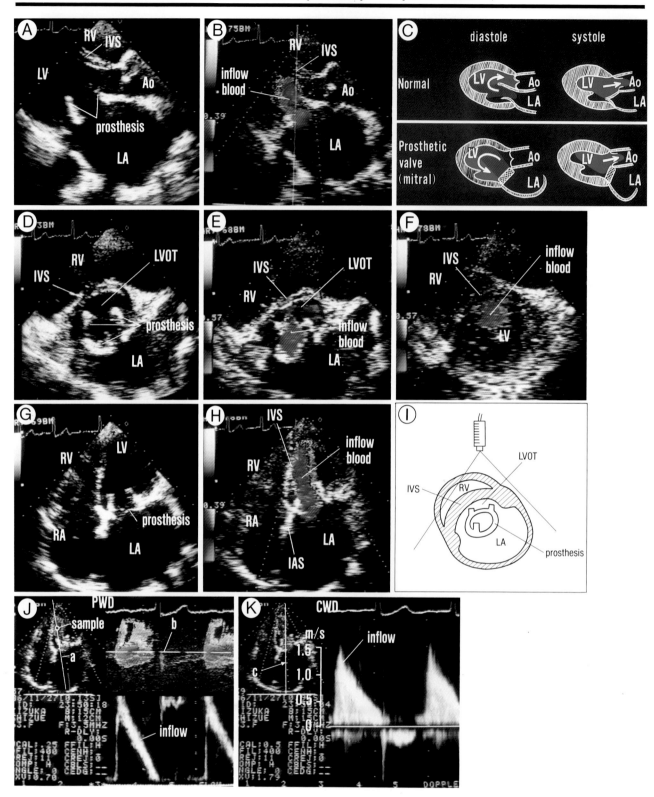

2-D Doppler images in a patient with a prosthetic valve in mitral position (MVR).
Ⓐ B-mode in long-axis view in diastole. Ⓑ 2-D Doppler same view, diastole. During diastole, mitral inflow is directed toward the interventricular septum, occupying the left ventricular outflow tract while ventricular outflow velocities are directed posteriorly toward the inflow tract. Ⓒ Diagram showing that ventricular diastolic flow patterns are reversed anteriorly-posteriorly from normal. Ⓓ B-mode in short-axis view at the level of the mitral valve in diastole. Ⓔ 2-D Doppler same view, diastole. Ⓕ 2-D Doppler in short-axis view at the level of the papillary muscles in diastole. Ⓖ B-mode in apical four-chamber view in diastole. Ⓗ 2-D Doppler same view, diastole. Inflow blood through the prosthesis strikes the interventricular septum. Ⓘ Diagram of Ⓓ and Ⓔ. Ⓙ Simultaneous display of flow-mapping M-mode and pulsed-wave Doppler (beam line: a, sample volume: sample (b)). Ⓚ Continuous-wave Doppler of antegrade transprosthetic flow velocity (beam line: c)
[Evaluation of blood flow dynamics in mitral valve prosthesis]
　max V=1.5 m/s, mean V=0.71 m/s, mean ΔP=2 mmHg, P 1/2 T=0.11 sec, MVA=2.0 cm².

Case 21　Prosthetic Valve (2): Aortic Position (St. Jude) and Mitral Position (St. Jude) 48-year-old male

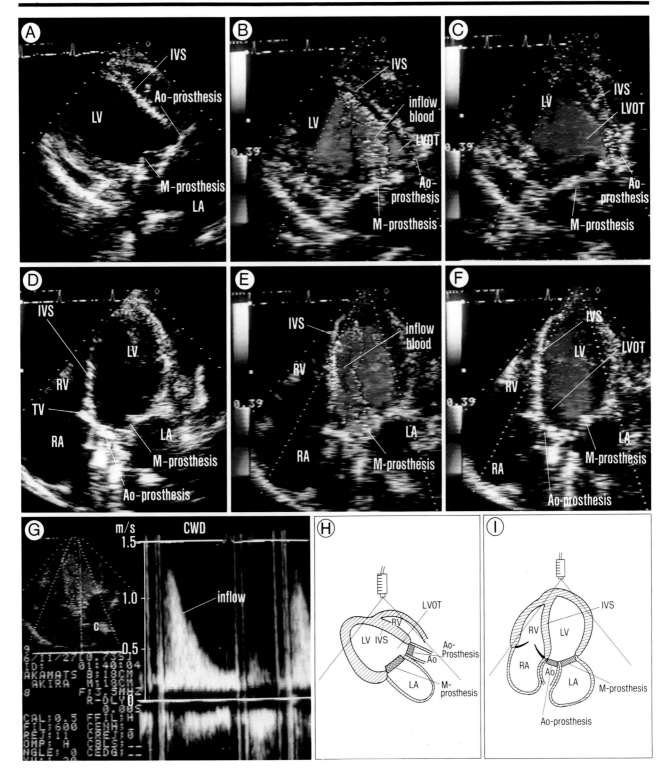

2-D Doppler images in a patient with prosthetic valves in aortic and mitral positions (AVR+MVR).
Ⓐ B-mode in long-axis view in diastole. Ⓑ 2-D Doppler same view, diastole. Ⓒ 2-D Doppler same view, systole. Ⓓ B-mode in apical five-chamber view in diastole. Ⓔ 2-D Doppler same view, diastole. Inflow blood through mitral prosthetic valve is directed anteriorly toward the interventricular septum. Ⓕ 2-D Doppler same view, systole. Ⓖ Continuous-wave Doppler of transprosthetic flow velocity in mitral position (beam line: c). Ⓗ Diagram of Ⓓ, Ⓔ, and Ⓕ.

[Evaluation of blood flow dynamics in mitral valve prosthesis]
　max V=1.39 m/s, mean V=0.71 m/s, mean ΔP=3 mmHg, MVA=2.4 cm^2

Case 22　Prosthetic Valve(3):Mitral Position (Björk-Shiley)　50-year-old female

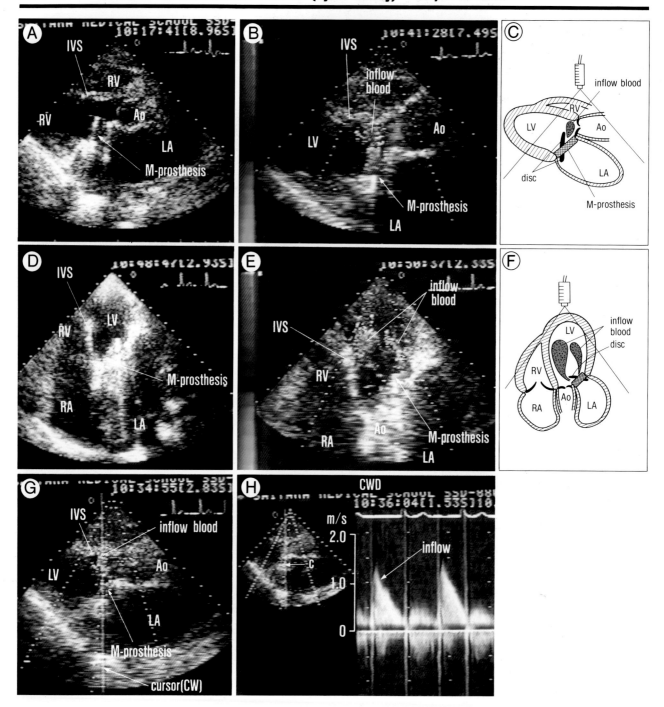

2-D Doppler images in a patient with mitral valve prosthesis (MVR).

Ⓐ B-mode in long-axis view in diastole. Ⓑ 2-D Doppler same view, diastole. In this case, major orifice of Björk-Shiley disc valve is directed anteriorly. Ⓒ Diagram of Ⓑ. Ⓓ B-mode in apical five-chamber view in diastole. Ⓔ 2-D Doppler same view, diastole. Two streams of inflow blood through major and minor orifices of the disc valve are demonstrated in diastole. Ⓕ Diagram of Ⓔ. Ⓖ 2-D Doppler in long-axis view in diastole. Ⓗ Continuous-wave Doppler of transprosthetic flow velocity (beam line: c).

[Evaluation of blood flow dynamics in mitral valve prosthesis]
　max V=1.4 m/s, mean V=0.71 m/s, mean Δ =2 mmHg, P 1/2 T=0.10 sec, MVA=2.2 cm²

Case 23　Paravalvular Leak:Aortic Valve Prosthesis (St. Jude)　51-year-old male

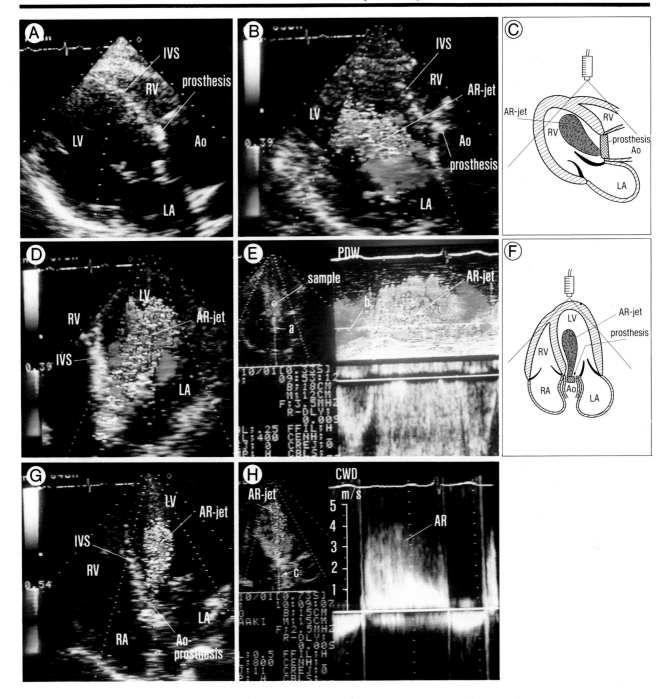

2-D Doppler image in a patient with paravalvular leak after aortic valve replacement.
A B-mode in long-axis view in diastole. **B** 2-D Doppler same view, diastole. AR-jet due to paravalvular leak of aortic valve prosthesis reaches the level of the papillary muscles (Sellers' grade 3). **C** Diagram of **B**. **D** 2-D Doppler in apical five-chamber view in diastole. **E** Simultaneous display of flow-mapping M-mode and pulsed-wave Doppler (beam line : a, sample volume : sample (b)). **F** Diagram of **D**, **E**, **F**, **G**, and **H**.
G 2-D Doppler in apical five-chamber view in diastole. **H** Continuous-wave Doppler of aortic regurgitant flow (beam line : c).

Case 24　Prosthetic Valve Failure (1): Mitral Position　46-year-old female

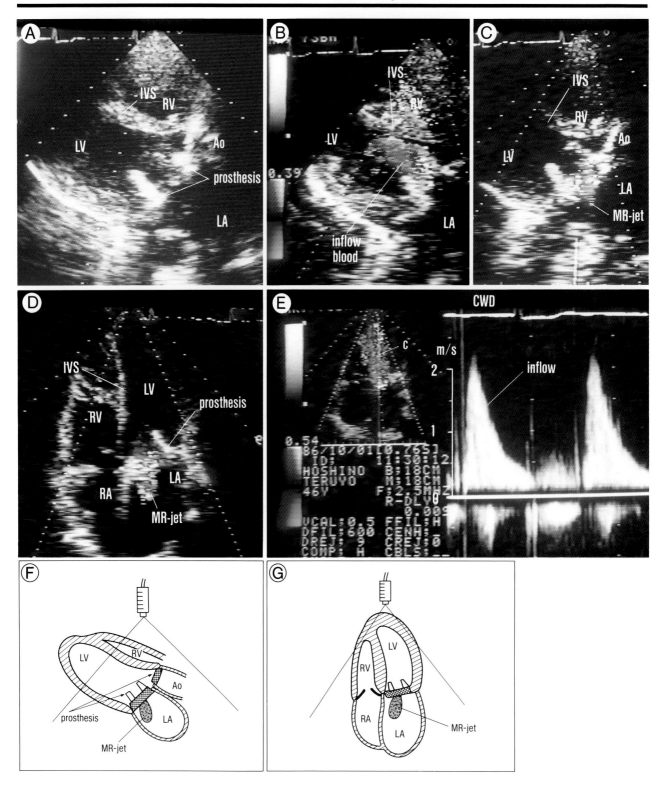

2-D Doppler images in a patient with prosthatic valve failure in the mitral position after aortic valve (Carpentier-Edwards) and mitral valve (Björk-Shiley) replacement.
Ⓐ B-mode in long-axis view in diastole. Ⓑ 2-D Doppler same view, diastole. Ⓒ 2-D Doppler same view, systole. Ⓓ 2-D Doppler in apical four-chamber view in systole. In Ⓒ and Ⓓ, moderate prosthetic regurgitation (MR-jet) is demonstrated (Sellers' grade 2).
Ⓔ Continuous-wave Doppler of inflow blood through the mitral prosthesis (beam line: c).
[Evaluation of mitral prosthetic valve]
　max V=2.3 m/s, mean V=1.0 m/s, P 1/2 T=0.07 sec, MVA=3.0 cm². An increase in diastolic flow volume due to the regurgitation may produce high velocities in the left ventricular inflow blood.

Case 25　Prosthetic Valve Failure (2): Mitral Position　62-year-old male

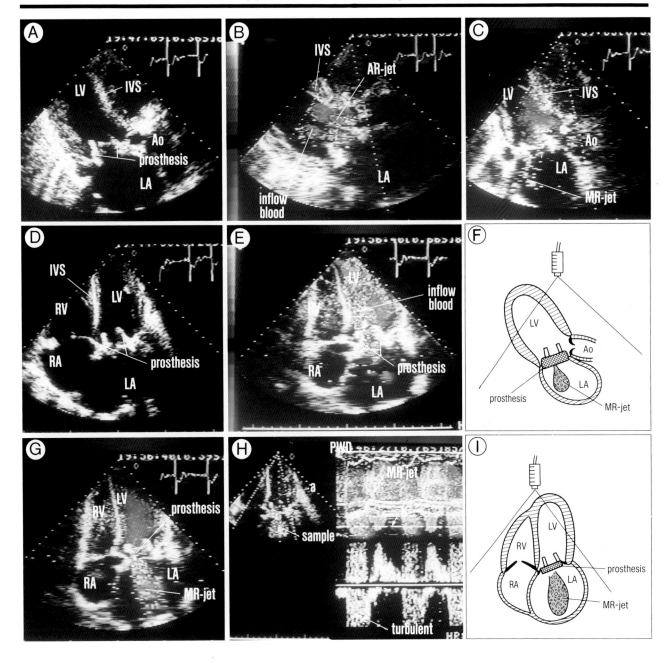

2-D Doppler images in a patient with prosthetic valve failure (Hancock) in the mitral position.
Ⓐ B-mode in long-axis view in systole. Ⓑ 2-D Doppler same view, diastole. Coexisting moderate aortic regurgitation (AR-jet) is shown (Sellers' grade 2). Ⓒ 2-D Doppler same view, systole. Severe prosthetic regurgitation (MR-jet) is shown (Sellers' grade 3). Ⓓ B-mode in apical four-chamber view in systole. Ⓔ 2-D Doppler same view, diastole. Inflow blood through malfunctiong mitral prosthesis is imaged in mosaic patterns indicating turbulent blood flow. Ⓕ Diagram of Ⓒ. Ⓖ 2-D Doppler in apical four-chamber view in systole. Severe mitral regurgitation is clearly demonstrated. Ⓗ Simultaneous display of flow-mapping M-mode and pulsed-wave Doppler (beam line : a, sample volume : sample (b)). Ⓘ Diagram of Ⓖ and Ⓗ.

Intraoperative 2-D Doppler

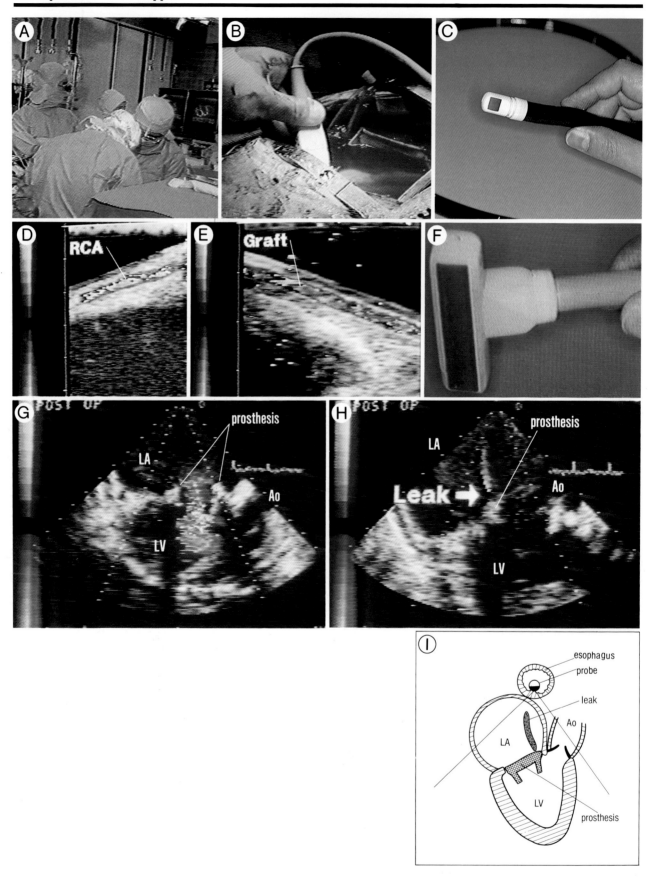

Intraoperative use of 2-D Doppler technique.
A Intraoperative use of 2-D Doppler during open heart surgery. **B** Epicardial approach using a regular probe. **C** Transesophageal probe.
D Visualization of a right coronary artery (epicardial approach). **E** Visualization of a saphenous vein graft (epicardial approach). **F** 7.5 MHz linear array transducer for visualization of coronary arteries. **G** 2-D Doppler in a patient with mitral prosthesis in transesophageal long-axis view in diastole. **H** 2-D Doppler same view, systole. Slight paravalvular leak from the edge of the prosthesis is imaged. **I** Diagram of **H**.

Chapter 10   Ischemic Heart Disease and Cardiac Masses

10—1   **Ischemic Heart Diseases: Ventricular septal perforation, dysfunction of papillary muscle, and left ventricular aneurysm**

Conventional 2-D echocardiography has been known to be effective in segmental wall motion analysis, and in the diagnosis of ventricular aneurysm[1-3] and parietal thrombosis in ischemic heart disease. Since the 2-D Doppler allows easy diagnosis of abnormal blood flow such as that from a ventricular septal perforation[4] as well as analysis of left ventricular blood flow[5,6] in real time, the clinical significance of the 2-D Doppler is profound.

○ P.133 **Case 26** is an example of ventricular septal perforation occurring secondarily to a myocardial infarction. A jet of shunt blood flow travels from the left ventricular lumen to the right ventricular lumen at the perforation in the ventricular septum. When the ventricular septal perforation is small this may form a tortuous tunnel. In such cases it may be difficult to define the site of the perforation in the conventional B-mode : however, this kind of shunt blood flow is imaged easily with 2-D Doppler.

In ischemic heart disease, mitral regurgitation due to ischemia or infarction of the ventricular wall involving the papillary muscle can be observed at times. **Case 27** shows an ○ P.133 example of mitral regurgitation due to dysfunction of the anterior papillary muscle. The anterior cusp of the mitral valve is displaced towards the left atium.

When part of the left ventricular wall fails to contract because of myocardial infarction, an abnormality is detected in the behavior of the blood in the left ventricle during expansion of the left ventricular lumen. In particular, when part of the wall forms a ventricular aneurysm that exhibits paradoxical movement in systole, the abnormality in the left ventricular blood flow becomes more marked. The analysis of the blood flow pattern in the left ventricle by the 2-D Doppler seems to open up a very interesting new horizon. The authors studied cases[5] that exhibited abnormal wall motion of the left ventricle secondary to anteroseptal myocardial infarction (confirmed by angiography) with 2-D Doppler. Two typical blood

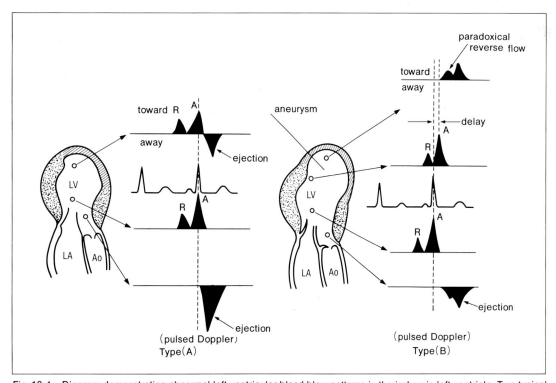

Fig. 10-1   Diagram demonstrating abnormal left ventricular blood blow patterns in the ischemic left ventricle. Two typical patterns are observed : Pattern (A) associated with akinesis and dyskinesis of segments 1-2 ; and pattern (B) identified with ventricuar aneurysms in segments 1-3. Note that in pattern (B) flood flow in the opposite direction to normal is detected due to bulging at the apex during systole.

flow patterns in the left ventricle were observed. Pattern (A) was observed mainly in akinesis and dyskinesis of segments 1-2. In pattern (A) the height of the A wave by atrial contraction is high in the diastolic left ventricular inflow pattern and, at the same time, the ratio of the A wave to the R wave increases. this is understood to mean a drop in compliance due to scarring and/or ischemia in the left ventricular wall[7]. The systolic blood flow pattern is kept normal in pattern (A).

On the other hand, in pattern (B), blood flow in the opposite direction to normal, that is, towards the transducer, is detected due to bulging at the apex during systole. The velocity of the left ventricular outflow blood is also significantly lowered. Our study revealed that pattern (A) is mainly detected in akinesis and dyskinesis of segments 1-2 while pattern (B) is observed mainly in ventricular aneurysms in segments 1-3. Analysis of the ventricular blood flow pattern is an area that requires more detailed study in the future. **Case 28** is an example of a small ventricular aneurysm at the apex while **Case 29** gives an example of a large apical ventricular aneurysm. **Case 28** shows a typical ventricular blood flow pattern belonging to pattern (A). Probably due to the smallness of the ventricular aneurysm, pattern (A) is observed in **Case 28**(Fig. 10-1).

○ P.134
○ P.135

10-2 Cardiac Masses : Left atrial and left ventricular myxomas

Myxoma of the left atrium is the most frequently encountered heart tumor and its clinical symptoms and hemodynamics are extremely similar to those of mitral stenosis. With the development of echocardiography, diagnosis has become possible based on characteristic findings and has facilitated differential diagnosis with mitral stenosis. A characteristic hemodynamic is found for tumors that show pendular motion, particularly with pedunculated tumors, because they become imbedded at the mitral opening during diastole. Observation by 2-D Doppler (**Case 30**) reveals an inflow blood from the left atrium to the left ventricle during diastole in jet form. From the evaluation of mitral blood inflow by CWD, the area of the mitral valve opening is calculated at 0.9 cm^2.

○ P.136

Compared to the left atrial myxoma, the left ventricular myxoma is very rarely encountered, but the diagnosis, using echocardiography, is extremely simple. The hemodynamics in the left atrial myxoma is found to be similar to mitral stenosis ; however, in the cases of left ventricular myxoma it is similar to stenosis of the aortic valve. **Case 31** shows the 2-D Doppler findings of the left ventricular myxoma. The blood flow at the aortic root indicates a marked turbulent pattern such as occurs in aortic valve stenosis, due to obstruction of the left ventricular outflow tract by a myxoma.

○ P.137

References

1) Wong, M., Shah, P. M. : Accuracy of two-dimensional echocardiography in detecting left ventricular aneurysm. Cardiol., 6 : 250-254, 1983.

2) Barrett, M. J., Charuzi, Y., and Corday, E. : Ventricular aneurysm : Cross-sectional echocardiographic approach. Am. J. Cardiol., 46 : 1133-1137, 1980.

3) Visser, C. A., Kan, G., Meltzer, R. S., Koolen, J. J., and Dunning, A. J. : Incidence, timing and prognostic value of left ventricular aneurysm formation after myocardial infarction : A prospective, serial echocardiographic study of 158 patients. Am. J. Cardiol., 57 : 729-732, 1986.

4) Yoshida, K., Yoshikawa, J., Akasaka, T., Shono, H., Shakudo, M., Asaka, T., Shiratori, K., Koizumi, K., Okumachi, F., Takao, S., Maenishi, F., Yagi, T., Kato, H. : Ultrasonic features of cardiac rupture. Proceedings of the 48th Meeting of the Japan Society of Ultrasonics in Medicine, 37-38, 1986. Abstract

5) Omoto, R., Wong, M., Matsumura, M., Yamagata, S., and Ishiguro, T. : Noninvasive analysis of left ventricular blood-flow dynamics in left ventricular aneurysm by color flow mapping. J. Am. Coll. Cardiol., 9(2) : 66 A, 1987.

6) Hirai, H., Suzuki, M. : Left ventricular flow patternes in ischemic heart disease - Assessment by two-D color flow mapping. Proceedings of the 48th Meeting of the Japan Society of Ultrasonics

in Medicine, 45-46, 1986. Abstract

7) Kuwako, K., Isobe, M. : Two-dimensional doppler echocardiographic assessment of diastolic function of the left and right ventricle in coronary heart disease. Proceedings of the 48th Meeting of the Japan Society of Ultrasonics in Medicine, 41-42, 1986. Abstract

Chapter 11 Diseases of the Aorta and the Peripheral Vessels

11—1 Introduction

The first clinical application of the Doppler effect was by Satomura[1] in 1956, and its initial application to blood flow measurement was performed on the peripheral vessels. Noninvasive two-dimensional blood flow visualization using the Doppler technique has developed mainly in the peripheral vessels and the carotid artery. In 1971 Hokanson et al.[2] reported "ultrasonic arteriography" using the pulsed-wave Doppler technique. Then Reid and Spencer[3] in 1972 displayed the carotid artery flow by the continuous-wave Doppler technique. A report of color-coded flow visualization of the carotid artery by Curry and White[4] followed in 1978. Brandestini[5] displayed the carotid artery using the color-coded multi-gate M-mode. However, no attempts at real-time noninvasive flow visualization were made.

It was not until the development of the blood flow imaging system by Namekawa et al.[6] in 1982 that real-time noninvasive flow visualization without enhancement was performed. The authors[7] have reported the clinical application of 2-D Doppler to aortic disease, in particular to dissecting aortic aneurysm, and thoracic and abdominal aortic aneurysm. Since 2-D Doppler systems with phased-array sector scanning had been developed mainly for the heart and the great vessels, their capacity for displaying more detailed structures and organs close to the transducer was not sufficient for application to the peripheral vessels except in the case of dilated lesions such as femoral artery aneurysms.

However, a linear array color flow mapping system with improved resolution was developed in 1985, and has been applied to the mapping of the peripheral vessels[8]. The term "2-D Doppler" covers not only real-time two-dimensional Doppler echocardiography of the heart and the great vessels but also real-time two-dimensional Doppler echography of the peripheral vessels.

In this chapter, transesophageal 2-D Doppler for thoracic aortic aneurysms, intraoperative 2-D Doppler for aortic disease, and curved linear arrayed 2-D Doppler for peripheral vascular disease are discussed.

11—2 Diseases of the Aorta

1. Dissecting aortic aneurysm

Since dissecting aortic aneurysm is a serious disorder which may be fatal soon after onset, early accurate diagnosis is mandatory for saving life. Although noninvasive diagnostic methods such as echocardiography, CT[9] and MRI[10] have been available clinically, their dependability in terms of diagnostic accuracy has been inferior to that of invasive aortography. However, the recent progress in the area of echocardiography has increased its clinical reliability.

It was Millward et al.[11] who first observed dissecting aortic aneurysm by echocardiography. He reported on the use of M-mode echocardiography to examine the intimal flap in the aortic root in 1972. In 1973 Nanda et al.[12] reported on a diagnostic index for dissecting aortic aneurysm with M-mode echocardiography. Matsumoto et al.[13] were the first, in 1978, to report on the application of two-dimensional echocardiography (2-D echo) for the observation of dissecting aortic aneurysm. The clinical significance of using two-dimensional echocardiography for this disorder was subsequently discussed by several investigators[14]-[16]. Mathew & Nanda[17], and Okamoto et al.[18] applied the pulsed-wave Doppler method to its diagnosis. After the development of real-time two-dimensional Doppler echocardiography (2-D Doppler), the present authors reported on their observation of dissecting aortic aneurysm by 2-D Doppler in 1984[7]. Then, in 1984 the authors[19] reported intraoperative use of 2-D Doppler during surgery for the same condition. In 1984, Börner et al.[20] applied transesophageal two-dimensional echocardiography to the diagnosis of type III dissecting aortic aneurysm. The authors[21] reported total visualization of a thoracic dissecting aortic aneurysm with transesophageal 2-D Doppler, indicating the possibility of visualizing total images of dissecting aortic aneurysm with combined use of transesophageal and transcutaneous approaches.

1) Transcutaneous approach

The conventional approaches to dissecting aortic aneurysm using echocardiography are transcutaneous. Systematic approaches toward extensive thoracic and abdominal lesions are needed[22]. The transcutaneous approaches to dissecting aortic aneurysm by 2-D Doppler indicated in Tab. 11-1 are almost the same as those of two-dimensional echocardiography. The heart and the aortic root were examined by the left parasternal approaches in the left semi-decubitus position. In that approach the descending aorta is seen in sagittal scanning.

Tab. 11-1   Transcutaneous approaches of 2-D Doppler to dissecting aortic aneurysm

Heart ⎫ Aortic root ⎭	Left parasternal approach
Ascending aorta	Rght parasternal approach
Aortic arch	Suprasternal approach
Descending aorta	⎧ Left parasternal approach ⎩ Left paravertebral approach
Thoraco-abdominal aorta around the Diaphragm	Subxyphoidal approach
Abdominal aorta ⎫ Iliac artery ⎭	Ventral approach

However, since the descending aorta is at a deep site and the Doppler beam meets the descending aorta almost at a right angle, visualization of its flow is difficult. The short-axis and long-axis views of the ascending aorta are obtained by the right parasternal approach in the right decubitus position. The ascending aorta is a key point for differentiation between DeBakey I or II, and III. Since the upper aorta cannot be visualized by a transesophageal approach, this transcutaneous approach is very important. In DeBakey type I or II, when the ascending aorta is involved in dissection and dilation, the right parasternal approach can be used for easy visualization of the dilated ascending aorta. The suprasternal approach is good for showing the aortic arch and the arch vessels. The descending aorta is also approached by the left paravertebral approach from the back when the descending aortic aneurysm is in contact with the chest wall, or when pleural effusion fills the space between the descending aorta and the chest wall, thus keeping the lung aside.

The thoraco-abdominal aorta around the diaphragm can be visualized well by the subxyphoidal approach. Although an abdominal aortic aneurysm may be visualized by the ventral approach, special Doppler approaches are also employed. The Doppler method is very sensitive to the angle made by the blood flow with the beam, and approaches to the abdominal aorta from a proximal or a distal location are advantageous for visualization of the blood flow (Fig. 11-1). The authors have named these approaches the proximal approach and the distal approach, respectively[7]. A frontal 2-D Doppler view obtained by

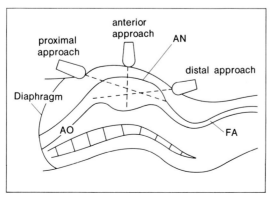

Fig. 11-1   Approaches of 2-D Doppler to the abdominal aortic aneurysm (AN).

scanning in the frontal plane is compatible with an antero-posterior view by aortography, as shown in **Case 38**, and a sagittal view by 2-D Doppler is compatible with a lateral view by aortography.

Since the diagnostic criterion of dissection is the presence of an intimal flap in any portion of the aorta that is visualized by any approach, diagnosis of this condition may be obtained by transcutaneous 2-D echogram. However, visualization of the total aorta by the transcutaneous approach alone is difficult owing to weak echo penetration of the lung and of the bones in the thorax, and to the intestinal gas in the abdomen. Accordingly, it is difficult to differentiate between types of dissection, and thus to determine the therapeutic approach. However, since transcutaneous echocardiography can be performed simply and efficiently enough to allow its use even in an intensive care unit without any pain to the patient, it should be included in the routine examination performed just after admission to the intensive care unit. Even though aortography or transesophageal 2-D Doppler (see below) is performed as the final diagnostic procedure, transcutaneous approaches are of clinical significance since they can supplement the findings of other techniques. Accordingly, in the examination of dissecting aortic aneurysm, each of the transcutaneous approaches mentioned above should be used in order to obtain as much information as possible.

Artifact signals due to side lobes are sometimes mistaken for an intimal flap in the interpretation of 2-D echocardiograms. Usually the intimal flap moves in synchrony with the cardiac cycle and 2-D Doppler can demonstrate different patterns of blood flow in the true and false lumina that are separated by the intimal flap.

2) Transesophageal 2-D Doppler

It is very difficult to visualize the totality of an extensive dissecting aortic aneurysm by the conventional transcutaneous approaches. In particular, the descending aorta is a weak point for transcutaneous echography owing to its deep situation in the thorax and to the prevention of echo penetration by the ribs and the left lung. Despite the development of 2-D Doppler, color flow visualization in the deep thorax has been impossible. Transesophageal echography facilitates both precise observation of the descending aorta from the adjacent esophagus, and visualization of the whole thoracic aorta apart from the upper ascending portion, which is not shown owing to the intervention of the bronchus between it and the esophagus and the consequent interruption of the ultrasound echo. Short-axis scanning by transesophageal 2-D Doppler displays the short-axis view of the aorta at all levels. Simultaneous displays of serial short-axis views of the aorta, similar to serial CT displays, offer a three-dimensional picture of the thoracic aorta **(Case 32, E-L)**.

○ P.138
○ P.139

Although structural information on dissecting aortic aneurysms obtained by 2-D Doppler in the gray scale is very useful, additional blood flow data derived from color flow mapping with 2-D Doppler permit differentiation of the true and the false lumina, diagnosis of the

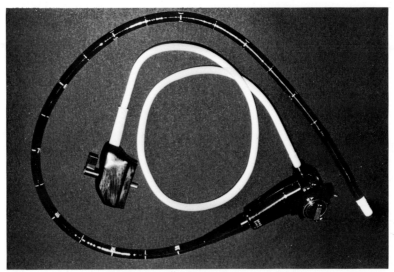

Fig. 11-2 The transesophageal 2-D Doppler transducer. Short-axis scanning, diameter

severity of aortic regurgitation, identification of tiny entry and reentry sites that may be overlooked on the 2-D echogram, diagnosis of leakage from the sites of anastomosis, and so on. In all twelve cases who had been examined by transesophageal 2-D Doppler after the onset of dissection and have been reported by the authors[23], differentiation of DeBakey types and identification of the sites, sizes and number of entries could be made. In seven of these cases reentry information was obtained, but in the other five, reentry was located distal to the abdominal aorta, and so could not be visualized. In two of three cases with aortic regurgitation, prolapse of the intimal flap from the aortic ring is visualized.

The principal shortcoming of transesophageal 2-D Doppler, however, is that its visualization of the arch vessels, abdominal visceral vessels, upper ascending aorta and distal abdominal aorta is poor. Supplementary information on these regions must be obtained by transcutaneous 2-D Doppler. Accordingly, a highly useful picture of an entire dissecting aortic aneurysm may in many cases be obtained merely via the transcutaneous and transesophageal 2-D Doppler approaches, so that surgery without aortography may be feasible.

The transesophageal 2-D Doppler images presented in this chapter are from short-axis scanning, and are shown as if viewed from below. Views of the descending aorta consequently show the right side on the left and vice versa, whereas those of the ascending aorta present the right side on the right.

3) Intraoperative 2-D Doppler

Intraoperative 2-D Doppler can perform the functions of both an intraoperative 2-D echogram and angiography noninvasively. Apart from its noninvasiveness, it is characterized by real-time color flow imaging, ease of echo penetration, a variety of feasible approaches, a good signal-to-noise ratio, a short examination time, ease of interpretation, and ease of operation. Preoperative angiographic and transcutaneous echographic examinations do not necessarily allow diagnosis and evaluation of the total lesion in complicated cases because the injection of the limited amount of contrast medium permissible in angiography of such cases allows only a restricted view of the lesion, and because the limitations of the approaches to the closed chest in echography restrict the length of aorta that can be displayed. Intraoperative 2-D Doppler is useful for confirming or correcting a preoperative diagnosis and in determining or confirming the extent of surgery necessary before aortic clamping. Within the region of the surgery, it also overcomes the shortcomings of the transesophageal approach mentioned above. After aortic unclamping, 2-D Doppler is also useful in evaluating the effects of the operation on the aortic structure and on the blood flow dynamics before chest closure. If 2-D Doppler discloses any significant defects, they can be repaired quickly before the patient's condition deteriorates.

Combinations of transcutaneous, transesophageal and intraoperative 2-D Doppler approaches are expected to permit more accurate and safer diagnosis and treatment. Diagnostic and therapeutic approaches used in our Department of Surgery in the acute phase of dissecting aortic aneurysm are indicated in Fig. 11-3. Although aortography is used

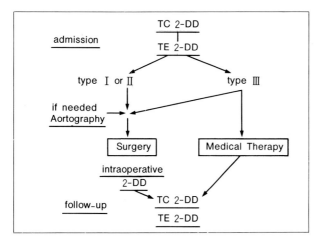

Fig. 11-3 Diagnostic and therapeutic approaches to the acute dissecting aortic aneurysm (Department of Surgery, Saitama Medical School). TC=transcutaneous; TE=transesophageal; 2-DD=two-dimensional Doppler.

to a golden standard for the final diagnosis of dissecting aortic aneurysm, transesophageal 2-D Doppler is sure to take its place, relegating aortography to the status of a supplementary method. Aortography will be performed only to obtain information that cannot be evaluated by transcutaneous and transesophageal 2-D Doppler.

❍P.138

Case 32 Dissecting aortic aneurysm, DeBakey type III b, 74-year-old male. Transesophageal 2-D Doppler

An entry in the descending aorta cannot usually be visualized by transcutaneous approaches, but the transesophageal approaches can clearly delineate it. Here, an entry 1 cm in width by 3 cm long, is located in the descending aorta 24 to 27 cm from the teeth. In systole, the flow from the lower, true lumen to the upper, false lumen is displayed in red (**Case 32, A**), and in diastole, that from the false lumen to the true lumen is displayed in blue (**Case 32, B**). Flow mapping M-mode indicates the timing of the flow through the entry (**Case 32, C**) and spectral analysis provides the velocity profile of the flow through the entry (**Case 32, D**). The flow through the entry often shows a biphasic pattern.

Total visualization of the dissecting aortic aneurysm was performed in this case (Fig. 11-4). At the aortic root can be seen mild aortic regurgitation of grade I reaching halfway to the tip of the mitral valve (**Case 32, E**). The ascending aorta is not involved in the dissection

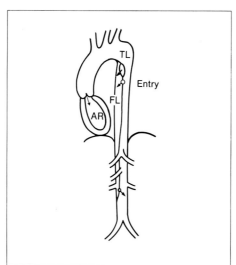

Fig. 11-4 Diagram of the dissecting aortic aneurysm in Case 32. TL =true lumen ; FL=false lumen.

and it is seen that aortic regurgitation is not correlated with the dissection (**Case 32, F**). The dissection in the descending aorta is shown to proceed distally from a point 23 cm from the ❍P.139 teeth (**Case 32, G**). Apart from the main entry (**Case 32, H**), a small entry, 1 mm in diameter, can be seen at 28 cm from the teeth (**Case 32, I**). It is very difficult to detect such a small entry even by transesophageal 2-D echography without color flow information. More distally, dissection proceeds spirally, so that at 30 cm from the teeth the true lumen is on the left side of the body (**Case 32, J**), but at 34 cm it is on the right (**Case 32, K**). At 48 cm from the teeth, in the abdominal aorta, three entries 1-2 mm in diameter were discovered (**Case 32, L**). Although the flow through the reentry is biphasic, like that through the entry, that from the false to the true lumen is greater than that from the true to the false lumen, in contrast to the pattern at the main entry.

❍P.140

Case 33 Dissecting aortic aneurysm, arch type with retrograde dissection, 46-year-old male.
Transesophageal 2-D Doppler (Fig. 11-5)

This case has a large entry at the aortic arch and retrograde dissection to the aortic ring. Transcutaneous 2-D Doppler displayed grade 2 aortic regurgitation but the precise mechanism of this was not seen. Transesophageal 2-D Doppler displays the intimal flap prolapsed from the aortic ring in diastole, and the relationship of the aortic regurgitation to

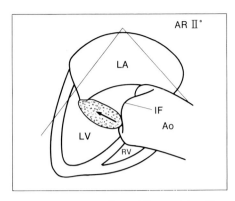

Fig. 11-5 Diagram of the aortic root of the dissecting aortic aneurysm in Case 33. Transesophageal view. IF=intimal flap.

this prolapsed flap (**Case 33, C**).

The aortic valve was resuspended, and the ascending aorta and aortic arch were replaced, reducing aortic regurgitation to grade I by transesophageal 2-D Doppler.

Case 34   Dissecting aortic aneurysm DeBakey type II, 60-year-old male.
Transcutaneous approach

The dilated ascending aorta is visualized well by transcutaneous 2-D Doppler from the right parasternal approach. The short-axis 2-D echocardiogram of the ascending aorta displays an intimal flap (**Case 34, A**) and 2-D Doppler displays fast flow in the true lumen and slight flow in the false lumen (**Case 34, B**). The long-axis 2-D echocardiogram of the aortic root shows an intimal flap at the aortic root (**Case 34, C**) and aortic regurgitation of grade 2 can be seen using 2-D Doppler (**Case 34, D**). Since this case was found by suprasternal 2-D echocardiography to exhibit neither dissection nor dilation at the aortic arch, a diagnosis of DeBakey type II was reached.

○ P.140

Case 35   Dissecting aortic aneurysm, DeBakey type I, 39-year-old male.
Intraoperative 2-D Doppler

An intraoperative 2-D Doppler display shows the long-axis view, with the left ventricle on the right side of the image and the aortic root on the left. Thus, for the operator, who usually stands on the right side of the patient on the operating table, there is a direct correspondence between the direction of manipulation of the transducer and that of the movement on the display image.

In this case, median sternotomy was performed, and the heart and the ascending aorta and aortic arch were scanned longitudinally. Figure 11-6 shows the condition prior to the surgical procedure. In **Case 35, C**, regurgitant flow from the aortic valve is displayed beyond the tip of the mitral valve. Aortic regurgitation is of grade 3. At the aortic root, an intimal flap and a large intimal tear (the entry) can be seen (**Case 35, B**); and both true and false lumina are displayed in color at the aortic arch (**Case 35, A**).

After replacement of the aortic valve and the ascending aorta (Fig. 11-7), a smooth flow of blood through the graft in the ascending aorta is shown in **Case 35, E**; and only the true

○ P.141

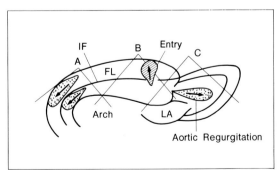

Fig. 11-6 Diagram of the dissecting aortic aneurysm in Case 35. Intraoperative view prior to surgical procedure. TL=true lumen; FL=false lumen; IF =intimal flap.

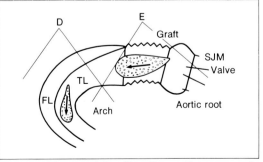

Fig. 11-7 Diagram of the dissecting aortic aneurysm in Case 35. Intraoperative view after replacement of the aortic valve and the ascending aorta.

lumen is displayed in color at the aortic arch (**Case 35, D**). The absence of any display of flow in the false lumen implies that the entry was completely closed.

Case 36 Dissecting aortic aneurysm, DeBakey type III b, 48-year-old male. Intraoperative 2-D Doppler (Fig. 11-8)

○ P.141

In this case, the aortic arch was directly scanned by 2-D Doppler through a left thoracotomy from the distal portion to the origin of the left subclavian artery. The site and size of the entry distal to the origin of the left subclavian artery are clearly displayed. In systole, a jet flow through the entry from the true to the false lumen is present (**Case 36, A**), and a reverse flow is present in diastole (**Case 36, B**). The flow mapping M-mode indicates the timing of the flow through the entry (**Case 36, D**) and spectral analysis shows that this flow through the entry is laminar during systole (**Case 36, E**).

Since the entry is small, the aortic wall of the false lumen was incised just at the entry with the aid of intraoperative 2-D Doppler, and the entry was closed by direct suturing. After aortic unclamping the false lumen was confirmed to have no flow, as in Case 35. Thus, intraoperative 2-D Doppler was very useful both for determining the precise operative procedure and for evaluating the results of surgery.

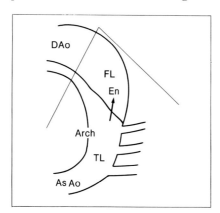

Fig. 11-8 Diagram of the dissecting aortic aneurym in Case 36. Intraoperative view. AsAo=ascending aorta; DAo=descending aorta; En=entry.

Case 37 Annuloaortic ectasia, Marfan syndrome, 59-year-old male.

○ P.142

The Marfan syndrome is often associated with annuloaortic ectasia. A long-axis view of the aortic root in the 2-D echocardiogram shows the dilated aortic ring root (**Case 37, A**). Two-dimensional Doppler displays grade 3 aortic regurgitation in diastole (**Case 37, B**).

Case 38 Dissecting abdominal aortic aneurysm, 77-year-old male (Fig. 11-9).

○ P.142

A proximal frontal view of the ventral approach to the abdominal aorta by 2-D Doppler yielded an image compatible with the anterior-posterior view of aortography. An intimal flap is present in the abdominal aortic aneurysm. In systole the true lumen is displayed by a blue-colored distal flow (**Case 38, A**), and in diastole a slow reverse flow from the false to the true lumen is depicted in red (**Case 38, B**). Dilation of both iliac arteries is also seen.

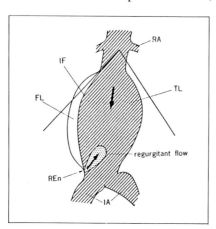

Fig. 11-9 Diagram of the dissecting abdominal aortic aneurysm in Case 38. Proximal frontal vew. REn=Reentry.

Case 39 Dissecting aortic aneurysm, DeBakey type III b, 48-year-old male. Transcutaneous approach to the abdominal aorta (Fig. 11-10).

The transcutaneous approach to the abdominal aorta in dissecting aortic aneurysm DeBakey type III b reveals different flow patterns in the two lumina of the abdominal aorta. In the upper lumen, in 2-D Doppler a red-colored normograde flow is displayed and in the lower lumen, a reverse flow colored blue (**Case 39, A**). The flow mapping M-mode shows a simultaneous pulsatility in the two lumina, though the directions of the flow are opposite ○ P.142 (**Case 39, C**). The flow patterns in two lumina of the aorta are a good clue for differentiating between the true and the false lumina.

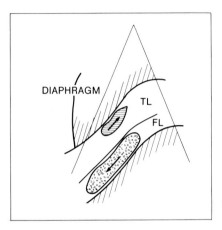

Fig. 11-10 Diagram of the abdominal aorta in dissecting aortic aneurysm, Case 39. Long-axis view of the abdominal aorta.

Case 40 Dissecting aortic aneurysm, DeBakey type III b, 65-year-old male. Intraoperative 2-D Doppler.

Since this case was associated with an infrarenal abdominal aortic aneurysm, replacement of the abdominal aorta with fenestration was performed, without any thoracic procedure. Intraoperative 2-D Doppler revealed the relationship between the dissection and the major abdominal visceral vessels and provided a three-dimensional understanding of the dissection.

At the level of the diaphragm, a short-axis 2-D Doppler view displays a small true lumen ○ P.143 with fast flow (red) and the surrounding false lumen in pale red (**Case 40, A**). The celiac axis is displayed as a red-colored flow from the false lumen, but the flow is not actually prevented (**Case 40, B**). These 2-D Doppler findings suggest that the closure of the entry in the thorax is not recommended in this case. The superior mesenteric artery exhibits some dissection at its origin from the aorta but is fed from the true lumen (**Case 40, C**). The left renal artery is also dissected at its root, and the dissected intimal flap forms a narrow channel like a bridge, a condition termed "bridge formation" by the authors (**Case 40, D**).

2. True aneurysm

Although 2-D echograms can display the dilation, extent and mural thrombus formations of a true aneurysm, 2-D Doppler shows the intraaneurysmal blood flow pattern. In an aneurysm the swirling flow phenomenon is invariably present and may be related to expansion of the aneurysm.

Two-dimensional techniques for a true aortic aneurysm are almost the same as those for a dissecting aortic aneurysm. Transcutaneous, transesophageal and intraoperative 2-D Doppler approaches may be used.

Case 41 Abdominal aortic aneurysm, 61-year-old male (Fig. 11-11).

In several ventral approaches described above, the distal frontal approach to an abdominal aortic aneurysm in 2-D Doppler showed its swirling flow from the distal ○ P.143 viewpoint (**Case 41, A**). Abdominal aortic aneurysms tend to deviate anteroposteriorly or laterally from the center line of the normal proximal aorta and this deviation causes the swirling flow phenomenon in the aneurysm. In the aneurysm, fast pulsatile flow in one direction from the proximal aorta exerts a shear stress on the wall in that direction, and

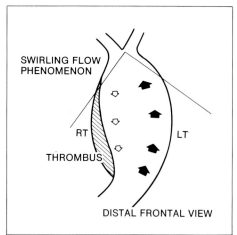

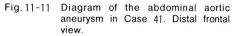

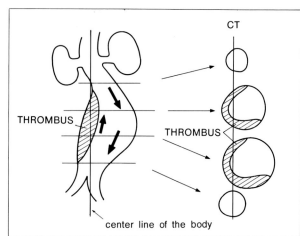

Fig. 11-11 Diagram of the abdominal aortic aneurysm in Case 41. Distal frontal view.

Fig. 11-12 Diagram of the serial CT images, which are arranged according to the actual relationship with the center line of the body in Case 41.

prevents mural thrombus formation in that portion of the aneurysm. However, there is a slow, continuous reverse flow in which a mural thrombus has formed. Consequently, the side of the aneurysm where the pulsatile flow is fast is more convex than the opposite side[24].

The serial CT images in Fig. 11-12, which are arranged according to the actual relationship with the center line of the body, show some deviation and expansion of the aneurysm to the side with the fast pulsatile flow. The factors at work in expansion of an aortic aneurysm include not only the weakness of the wall and the increased wall tension due to LaPlace's law, but also this shear stress caused by the high-velocity, high-energy flow. Spectral analysis of pulsatile flow indicates a very fast rate **(Case 41, C)**; and that of the flow on the thrombus formation side shows a low, continuous reversed flow **(Case 41, D)**.

Case 42　Celiac axis aneurysm, 71-year-old female (Fig. 11-13).

Aneurysm of the celiac axis is a very rare condition[25]. Although angiography in this case did not reveal the three-dimensional structure details owing to overlapping by the contrast medium, 2-D Doppler clearly displayed the detail of the structure together with the flow pattern. A long-axis view of the abdominal aorta in 2-D echogram displays the aneurysm of the celiac axis with a thrombus, 5 cm in diameter **(Case 42, A)**. Two-dimensional Doppler shows the flow entering the aneurysm and the superior mesenteric artery **(Case 42, B)**. In the magnified 2-D Doppler image, it is possible to differentiate between the brighter red flow in the celiac axis and the paler yellow flow that is entering the aneurysm **(Case 42, C)**. This finding indicates that this aneurysm arises from the lower side of the wall of the superior end of the celiac axis.

◎ P.144

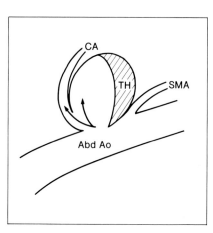

Fig. 11-13 Diagram of the celiac axis aneurysm in Case 42. Long-axis view of the abdominal aorta.
CA=celiac axis, SMA=superior mesenteric artery, TH= thrombus, abd Ao=abdominal aorta.

11-3 Diseases of the Peripheral Vessels

Disease of the peripheral vessels includes disease of the lower limb arteries, the carotid artery and the lower limb veins. Conventional noninvasive examination of these disorders by B-mode ultrasound, Doppler and RI has some limitations and the final diagnosis has depended on an invasive technique. Real-time two-dimensional Doppler echocardiography may eliminate the need for invasive catheterization in cases of cardiac disease. However, the initially developed 2-D Doppler system employs a phased-array sector scanning method which was very effective for visualizing the blood flow in the cardiac chamber and the aorta, but not in the peripheral vessels, which were comparatively small, superficial and had low-velocity flow, because its resolution of smaller structures was insufficient. In 1985, linear array 2-D Doppler was developed and was reported to be effective for visualizing the flow in the peripheral vessels[8),8a)]. The linear array 2-D Doppler is superior to the phased-array 2-D Doppler both in its resolution of smaller structures and for the visualization of the slow flows with a high-frequency transducer. The 2-D Doppler images in this section were displayed and recorded by the prototype instrument of this type, the Aloka XA-340, but this model was rather noisy. The transducer was of a convex type with frequency of 5 MHz and could provide good visualization of the flow by oblique orientation of the Doppler beam to the superficial vessels (Fig. 11-15). The pulse repetition frequency was 2 or 4 KHz and the theoretical minimal detectable velocity vector to the transducer that was capable of being displayed in color was 2 or 4 cm/sec, respectively. The various frequencies and pulse repetition frequencies of later models are applicable for visualization of the flows in the various vessels of the body, the velocities of which varied very widely.

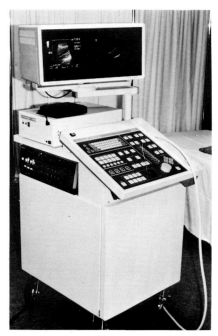

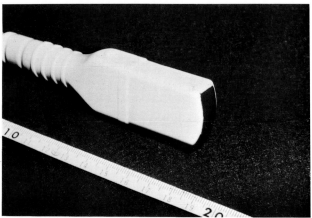

Fig. 11-15 The convex type transducer for the linear arrayed 2-D Doppler. Frequency of 5 MHz.

Fig. 11-14 The linear array 2-D Doppler system, Aloka SSD-350.

1. Disease of the lower limb arteries

Case 43 Normal lower limb artery

The femoral artery is approached from the anterior, and the popliteal artery is approached from the posterior. The long-axis view of the femoral artery in 2-D Doppler displays its bifurcation. The upper branch is the superficial femoral artery and the lower one, the deep femoral artery (**Case 43, A**). The superficial femoral artery can be scanned continuously as far as the root of the popliteal artery (**Case 43, B**), and the posterior tibial artery (**Case 43, C**), which is 2 mm in diameter, can be seen. The current linear array 2-D Doppler apparatus can display the flow in vessels of a minimum diameter of 1.5 mm.

⟳ P.144

Case 44 Leriche syndrome, 76-year-old female (Fig. 11-16).

○ P.144

Leriche syndrome is an occlusive disease of the aortic bifurcation. The long-axis 2-D Doppler view of the aortic bifurcation reveals complete occlusion of the iliac artery and the collateral flow through the lumbar artery (**Case 44, A**). Since the lumbar artery is usually slim and has a small blood flow, it is very difficult to visualize the flow in color with 2-D Doppler. In the Leriche syndrome the lumbar artery is large, has a high velocity flow, and is easily displayed in color by 2-D Doppler, as long as echo penetration is good.

Case 45 Arteriosclerosis of the femoral artery, 70-year-old male (Fig. 11-17).

○ P.145

The superficial femoral artery, the upper vessel displayed, has a stenosis formed of atheromatous plaque, half-way down the thigh (**Case 45, A**). The velocity of the flow through the stenosis is high and is displayed in red proximal to the stenosis, and with a mosaic pattern distal to the stenosis due to the high velocity. The direction of the flow is from left to right. The superficial femoral vein is the lower vessel; and the blue color of its flow is enhanced by calf pumping. The direction of the flow in the vein is from right to left. Thus, differentiation between the artery and the vein is easy.

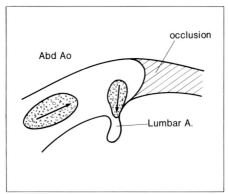

Fig. 11-16 Diagram of Leriche syndrome in Case 44. Long-axis view of the aorta.

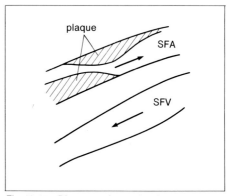

Fig. 11-17 Diagram of arteriosclerosis of the superficial femoral artery (SFA) in Case 45.

Case 46 Arteriosclerosis obliterans, occlusion of the common femoral artery, 72-year-old male (Fig. 11-18).

○ P.145

This case exhibited occlusion of the femoral artery, but without any ischemic symptoms in the leg. With 2-D Doppler, a collateral channel is visible extending from the pelvic artery to the deep femoral artery (**Case 46, A**). From the point of inflow of the collateral channel, which is displayed in the brighter color, the flow bifurcates into proximal and distal directions. The flow running proximally meets the occlusion and turns at the bifurcation of the femoral artery to enter the superficial femoral artery. The deep femoral artery becomes an important collateral channel arising from the pelvic artery when the common femoral artery and the iliac artery are occluded.

Case 47 Pseudoaneurysm of the internal shunt, 55-year-old female (Fig. 11-19).

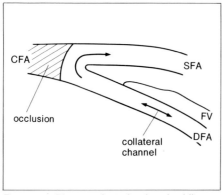

Fig. 11-18 Diagram of arteriosclerosis obliterans in Case 46. Long-axis view of the bifurcation of the femoral artery.

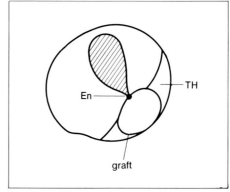

Fig. 11-19 Diagram of the pseudoaneurysm of the internal shunt in Case 47. Short-axis view of the graft.

○ P.145

In this case, there was an internal shunt for hemodialysis made of a Gore-Tex graft in the inguinal region but a pseudoaneurysm had formed in this shunt owing to puncture. The short-axis 2-D echogram of the graft shows a small entry to the pseudoaneurysm, as well as a thrombus in the pseudoaneurysm **(Case 47, A)**. Two-dimensional Doppler displays a jet flow from the entry with a mosaic pattern **(Case 47, B)**. The entry was closed by direct suturing.

2. Disease of the carotid artery

Although invasive angiography plays an important preoperative role in precise diagnosis, it may induce complications in the brain and cannot be used for screening. Hopes have rested, over the years, on a number of noninvasive methods, especially on two-dimensional flow visualization, in the search for a means of eliminating this inconvenience. However, none were able to offer the level of accuracy of angiography[26]. The authors expect that real-time color flow mapping by 2-D Doppler may well improve the accuracy of diagnosis without involving any difficulty in operation[27].

Case 48   Normal carotid artery

○ P.146

The carotid artery is visualized in color by 2-D Doppler from its root to a point about 3 cm distal to the bifurcation. Two-dimensional Doppler displays the proximal common carotid artery in red **(Case 48, F)**, and the middle common carotid artery changing from red to black to blue as it proceeds distally **(Case 48, E)** (cf. Chapter 6-6). The distal common carotid artery and the internal and external carotid arteries are displayed in blue **(Case 48, D)**. At the carotid sinus, a yellowish reverse flow known as a boundary layer flow separation[28] is seen.

The internal and external carotid arteries may be differentiated as follows:

1) The internal carotid artery is in the postero-lateral region of the neck, the external carotid, at the antero-median side.

2) Diastolic flow is visualized in color more clearly and longer in the internal carotid artery than in the external.

3) At its root, the external carotid artery has branches, while the internal carotid artery has none.

Case 49   Normal carotid artery and vertebral artery

Branches of the external carotid artery **(Case 49, A)**(Fig. 11-20).

The external carotid artery is shown to have branches. The first is the superior thyroidal artery and the second, the lingual artery.

○ P.146

The vertebral artery **(Case 49, B)** (Fig. 11-21).

Two-dimensional Doppler displays the vertebral artery behind the carotid artery, which runs through the transverse processes of the vertebrae. The pulsatile flow to the brain is displayed. This vertebral artery can be followed to its origin at the subclavian artery.

Case 50   Carotid artery stenosis, 75-year-old male (Fig. 11-22).

If the common carotid artery is approached from the postero-lateral aspect of the neck,

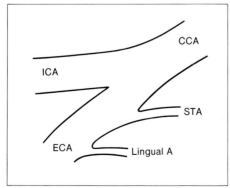

Fig. 11-20   Diagram of the normal external carotid artery (ECA) and its branches in Case 49. ICA=internal carotid artery; CCA=common carotid artery.

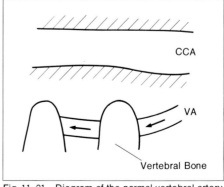

Fig. 11-21   Diagram of the normal vertebral artery (VA) in Case 49.

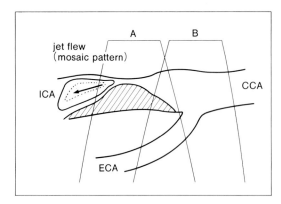

Tab. 11-2 Stenosis and color flow pattern in the internal carotid artery

Stenosis		Color Flow Pattern	
		systole	diastole
Normal	0%	aliasing (±)	blue (±)
Mild	1～49%	aliasing (±)	blue (±)
Moderate	50～79%	mosaic	blue
Severe	80～99%	mosaic	aliasing or mosaic
Occlusion	100%	none	none

Fig. 11-22 Diagram of the stenosis of the internal carotid artery in Case 50.

○ P.146

the internal carotid artery is displayed anteriorly and the external carotid artery is displayed posteriorly. Two-dimensional Doppler displays atheromatous plaque forming a 90% stenosis in the internal carotid artery just distal to the bifurcation. Post-stenotic flow shows a mosaic pattern in both systole and diastole (**Case 50, A**). Continuous-wave Doppler shows a maximum velocity 3.5 m/sec in systole and a velocity of 2 m/sec at the end of diastole (**Case 50, C**). Since the maximum velocity measured by continuous-wave Doppler corresponds well with the severity of stenosis, the severity of a stenosis may be assessed by a combined consideration of the flow patterns in systole and in diastole, as Tab. 11-2 indicates[29]. At a frequency of 5 MHz and a pulse repetition frequency of 4 KHz, stenosis of over 50% (but not occlusion) of the lumen of the internal carotid artery, the color flow pattern in systole is mosaic; and when the vessel is over 80% stenosed, the pattern in diastole shows either aliasing or a mosaic appearance.

3. Disease of the lower limb veins

The various conventional noninvasive diagnostic methods for venous disorders of the lower extremity, such as Doppler[30], ultrasound[31] and plethysmography[32], all have limitations. The authors[33], in 1986, were the first to report that real-time 2-D Doppler was very useful for the noninvasive diagnosis of venous diseases of the lower extremity, giving both functional and structural data simultaneously. The application of 2-D Doppler to the lower limb veins is expected to contribute to the understanding of the pathophysiology of venous disorders of the lower limb.

Two-dimensional Doppler examination is performed by the anterior approach to the iliac, femoral and greater saphenous veins (Fig. 11-23). A supine posture is recommended for the

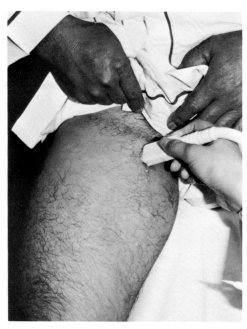

Fig. 11-23 2-D Doppler examination for the venous disease of the lower extremity. The inguinal region is approached in a patient who is in a sitting position.

examination of acute deep vein thromboses, and a sitting or standing position for chronic deep vein thromboses and varicoses. Although the low flow velocity in the lower limb veins is a disadvantage for color flow visualization, flow enhancement by deep respiration, especially expiration and manual calf pumping (alternating compression and release of the calf muscle with the hands) facilitate the clear display of even minor abnormalities of flow in 2-D Doppler.

◯ P.147 **Case 51 Normal lower limb vein, 70-year-old male.**

In the normal lower limb veins, blood is allowed to flow only proximally, on account of the function of the venous valves. If these are normal, no reflux flow at all occurs. Blood flow in the lower limb veins is in stasis during inspiration, because of the elevated pressure in the abdominal cavity, and it flows proximally during expiration for the converse reason. The 2-D Doppler images of Case 51 display the lower limb veins while manual calf pumping was carried out in order to facilitate continuous visualization from the iliac to the popliteal vein **(Case 51, E, F, G, H)**.

Case 52 Varicose vein, 38-year-old-male (Fig. 11-24).

The majority of varicose veins are due to valve incompetency at the saphenofemoral junction. During inspiration and at the release of calf compression, reflux flow from the venous valve at the saphenofemoral junction occurs in varicose veins. During calf compression the flow from the greater saphenous vein to the femoral vein appears in blue in **◯ P.147** 2-D Doppler **(Case 52, A)**, and at the release of the compression, the reflux flow from the femoral vein into the greater saphenous vein is displayed in red **(Case 52, B)**.

Severity index : Index of valve incompetency at the saphenofemoral junction (Tab. 11-3)[33].

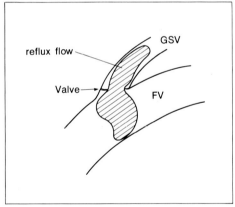

Fig. 11-24 Diagram of valve incompetency at the saphenofemoral junction in the varicose vein of Case 52.

GSV=greater saphenous vein ; FV=femoral vein ; ILV=iliac vein

Tab. 11-3 Severity index of valve incompetency at the saphenofemoral junction.
Reflux flow by calf pumping

	Width/GSV Diameter	Brightness	Pre-Valvular Area
Grade I	<1/2	low	(−)
Grade II	>1/2	high	small
Grade III	≒1	high(mosaic)	large

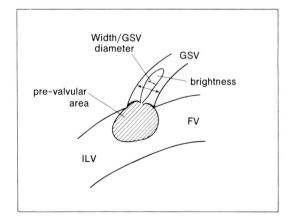

Valve incompetency at the saphenofemoral junction is graded by the severity index from **◯ P.147** I to III in 2-D Doppler **(Figs. X, Y, Z, under Case 52)**. Two-dimensional Doppler images of the saphenofemoral junction at the point of reflux just after the release of the calf compression in the sitting position were used for analysis. The two-dimensional Doppler was performed at a frequency of 5 MHz with a pulse repetition frequency of 4 KHz. Three good criteria for severity grading of valve incompetency at the saphenofemoral junction are the following: the ratio between width of the reflux flow from the valve and the diameter of the greater saphenous vein; the brightness of the regurgitant flow; and the area of the prevalvular regurgitant flow in the femoral vein.

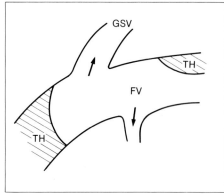
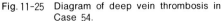

Fig. 11-25 Diagram of deep vein thrombosis in Case 54.

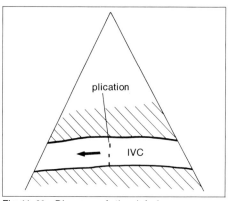

Fig. 11-26 Diagram of the inferior vena cava plicated after pulmonary embolism in Case 55.

⊙ P.148

Case 53 Deep vein thrombosis, 76-year-old male.

In deep vein thrombosis, the occluded vein is shown with a thrombus echo inside, and without any flow even on calf pumping. In the authors' experience, 2-D Doppler diagnoses concerning site of occlusion in the vein are compatible with those of RI venography[33]. Although contrast venography has been considered to be a golden standard for the diagnosis of deep vein thromboses, the injection of contrast medium may aggravate the symptoms. A reliable and accurate noninvasive diagnostic method is needed. Two-dimensional Doppler is a powerful technique for noninvasively visualizing a thrombus or a slight flow of blood.

During follow-up, the vein occluded by the thrombus may have partially recanalized. Two-dimensional Doppler images of Case 53 display the thrombus and the flow promoted by calf pumping through the narrow channel between the thrombus and the venous wall **(Case 53, B)**. From the greater saphenous vein, a blue-colored flow enters the femoral vein, and recanalization is also displayed **(Case 53, A)**.

⊙ P.148

Case 54 Deep vein thrombosis, 57-year-old female (Fig. 11-25).

The edema of the leg in this case disappeared completely after thrombolytic treatment. The two-dimensional Doppler images show occlusion of the common femoral vein and of the external iliac vein **(Case 54, A)**. This occlusion results in collateral flow from the femoral vein through the branches of the femoral vein, such as the saphenous vein, to the pelvic vein **(Case 54, A, B)**. Two-dimensional Doppler is useful for follow-up study in deep vein thrombosis.

⊙ P.148

Case 55 Pulmonary embolism, after plication of the inferior vena cava, 44-year-old male (Fig. 11-26).

Deep vein thrombosis may cause severe pulmonary embolism. In this case, in which there have been multiple episodes of embolism, the inferior vena cava is interrupted beneath the renal vein by plication procedure. Distal to the plication, the flow is not visualized in color owing to stasis, but proximal to it, a flow of higher velocity is displayed in blue **(Case 55, A)**.

References

1) Satomura, S., Matsubara, S., and Yoshioka, M.: A new method of mechanical vibration measurement and its application. Memoirs of the Institute of Scientific and Industrial Research, Osaka University, 13: 125, 1956.

2) Hokanson, D.E., Mozersky, D., Sumner, D.S., and Strandness, D.E., Jr.: Ultrasonic arteriography: a new approach to arterial visualization. Biomed. Engng., 6: 420, 1971.

3) Reid, J.M., and Spencer, M.P.: Ultrasonic Doppler technique for imaging blood vessels. Science, 176: 1235, 1972.

4) Curry, G.R., and White, D.N.: Color-coded ultrasonic differential velocity arterial scanner (Echoflow). Ultrasound Med. Biol., 4: 27, 1978.

5) Brandestini, M.A., Howard, E.A., Weile, E.B., Stevenson, J.G., and Eyer, M.K.: The synthesis of echo and Doppler in M-mode and sector scan. Proceedings of the 24th Annual Meeting of AIUM, 125, 1979.

6) Namekawa, K., Kasai, C., Tsukamoto, M., and Koyano, A. : Imaging of blood flow using autocorrelation, Ultrasound Med. Biol., 8 : 138, 1982.

7) Takamoto, S. : Aortic disease. *In* Color Atlas of Real-Time Two-Dimensional Doppler Echocardiography. 1st Ed. Edited by R. Omoto. Tokyo, Shindan-to-Chiryo Co., 1984.

8) Takamoto, S., Umaki, K., Otani, S., Irie, T., Kasai, C., Koyano, A., Matsumura, M., Kyo, S. and Omoto, R. : Real-time color flow mapping of the carotid, femoral and tibial arteries by new 2-D Doppler with a convex transducer. Proceedings of the 30th Annual Meeting of AIUM, 62, 1985.

8a) Takamoto, S., Umaki, K., Otani, T., Irie, C., Kasai, A., Koyano, S., Kyo, S. and Omoto, R. : Real-Time color flow mapping of the peripheral arteries by new 2-D Doppler echography system. Proceedings of the 46th Meeting of the Japan Society of Ultrasonics in Medicine, 913, 1985.

9) Moncada, R., Salinas, M., Churchill, R., Love, L., Reynes, C., Demos, T.C., Gunnar, R.M., and Pifarre, R. : Diagnosis of dissecting aortic aneurysm by computed tomography. Lancet, 1 : 238, 1981.

10) Amparo, E.G., Higgins, C.B., Hricak, H., and Sollitto, R. : Aortic dissection : Magnetic resonance imaging. Radiology, 155 : 399, 1985.

11) Millward, D.K., Robinson, N.J., and Craige, E. : Dissecting aortic aneurysm diagnosed by echocardiography in a patient with rupture of the aneurysm into the right atrium. Am. J. Cardiol., 30 : 427, 1972.

12) Nanda, N.C., Gramiak, R., and Shah, P.M. : Diagnosis of aortic root dissection by echocardiography, Circulation, 48 : 506, 1973.

13) Matsumoto, M., Matsuo, H., Ohara, T., Yoshioka, Y., and Abe, H. : A two-dimensional echoaortocardiographic approach to dissecting aneurysms of the aorta to prevent false-positive diagnoses. Radiology, 127 : 491, 1978.

14) Mintz, G.S., Kotler, M.N., Segal, B.L., and Parry, W.R. : Two-dimensional echocardiographic recognition of the descending thoracic aorta. Am. J. Cardiol., 44 : 232, 1979.

15) DeMaria, A.N., Bommer, W., Neumann, A., Weinert, L., Bogren, H., and Mason, D.T. : Identification and localization of aneurysms of the ascending aorta by cross-sectional echocardiography. Circulation, 59 : 755, 1979.

16) Victor, M.F., Mintz, G.S., Kotler, M.N., Wilson, A.R., and Segal, B.L. : Two-dimensional echocardiographic diagnosis of aortic dissection. Am. J. Cardiol., 48 : 1155, 1981.

17) Mathew, T. and Nanda, N.C. : Two-dimensional and Doppler echocardiographic evaluation of aortic aneurysm and dissection. Am. J. Cardiol., 54 : 379, 1984.

18) Okamoto, M., Kinoshita, N., Miyatake, K., Beppu, S., Sakakibara, H. and Nimura, T. : Detection and analysis of blood flow in aortic dissection with two-dimensional echo Doppler technique. Ultrasound Med. Biol., Suppl 2 : 331, 1983.

19) Takamoto, S., Kondo, Y., Yoshikawa, Y., Kasai, C., Koyano, A., Kyo, S., Yokote, Y. and Omoto, R. : The first clinical experiences of intraoperative real-time two-dimensional Doppler echocardiography in the dissecting aneurysm of the aorta. Proceedings of the 29th Annual Meeting of AIUM. 167, 1984.

20) Börner, N., Erbel, R., Braun, B., Henkel, B., Meyer, J. and Rumpelt, J. : Diagnosis of aortic dissection by transesophageal echocardiography. Am. J. Cardiol., 54 : 1157, 1984.

21) Takamoto, S., Kyo, S., Matsumura, M., Hojo, H., Yokote, Y. and Omoto, R. : Total visualization of thoracic dissecting aortic aneurysm by trans-esophageal Doppler color flow mapping. Circulation 74 : Suppl.-II : 132, 1986.

22) Bubenheimer, P., Schmuziger, M. and Roskamp, H. : Ein-und zweidimensionale Echographie bei Aneurysmen und Dissektionen der Aorta. Herz, 5 : 226, 1980.

23) Takamoto, S., Kyo, S., Adachi, H., Matsumura, M., Yokote, Y. and Omoto, R. : Intraoperative color flow mapping by real-time two-dimensional Doppler echocardiography for evaluation of valvular and congenital heart disease and vascular disease. J. Thorac. Cardiovasc. Surg., 90 : 802, 1985.

24) Tamura, H., Takamoto, S., Asano, H., Adachi, H., Kyo, S., Yokote, Y. and Omoto, R. : Swirling flow phenomenon in the abdominal aortic aneurysm analyzed by 2-D Doppler. Proceedings of the 45th Meeting of the Japan Society of Ultrasonics in Medicine, 429, 1984.

25) Haimovici, H., Sprayregen, S., Eckstein, P., and Veith, F.J. : Celiac artery aneurysmectomy : Case report with review of the literature. Surgery, 79 : 592, 1976.

26) Sumner, D.S., Russell, J.B., Ramsey, D.E., Hajjar, W.M., and Miles, R.D. : Noninvasive diagnosis of extracranial carotid arterial disease. Arch. Surg., 114 : 1222, 1979.

27) Takamoto, S., and Omoto, R. : Clinical application of real-time Doppler color flow mapping to the carotid artery. *In* Ultrasonic diagnosis of cerebrovascular disease. Edited by M.P. Spencer. The Netherlands, Martinus Nijhoff Publishers, (in press).

28) LoGerfor, F.W., Nowak, M.D., Quist, W.C. : Structural details of boundary layer separation in a model human carotid bifurcation under steady and pulsatile flow conditions. J. Vasc. Surg., 2 : 263, 1985.

29) Takamoto, S., Hojo, H., Matsumura, M., Matsuda, T., Kyo, S., Yokote, Y., and Omoto, R. : Color flow mapping of the carotid artery by real-time two-dimensional Doppler echography, relationship between color flow patterns and the stenosis. Proceedings of the 5th Conference of the Japan Academy of Neurosonology (Tokyo), 54, 1986.

30) Barnes, R.W., Russell, H.E., and Wilson, M.R. : Doppler Ultrasonic Evaluation of Venous Disease : A Programmed Audiovisual Instruction. 2nd Ed. Iowa City, University of Iowa, 1975,

31) Talbot, S.R. : Use of real-time imaging in identifying deep venous obstruction : A preliminary report. Bruit 6 : 41-42, 1982.

32) Sumner, D.S. : Plethysmography in arterial and venous diagnosis. An introduction to vascular ultrasonography. Edited by W.J. Zwiebel, Orlando, Grune & Stratton, Inc., 1986.

33) Takamoto, S., Hojo, H., Kyo, S., Yokote, Y. and Omoto, R. : New non-invasive diagnostic technique for the venous disease of the lower extremity by real-time two-dimensional Doppler echography. Proceedings of 9th World Congress of Phlebology (Kyoto, 1986) (in press).

Case 26 Ventricular Septal Perforation secondary to Myocardial Infarction 62-year-old male

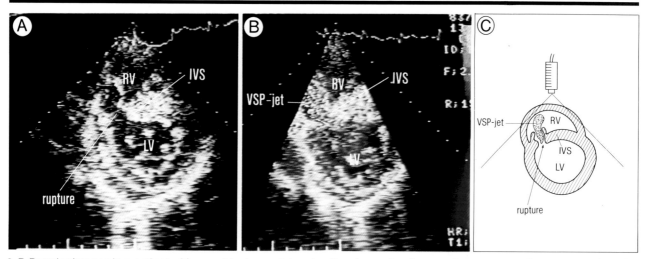

2-D Doppler images in a patient with a ventricular septal perforation (or rupture) secondary to myocardial Infarction (VSP).
Ⓐ B-mode in short-axis view at the level of the papillary muscles in diastole .The ruptured interventricular septum is directly visualized. (Courtesy of DR. J. Yoshikawa, Kobe General Hospital, Kobe, Japan). Ⓑ 2-D Doppler same view, systole. Turbulent, high velocity flow from left to right through the ruptured septum is imaged in mosaic patterns (VSP-jet). (Courtesy of DR. J. Yoshikawa, Kobe General Hospital, Kobe, Japan).

Case 27 Papillary Muscle Dysfunction secondary to Myocardial Infarction 78-year-old female

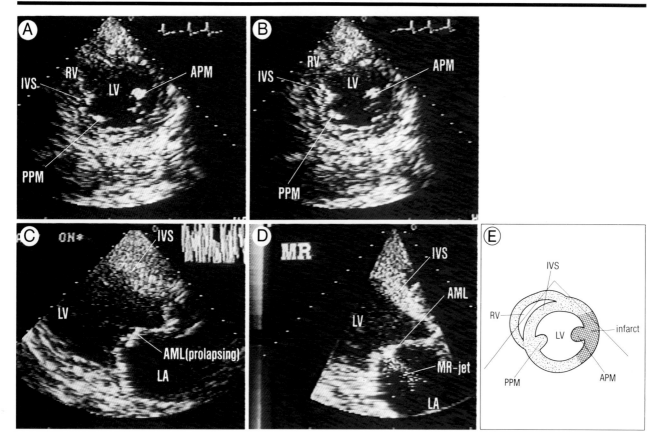

2-D Doppler images in a patient with papillary muscle dysfunction secondary to myocardial infarction.
Ⓐ B-mode in short-axis view at the level of the papillay muscles in diastole. Ⓑ B-mode same view, systole. Scarring of the anterior papillary muscle and the surrounding anterior wall of the left ventricle is observed. Ⓒ B-mode in long-axis view in systole. Protrusion of the anterior mitral leaflet, compatible with mitral valve prolapse, is shown. Ⓓ 2-D Doppler same view, systole. Mild mitral regurgitation due to papillary muscle dysfunction is demonstrated.

Case 28　Anteroseptal Myocardial Infarction with Apical Aneurysm　63-year-old male

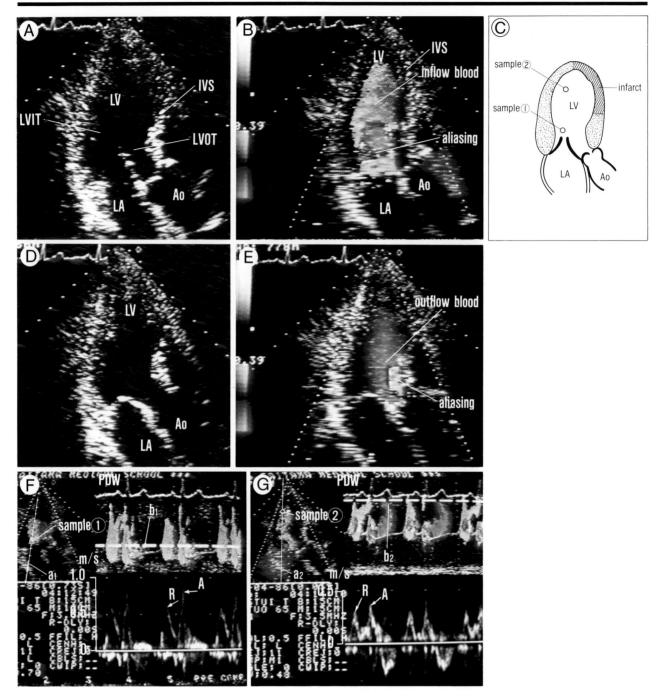

2-D Doppler images in a patient with a small apical aneurysm secondary to anteroseptal myocardial infarction（LV Aneurysm）.
A B-mode in apical long-axis view in diastole.**B** 2-D Doppler same view, diastole. **C** Diagram illustrating long-axis slice and sample sites of pulsed-wave Doppler recordings. **D** B-mode in apical long-axis view in systole. **E** 2-D Doppler same view, systole. **F** Simultaneous display of flow-mapping M-mode and pulsed-wave Doppler（beam line : a₁, sample volume : sample ①(b₁)）. **G** Ditto（beam line : a₂, sample volume : sample ②(b₂)）.

[Analysis of left ventricular flood flow dynamics]　(Inflow tract) R wave=0.55 m/s, A wave=0.86 m/s, A/R=1.56 (in diastole).
　　　　　　　　　　　　　　　　　　　(Apex) R wave=0.28 m/s, A wave=0.41 m/s, A/R=1.46 (in diastole).
　　　　　　　　　　　　　　　　　　　(Outflow tract) max V=0.85 m/s (in systole).

In mitral diastolic flow velocity pattern, the A wave is abnormally elevated and greater in amplitude than R wave, with an A to R ratio greater than 1.0. At the apex, R and A wave velocities are both decreased. In contrast, left ventricular systolic outflow is maintained at normal peak velocities.

Case 29 Anteroseptal Myocardial Infarction with Apical Aneurysm 56-year-old female

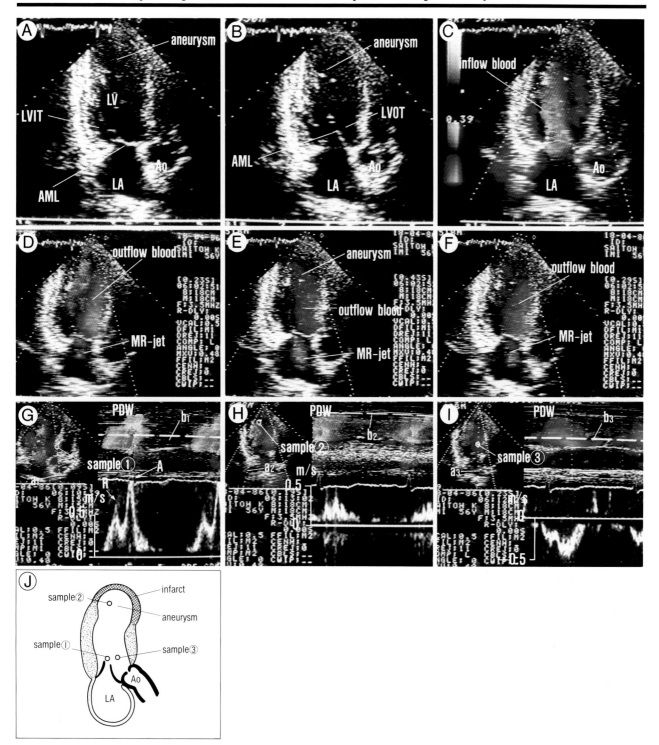

2-D Doppler images in a patient with a large apical aneurysm secondary to anteroseptal myocardial infarction (LV Aneurysm).
A B-mode in apical long-axis view in systole. **B** B-mode same view, diastole. **C** 2-D Doppler same view, diastole. **D** 2-D Doppler same view, early systole. Mild mitral regurgitation (MR-jet) is shown. **E** 2-D Doppler same view, mid-systole. **F** 2-D Doppler same view, late systole. **G** Simultaneous display of flow-mapping M-mode and pulsed-wave Doppler (beam line : a₁, sample volume : sample ①(b₁)). **H** Ditto (beam line : a₂, sample volume : sample ②(b₂)). **I** Ditto (beam line : a₃, sample volume : sample ③(b₃)). **J** Diagram illustrating long-axis slice, beam lines, and sample sites.

[Analysis of left ventricular blood flow dynamics] (Inflow tract) R wave=0.51 m/s, A wave=0.92 m/s, A/R=1.80 (in diastole).
(Apex) max V=0.42 m/s (in systole within the apical aneurysm).
(Outflow tract) max V=0.42 m/s (in systole)
At the apex, in the aneurysm, systolic flow is red and outward, toward the transducer. This pattern (paradoxical reverse flow) is completely opposite to normal systolic flow in the left ventricle.

Case 30   Left Atrial Myxoma   50-year-old male

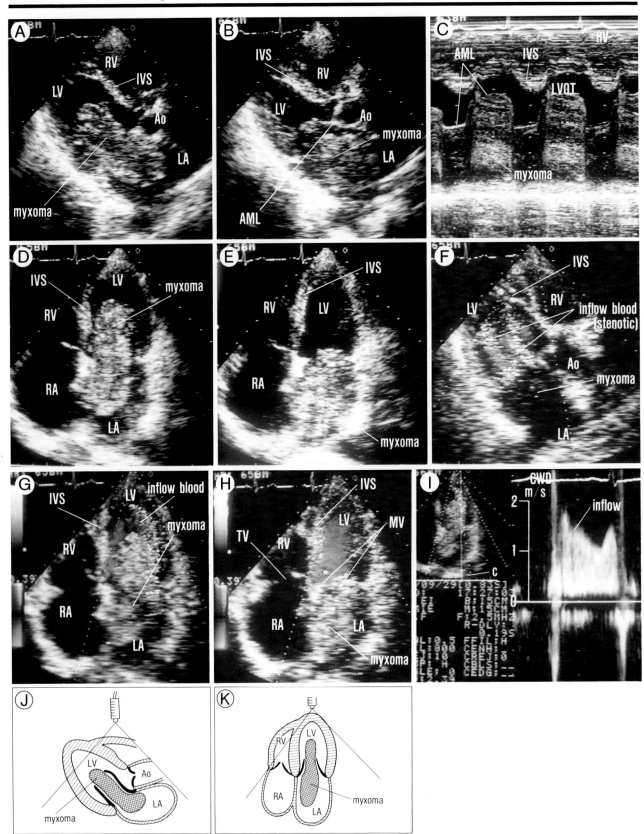

2-D Doppler images in a patient with a left atrial myxoma (LA Myxoma).
Ⓐ B-mode in long-axis view in diastole. **Ⓑ** B-mode same view, systole. **Ⓒ** M-mode echocardiogram. The left atrial myxoma appears posterior to the anterior mitral leaflet in diastole. **Ⓓ** B-mode in apical four-chamber view in diastole. **Ⓔ** B-mode same view, systole. **Ⓕ** 2-D Doppler in long-axis view in diastole. Mitral inflow flood appears to be forming two streams. **Ⓖ** 2-D Doppler in apical four-chamber view in diastole. Mitral inflow blood appears mainly posterior to the myxoma. **Ⓗ** 2-D Doppler same view, systole. **Ⓘ** Continuous-wave Doppler of mitral valve flow (beam line : c). The velocity curves are similar to those obtained in mild mitral stenosis.
[Evaluation of mitral valve flow]
  max V=1.6 m/s, mean V=1.1 m/s, mean ΔP=5 mmHg, P 1/2 T=0.23/sec, MVA=0.9 cm².

Case 31 Left Ventricular Myxoma 35-year-old male

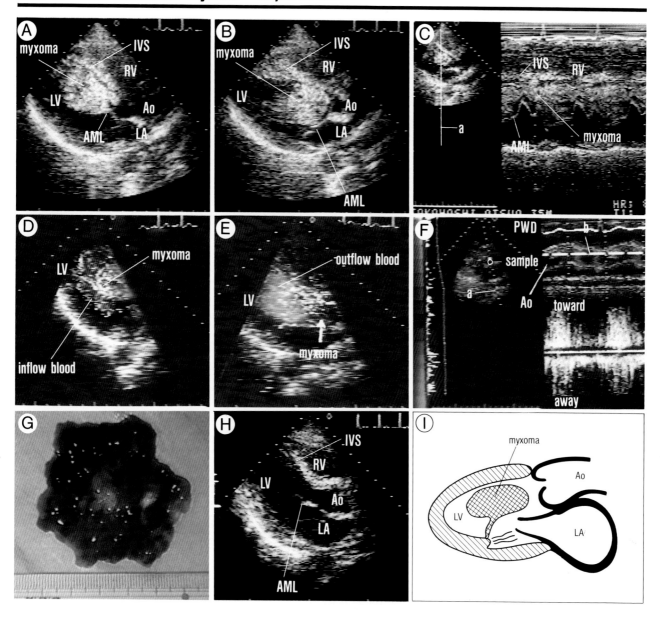

2-D Doppler images in a patient with a left ventricular myxoma (LV Myxoma).
Ⓐ B-mode in long-axis view in diastole. Ⓑ B-mode same view, systole. Ⓒ M-mode echocardiogram. The left ventricular myxoma appears anterior to the anterior mitral leaflet in both diastole and systole. Ⓓ 2-D Doppler in long-axis view in diastole. Inflow blood is imaged posterior to the myxoma. Ⓔ 2-D Doppler same view, systole. Ⓕ Simultaneous display of flow-mapping M-mode and pulsed-wave Doppler (beam line : a, sample volume : sample(b)). Blood flow through the aortic valve is turbulent owing to left ventricular outflow obstruction. Ⓖ Pathologic specimen. Ⓗ Explanatory illustration of a left ventricular myxoma. The myxoma was attached to the posterior papillary muscle.

138

Case 32 Dissecting Aortic Aneurysm (DeDakey type III b) 74-year-old male

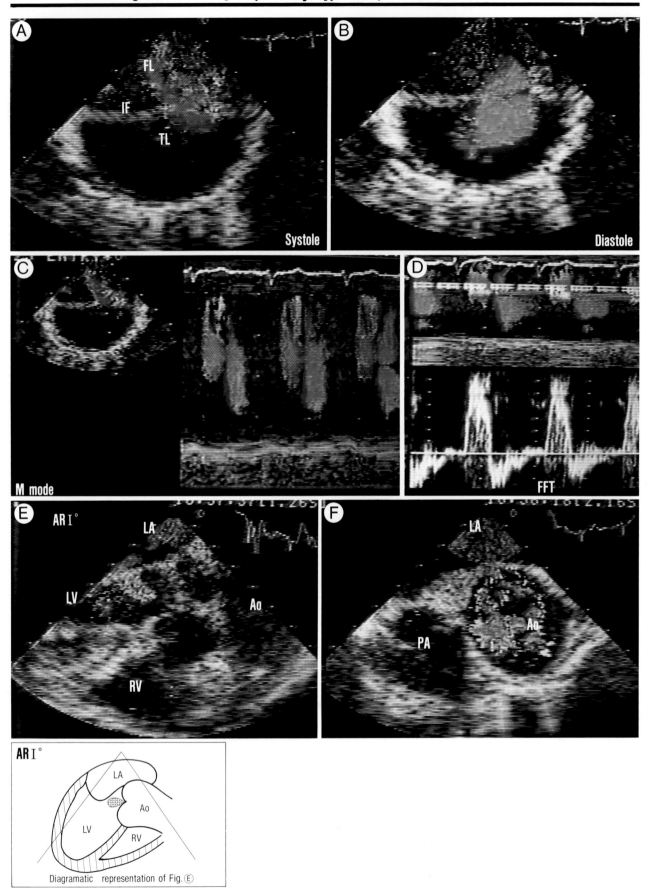

Transesophageal 2-D Doppler images of dissecting aortic aneurysm. Entry ⒶⒷⒸⒹ.
Entry exists at 24—27 cm from the teeth in the descending aorta.
Ⓐ 2-D Doppler, in systole. Ⓑ 2-D Doppler, in diastole. Ⓒ Flow mapping M-mode. Ⓓ Spectral analysis, Max V≒90 cm/sec.
TL=true lumen ; FL=false lumen ; IF=intimal flap.

Transesophageal 2-D Doppler

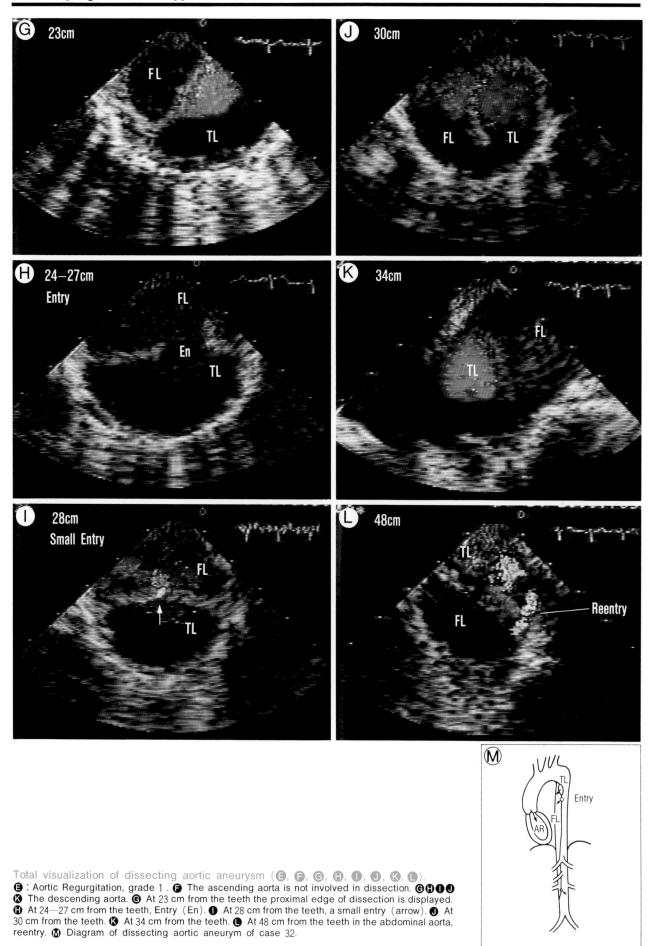

Total visualization of dissecting aortic aneurysm (**E**, **F**, **G**, **H**, **I**, **J**, **K**, **L**).
E : Aortic Regurgitation, grade 1 . **F** The ascending aorta is not involved in dissection. **G H I J**
K The descending aorta. **G** At 23 cm from the teeth the proximal edge of dissection is displayed.
H At 24—27 cm from the teeth, Entry (En). **I** At 28 cm from the teeth, a small entry (arrow). **J** At
30 cm from the teeth. **K** At 34 cm from the teeth. **L** At 48 cm from the teeth in the abdominal aorta,
reentry. **M** Diagram of dissecting aortic aneurym of case 32.

Case 33 Dissecting Aortic Aneurysm (arch type with retrograde dissection) 46-year-old male
Transesophageal 2-D Doppler

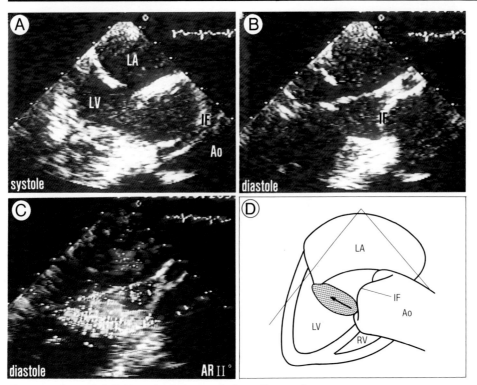

Transesophageal 2-D Doppler images of dissecting aortic aneurysm.
Ⓐ 2-D echo in systole. Ⓑ 2-D echo displays intimal flap (IF) prolapsed from the aortic ring in diastole. Ⓒ 2-D Doppler, grade 2 of aortic regurgitation. Ⓓ Diagram of Fig. Ⓒ.

Case 34 Dissecting Aortic Aneurysm (DeBakey type II) 60-year-old male

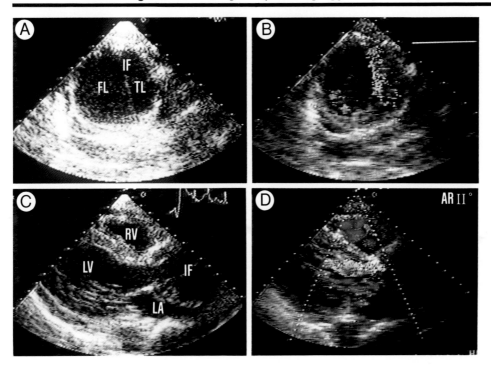

2-D Doppler images of dissecting aortic aneurysm with a precordial approach.
Ⓐ Short-axis 2-D echo obtained by a right parasternal approach shows intimal flap in the ascending aorta. Ⓑ 2-D Doppler, short-axis view of the ascending aorta. Ⓒ Long-axis view of the aortic root in 2-D echo. Ⓓ 2-D Doppler shows grade 2 of aortic regurgitation.

Case 35　Dissecting Aortic Aneurysm (DeBakey type I) 39-year-old male　**Intraoperative 2-D Doppler**

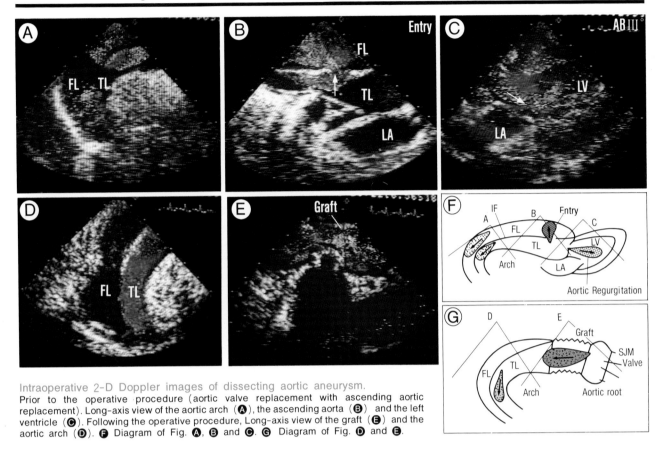

Intraoperative 2-D Doppler images of dissecting aortic aneurysm.
Prior to the operative procedure (aortic valve replacement with ascending aortic replacement). Long-axis view of the aortic arch (Ⓐ), the ascending aorta (Ⓑ) and the left ventricle (Ⓒ). Following the operative procedure, Long-axis view of the graft (Ⓔ) and the aortic arch (Ⓓ). Ⓕ Diagram of Fig. Ⓐ, Ⓑ and Ⓒ. Ⓖ Diagram of Fig. Ⓓ and Ⓔ.

Case 36　Dissecting Aortic Aneurysm (DeBakey type IIIb)　48-year-old male
Intraoperative 2-D Doppler

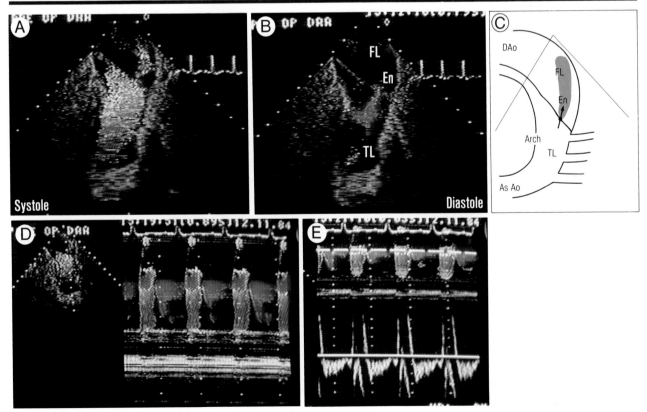

Intraoperative 2-D Doppler images of dissecting aortic aneurysm.
Entry just distal to the subclavian artery in the descending aorta.
Ⓐ Systole. Ⓑ Diastole. Ⓒ Diagram of the dissecting aortic aneurysm and the small entry. Ⓓ Flow mapping M-mode. Ⓔ Spectral analysis of the flow through the entry.

Case 37　Annuloaortic Ectasia, Marfan Syndrome　59-year-old male

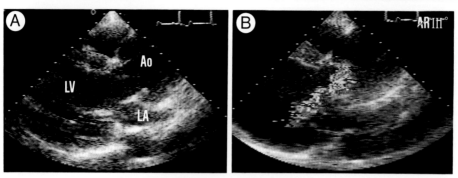

2-D Doppler images of annuloaortic ectasia by a precordial
approach.
Ⓐ Long-axis view of the aortic root,
2-D echo. Ⓑ 2-D Doppler, grade 3 of
aortic regurgitation.

Case 38　Dissecting Abdominal Aortic Aneurysm　77-year-old male

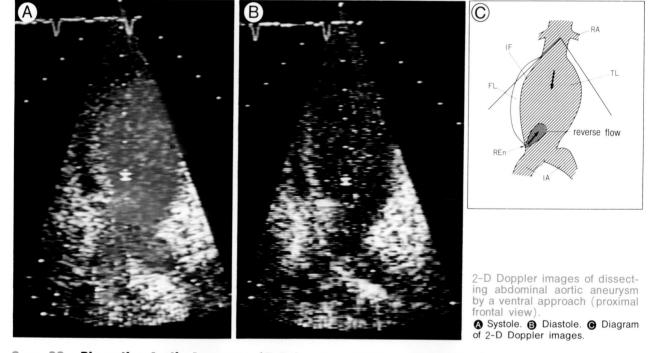

2-D Doppler images of dissecting abdominal aortic aneurysm
by a ventral approach (proximal
frontal view).
Ⓐ Systole. Ⓑ Diastole. Ⓒ Diagram
of 2-D Doppler images.

Case 39　Dissecting Aortic Aneurysm (DeBakey type Ⅲb)　48-year-old male

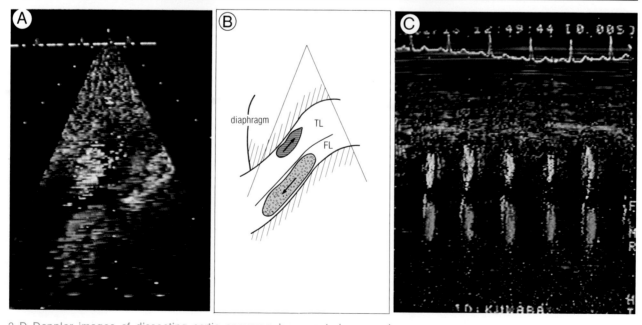

2-D Doppler images of dissecting aortic aneurysm by a ventral approach.
Ⓐ Long-axis view of the abdominal aorta. Ⓑ Diagram of Fig. Ⓐ. Ⓒ Flow mapping M-mode.

Case 40 Dissecting Aortic Aneurysm (DeBakey type IIIb) 65-year-old male
Intraoperative 2-D Doppler

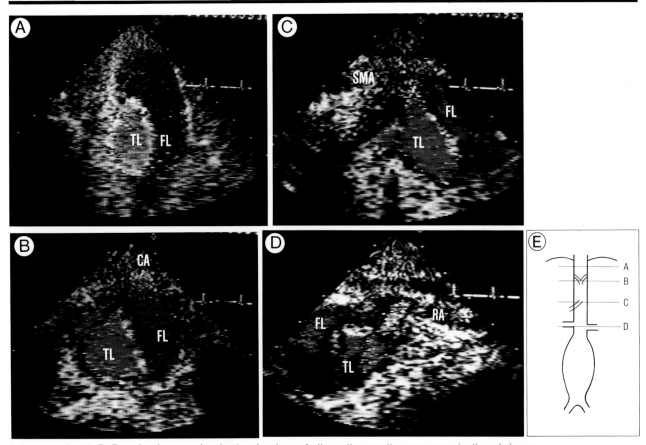

Intraoperative 2-D Doppler images in short-axis view of dissecting aortic aneurysm in the abdomen.
Ⓐ Level of the diaphragm. Ⓑ The celiac axis (CA) fed through the false lumen. Ⓒ The superior mesenteric artery (SMA). Ⓓ The left renal artery (RA), bridge formation (+). Ⓔ Diagram of the aorta of case 40.

Case 41 Abdominal Aortic Aneurysm 61-year-old male

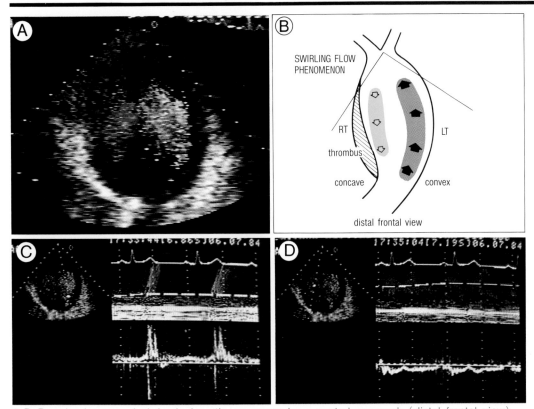

2-D Doppler images of abdominal aortic aneurysm by a ventral approach (distal frontal view).
Ⓐ Swirling flow phenomenon in the abdominal aortic aneurysm. Ⓑ Diagram of the abdominal aortic aneurysm. Ⓒ Spectral analysis of the flow at the convex side, distal-directed pulsatile flow. Ⓓ Spectral analysis of the flow at the concave side, reversed continous flow.

Case 42　Celiac Axis Aneurysm　71-year-old female

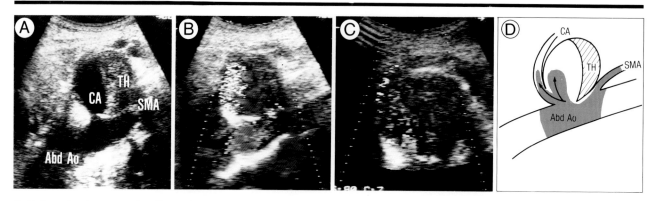

2-D Doppler images of celiac axis aneurysm.
Ⓐ 2-D echo, long-axis view of the abdominal aorta. Ⓑ 2-D Doppler. Ⓒ A magnified 2-D Doppler image shows aneurysm arising from the partial wall of the celiac axis (CA). SMA=superior mesenteric artery ; TH=thrombus ; Abd Ao=abdominal aorta.

Case 43　Normal Lower Limb Artery

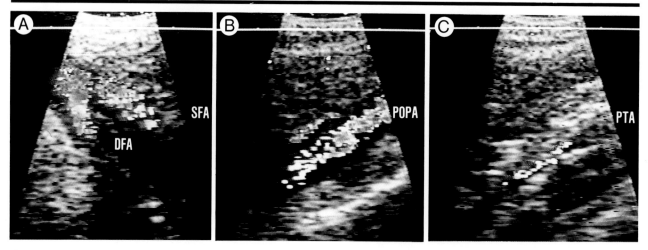

2-D Doppler images of normal lower limb artery in long-axis view.
Ⓐ Bifurcation of the femoral artery. SFA=superficial femoral artery ; DFA=deep femoral artery. Ⓑ The popliteal artery (POPA). Ⓒ The posterior tibial artery (PTA).

Case 44　Leriche Syndrome　76-year-old female

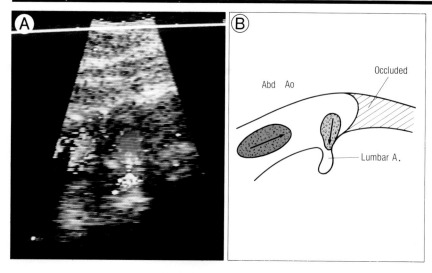

2-D Doppler image of Leriche syndrome.
Ⓐ Long-axis view of the aortic bifurcation. Collateral flow through the lumbar artery and the occluded iliac artery are displayed. Ⓑ Diagram of Fig. Ⓐ.

Case 45 Arteriosclerosis of the Femoral Artery 70-year-old male

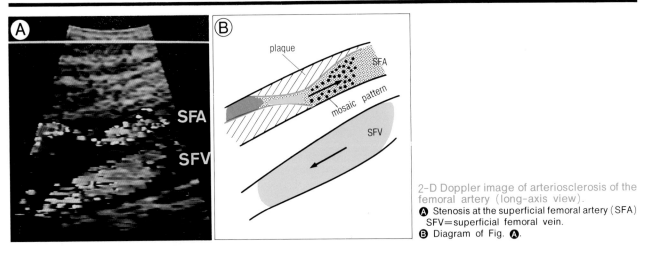

2-D Doppler image of arteriosclerosis of the femoral artery (long-axis view).
Ⓐ Stenosis at the superficial femoral artery (SFA) SFV=superficial femoral vein.
Ⓑ Diagram of Fig. Ⓐ.

Case 46 Arteriosclerosis Obliterans (ASO), Occlusion of the common femoral artery 72-year-old male

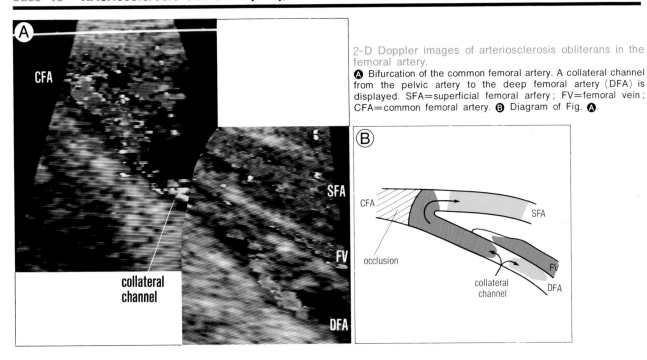

2-D Doppler images of arteriosclerosis obliterans in the femoral artery.
Ⓐ Bifurcation of the common femoral artery. A collateral channel from the pelvic artery to the deep femoral artery (DFA) is displayed. SFA=superficial femoral arfery ; FV=femoral vein ; CFA=common femoral artery. Ⓑ Diagram of Fig. Ⓐ.

Case 47 Pseudoaneurysm of tbe Internal Shunt 55-year-old female

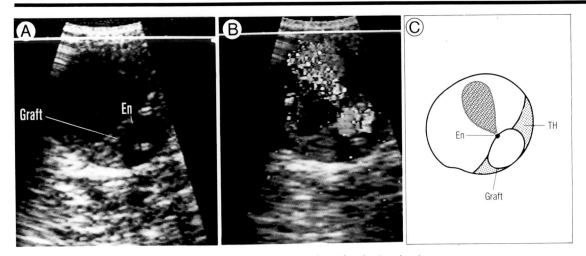

2-D Doppler image of pseudoaneurysm of the internal shunt in short-axis view.
Ⓐ 2-D echo. Ⓑ 2-D Doppler shows jet flow from the entry on the graft. En=Entry ; TH=thrombus. Ⓒ Diagram of Fig. Ⓑ.

Case 48 Normal Carotid Artery

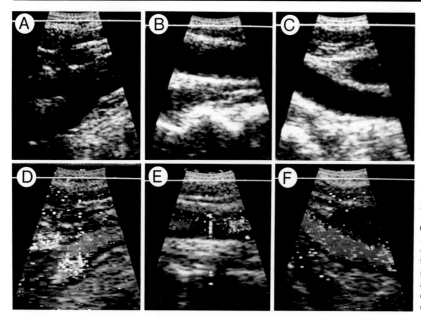

2-D echo and 2-D Doppler images of normal carotid artery.
A B C 2-D echo, long-axis view of the carotid artery. **D E F** 2-D Doppler, long-axis view of the carotid artery. **A D** The carotid bifurcation. Note that flow separation al the external side of the internal carotid artery. ECA=external carotid artery ; ICA=internal carotid artery. **B E** The common carotid artery (CCA). **C F** The proximal common carotid artery.

Case 49 Normal Carotid and Vertebral Arteries

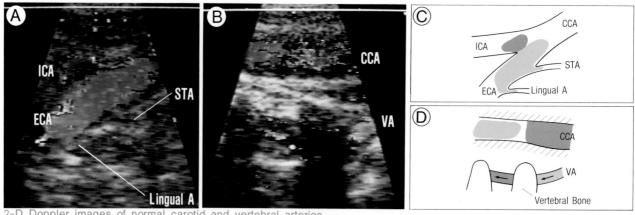

2-D Doppler images of normal carotid and vertebral arteries.
A Branches of the external carotid artery (ECA). STA=superior thyroidal artery. **B** The vertebral artery (VA) through the vertebral bone. CCA =common carotid artery. **C** Diagram of Fig. **A**. **D** Diagram of Fig. **B**.

Case 50 Carotid Artery Stenosis 77-year-old male

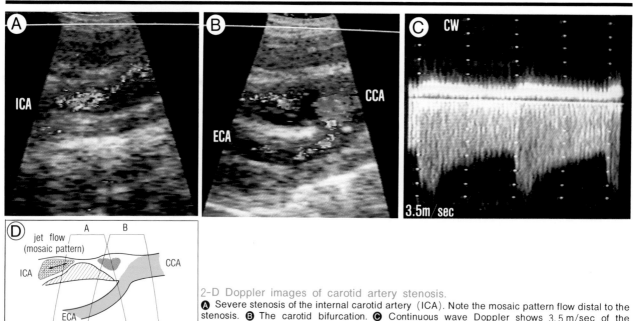

2-D Doppler images of carotid artery stenosis.
A Severe stenosis of the internal carotid artery (ICA). Note the mosaic pattern flow distal to the stenosis. **B** The carotid bifurcation. **C** Continuous wave Doppler shows 3.5 m/sec of the maximal velocity at the internal carotid stenosis. **D** Diagram of Fig. **A** and **B**.

Case 51 Normal Lower Limb Vein 70-year-old male

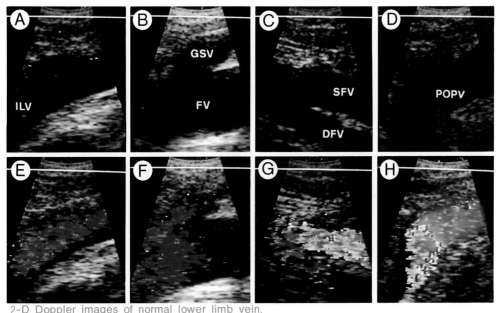

2-D Doppler images of normal lower limb vein.
A B C D 2-D echo. **E F G H** 2-D Doppler, calf pumping (+). **A E** The external iliac vein (ILV). **B F** The common femoral vein (FV) and the greater saphenous vein (GSV). **C G** Bifurcation of the common femoral vein. SFV=superficial femoral vein ; DFV=deep femoral vein. **D H** The popliteal vein (POPV).

Case 52 Varicose Vein 38-year-old male

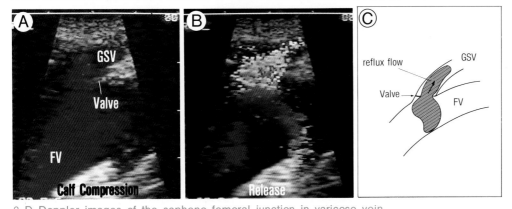

2-D Doppler images of the sapheno-femoral junction in varicose vein.
A At calf compression the proximal flow is displayed. **B** At release of calf compression valve incompetency, grade 3 at the sapheno-femoral junction is displayed. **C** Diagram of Fig. **B**.

Severity index of valve incompetency at the sapheno-femoral junction

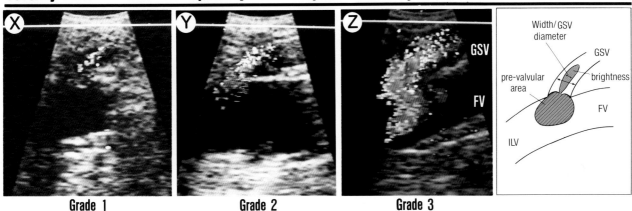

Grade 1   **Grade 2**   **Grade 3**

Severity index of valve incompetency at the sapheno-femoral junction
Reflux flow by calf pumping

	width/GSV diameter	brightness	pre-valvular area
grade 1	<1/2	low	(−)
grade 2	>1/2	high	small
grade 3	≒1	high (mosaic)	large

X Y Z 2-D Doppler images of the reflex flow at the sapheno-femoral junction.

Case 53 Deep Vein Thrombosis 76-year-old male

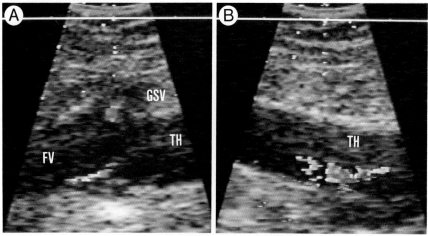

2-D Doppler images of deep vein thrombosis. Long-axis view of the femoral vein. Calf pumping (+).
Ⓐ The sapheno-femoral junction. Ⓑ The distal common femoral vein. Slight flow along the thrombus represents recanalization.

Case 54 Deep Vein Thrombosis 57-year-old female

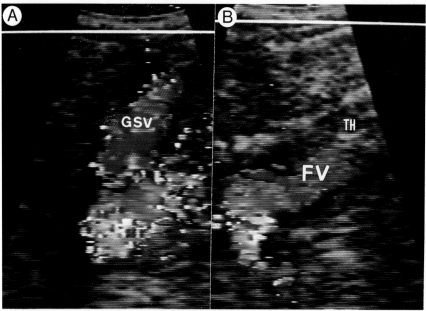

2-D Doppler images of deep vein thrombosis.
ⒶⒷ Long-axis view of the femoral vein. Calf pumping (+). Occlusion of the proximal femoral vein. Collateral channels through the branches of the femoral vein are displayed.
Ⓒ Diagram of Fig. Ⓐ and Ⓑ.

Case 55 Pulmonary Embolism, After Plication of the Inferior Vena Cava 41-year-old male

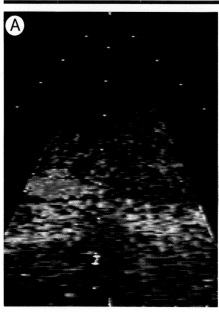
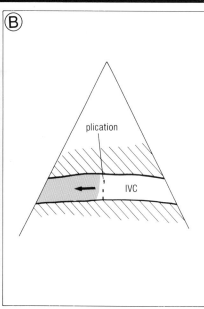

2-D Doppler image of the inferior vena cava after plication.
Ⓐ At the peripheral side of the plication no color flow is seen due to blood stasis, while at the central side velocity of blood flow is increased. Ⓑ Diagram of Fig. Ⓐ.

Chapter 12 Congenital Heart Disease

12—1 Introduction

The clinical significance of 2-D Doppler in congenital heart disease lies in its ability to produce real-time images of abnormal intracardiac blood flow, a capacity that in many cases makes possible the noninvasive establishment of a clinical diagnosis[1-6]. Difficulties are often experienced in diagnosing atrial septal defects (ASD) by conventional two-dimensional echocardiography or by FFT pulsed Doppler echocardiography alone, because the imaging of the atrial septum is often obscure in the former, and because it is often difficult with the latter, even for a highly skilled examiner, to obtain a good sampling point when an ASD is small.

Moreover, it is easy using ordinary two-dimensional echocardiography both to misdiagnose a healthy child with a functional heart murmur as ASD, and to fail to detect a defect in the ventricular septum in a patient with a small VSD. The use of 2-D Doppler echocardiography facilitates correct diagnosis merely by detecting the abnormal intracardiac shunt flow through the septal wall defect with no more effort than is required by conventional 2-D echocardiography. It is also possible to make a semi-quantitative estimation of the intracardiac shunt flow and of the severity of the heart lesion. There may be an urgent need both to correctly diagnose infants with severe cyanosis accompanied by cardiorespiratory failure and to administer proper treatment, possibly including surgery. Even if cardiac angiography appears to be indicated, it may be lethal in such critical cases. We have therefore been seeking an adequate non-invasive diagnostic tool for these patients, and have become convinced that 2-D Doppler can take over the role of cardiac angiography in some areas of heart disease[7-9].

Two-dimensional Doppler can offer much more information than cardiac angiography in some complex congenital heart diseases[7], because it makes separate recognition of multiple abnormal intracardiac blood flows possible in such cases, even if multiple abnormalities coexist in the same cardiac cavity. Changes in intracardiac hemodynamics according to growth are dramatic in some infants, and so occasional examination by 2-D Doppler may be indispensable for patient follow-up[10]. For example, in infants with extreme cases of tetralogy of Fallot, the pulmonary arterial blood flow is maintained by the patent ductus arteriosus (PDA), and the patient must be treated with prostaglandin to prevent reduction of the PDA shunt flow. Some palliative shunt operation such as the Blalock-Taussig shunt procedure may also be required before the closure of the PDA. Being a non-invasive technique, 2-D Doppler is extremely useful both for the good timing of the shunt operation and for the evaluation of its effects[11], because it can be performed repeatedly under physiological conditions. Accordingly, 2-D Doppler is considered to be one of the most important diagnostic techniques for research work in the physiology of congenital heart disease. Changes of the intracardiac shunt flow direction through a VSD in the Eisenmenger syndrome can be easily visualized and analyzed with 2-D Doppler (as described in the later section of this chapter) in a way that is generally impossible by cardiac angiography[5].

In the monochrome diagrams in this chapter, the intracardiac blood flows are indicated, for ease of understanding, by the four types of shading shown on the left, without regard to the blood flow velocity and the velocity distribution. The color displays of the intracardiac shunt flows clearly differentiate between ASD and VSD turbulent flows toward the transducer, but for the sake of simplicity, both have been shown with the same shading.

The key to express blood-flow images in monochrome diagrams

 (a) laminar flow towards the transducer

 (c) turbulent flow towards the transducer

 (b) laminar flow away from the transducer

 (d) turbulent flow away from the transducer

12－2　Atrial Septal Defect (ASD)

1. ASD secundum type (Case 56, 8-year-old male) (Tab. 12-1)

○ P.177

Defects of the interatrial septum in secundum type ASD are usually detected by an apical four-chamber view or a parasternal four-chamber view (**Case 56, A**). The shunt flow through the ASD into the right atrium is observed from late systole until the end of diastole in the normal sinus rhythm patient (**Case 56, B**)[1]. The differentiation between ASD shunt flow and the normal blood inflow from the superior and inferior venae cavae is important in making correct diagnosis. The imaging of the ASD shunt flow is clearer in **Case 56, C**, which has been obtained by tilting the transducer probe slightly upward (lowering the ultrasound beam), from the position used for **Case 56, B**. We can now see the abnormal ASD shunt flow more directly with a smaller angle of incidence, and the abnormal ASD shunt flow can be depicted with the greatest clarity. **Case 56**, D demonstrates the M-mode color flow mapping and FFT pulsed Doppler spectral analysis with the Doppler beam direction aligned along the center of the ASD shunt flow. The FFT pulsed Doppler spectrum shows the so-called 'four-peak' pattern[12,13] of ASD shunt flow in a patient with a normal sinus rhythm. A moderate degree of pulmonary regurgitation is often observed during cardiac diastole in the case of ASD (**Case 56, F**), and a disturbed color flow pattern due to an increment of pulmonary systolic flow volume and to the enlargement of the main pulmonary artery is often observed during cardiac systole in cases of high-flow ASD. The turbulent systolic pulmonary arterial flow pattern of high-flow ASD cases should be differentiated from the turbulent flow pattern in the main pulmonary artery in PDA or valvular pulmonary stenosis.

Tab. 12-1　H. M., 8-year-old male.

	Pressure (mmHg)	Sat. O$_2$(%)
SVC	mean＝3	73.3
IVC	mean＝2.5	86.1
RA	mean＝2	84.2
RV	22/2(edp＝3)	88.3
PA	23/8(mean＝14)	89.2
LA	mean＝3	97.2
LV	105/0(edp＝6)	97.4
PV	mean＝4	97.6
		48.9%

2. ASD(secundum type)＋MR(grade 2)＋TR(grade 1)＋pulmonary hypertension (Case 57, 52-year-old female) (Tab. 12-2)

A mild to moderate grade of mitral regurgitation and/or tricuspid regurgitation is often observed in the case of ASD associated with the advancement of pulmonary hypertension[14]. In this case, an ASD 5 cm in diameter can be detected in the apical four-chamber view

○ P.178

(**Case 57, A**) and the shunt flow through the defect can be observed from the middle of cardiac systole until the end of the diastole (**Case 57, B**). A moderate mitral regurgitation (grade 2) and a mild tricuspid regurgitation (grade 1) are also seen during systole. The subcostal approach reveals a reversed right-to-left shunt flow[15] through the defect from the

Tab. 12-2　I. K., 52-year-old female.

	Pressure (mmHg)	Sat. O$_2$(%)
SVC	mean＝12	67.7
IVC	mean＝14	77.1
RA	mean＝13	85.1
RV	80/0(edp＝12)	89.5
PA	82/22(mean＝45)	86.2
LA	11.5	93.8
LV	118/−4(edp＝14)	94.5
PV	mean＝12.5	98.5
	lt → rt shunt ratio	52.9%
	rt → lt shunt ratio	15.3%

end of systole until early in the next systole as shown in **Case 57, D**. This subcostal view[16,17] is the most advantageous for visualizing the ASD shunt flow directly, because it gives the smallest angle of incidence between the Doppler beam and the ASD shunt flow. The bi-directional shunt flow at the time of the change of shunt flow direction through the ASD, can be seen in the same view. The duration of the reversed shunt flow through the ASD varies according to the patient's respiration (**Case 57, G**).

3. ASD (Secundum type) (Case 58, 52 year-old female)

Preoperative transesophageal 2-D Doppler diagnosis, and intra-and post-operative 2-D Doppler evaluation

(1) Transesophageal 2-D Doppler diagnosis

In some adult cases of ASD, 2-D Doppler fails to lead to a correct diagnosis owing to poor echo penetration in transthoracic echocardiography. In such a case, transesophageal 2-D Doppler is an effective approach[18,19]. The thoracic esophagus is located just behind the left atrium (Fig. 12-1, **Case 58, A**), so that an S/N level superior to that afforded by transthoracic echocardiography can be obtained from the transesophageal window for observation of the left and right atria and the pulmonary veins. It is particularly sensitive in the diagnosis of atrial septal defects, because the atrial septum is close to the front of the scanning field without the dropout of the midportion of the atrial septum commonly seen in the apical four-chamber view of normal adult cases. **Case 58** had been diagnosed as a case

○ P.179

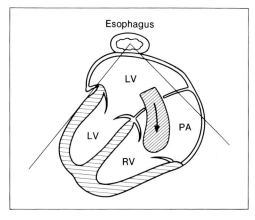

Fig. 12- 1　Diagrammatic representation of ASD (secundum type) in the transesophageal four-chamber view.

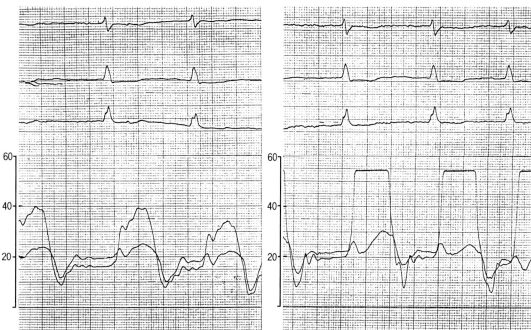

Fig. 12-2　The simultaneous pressure record of the right atrium (RA) and the right ventricle (RV) in Case 58. Note the typical dip-and-plateau pattern.

of mitral valve disorder before being referred to us, but transesophageal 2-D Doppler clearly demonstrated the ASD (**Case 58, A**) and indicated that the direction of the shunt flow through the defect was away from the transducer (**Case 58, B**).

(2) Intra-operative 2-D Doppler[11]

Intraoperative 2-D Doppler is also effective for the evaluation of the results of surgery. In **Case 58** a small residual shunt was detected just after the separation from the cardiopulmonary bypass (**Case 58, D**). Recurrent ASD is observed in about 2% of patients, and therefore intraoperative detection of dehiscence is important[20,21].

(3) Post-operative follow-up by 2-D Doppler

Case 58 developed constrictive pericarditis 3 months after corrective surgery[22,23]. **Case 58, E** shows the enlargement of the right atrium due to constrictive pericarditis and to impaired distensibility of the two ventricles. Cardiac catheterization also demonstrated the typical dip-and-plateau pattern in the right and left ventricular pressure (Fig. 12-2). As a result of the elevation of the ventricular end-diastolic pressure, atrioventricular regurgitation has become manifest. **Case 58, F** and **G** demonstrate moderate mitral and tricuspid regurgitation (MR=grade 2, TR=grade 2) after development of the constrictive pericarditis.

4. Endocardial cushion defect (ECD incomplete type)

○ P.180

ASD (primum) + ASD (secundum) + VSD (small) + MR (grade 2) (**Case 59**, 2 years old) (Tab. 12-3)

When multiple abnormalities exist in one cardiac chamber it is often difficult to detect all the abnormalities in anatomical structure and in blood flow circulation either by cardiac catheterization alone, even with multiple injection of radiographic contrast materials, or by conventional pulsed Doppler spectral analysis or continuous-wave Doppler with 2DE.

Case 59 has two defects in the atrial septum (primum and secundum ASD) and two channels through which mitral regurgitation occurs, one from the mitral valve through the primum ASD into the right atrium in systole. Three abnormal blood flows in the right atrium are easily detected using 2-D Doppler. Another abnormal shunt flow is also seen in the right ventricle due to a small VSD.

Tab. 12-3 I. K., 2-year-old female.

	Pressure (mmHg)	Sat. O₂(%)
SVC		65.3
IVC		69.8
RA	mean=7.5	89.4
RV	49/0(edp=11)	89.5
PA	43/10(mean=25)	88.9
LA	mean=6.5	96.2
PV		98.3
LV	108/2(edp=12)	94.5
Ao	115/65(mean=85)	95.7
	lt → rt shunt ratio	69.5%
	rt → lt shunt ratio	7.8%

Tab. 12-4 M. K., 36-year-old male.

	Pressure (mmHg)	Sat. O₂(%)
SVC	mean=2.0	70.8
IVC	mean=2.0	81.6
RA	mean=1.5	94.5
RV	25/0(edp=0)	94.5
PA	36/5(mean=15)	94.2
LA	mean=1.0	94.7
PV	mean=2.0	97.7
LV	100/0(edp=3.5)	93.0
Ao	120/65(mean=75)	93.9
	lt → rt shunt ratio	83.7%
	rt → lt shunt ratio	17.7%

5. Endocardial cushion defect (ECD incomplete type) (Case 60, 36-year-old male) (Tab. 12-4)

Preoperative 2-D Doppler diagnosis and intraoperative 2-D Doppler evaluation.

○ P.181

Case 60 is a case of incomplete ECD with a large primum ASD. Two-dimensional Doppler demonstrates a massive left to right shunt flow through the defect from late systole until the end of diastole (**Case 60, A**). The 2-D Doppler images also demonstrate a mild tricuspid regurgitation into the left atrium through the primum defect in systole. Cardiac catheterization indicates a right to left shunt at the atrial level (shunt ratio=17.7%), which is compatible with the above observations.

In some cases with severe cardiomegaly 2-D Doppler sensitivity is poor in the deep scanning field, and so in this case the severe mitral regurgitation (grade 3) is depicted only with a coarse color flow signal when the color flow gain is set at the ordinary level. When color flow gain is increased, the regurgitant flow can be detected in the area enclosed by the dotted line in **Case 60, C**.

However, intraoperative epicardial 2-D Doppler can clearly show the severe mitral regurgitation in this case at an ordinary gain level (**Case 60, E**). After mitral valvuloplasty intraoperative epicardial 2-D Doppler shows a marked decrease in the mitral regurgitation to grade 1 (**Case 60, F**).

6. Sinus venosus ASD (Case 61, 28-year-old female)

Sinus venosus ASD is rarely visualized from a transthoracic, parasternal or apical four-chamber view. It can be visualized in pediatric patients by careful scanning using the subcostal approach. In the adult, sinus venosus ASD is often missed by transthoracic echocardiography[24], so that transesophageal 2-D Doppler and intraoperative epicardial 2-D Doppler are important for confirmation of a preoperative diagnosis.

○ P.182

In this case, the intraoperative 2-D Doppler images clearly demonstrate the sinus venosus defect (**Case 61, A**) and the shunt flow through the sinus venosus defect (**Case 61, B**). The surgical result after patch suture closure of the defect can be confirmed by intraoperative epicardial 2-D Doppler (**Case 61, C**).

○ P.182

7. Supplement. quantitative assessment of ASD shunt flow by 2-D Doppler[1]

We postulated that, certain characteristics of the 2-D Doppler image of ASD shunt flow may be related to the shunt flow volume. To examine the validity of this hypothesis, we studied the correlation between the size of the 2-D Doppler shunt flow image of ASDs and the shunt ratios or the pulmonary/systemic flow volume ratios (Qp/Qs) obtained by cardiac catheterization in 30 consecutive cases of ASD without right to left shunt. Using a 3.5 MHz transducer with a 4 KHz pulse repetition frequency (PRF) and a rate of 15 frames per second, we recorded apical or parasternal four-chamber views of the ASD shunt flow in 2-D Doppler on video tape. The maximum shunt flow area (MSFA) of the 2-D Doppler image was measured by slow motion playback of the video tape, using the caliper system of the scanner (Supplement D, E, F). The MSFA was then normalized by dividing by the body surface area (BSA) and was expressed as the maximum shunt flow area index (MSFAI).

$$MSFAI = MSFA/BSA \cdots\cdots\cdots (1)$$

The shunt flow volume ($Qp-Qs$) was normalized using the cardiac output (Qs) and expressed as the normalized shunt flow volume (NSFV) (Fig. 12-3).

$$NSFV = (Qp-Qs)/Qs \cdots\cdots\cdots (2)$$

We assumed the correlation between NSFV and MSFAI according to our hypothesis.

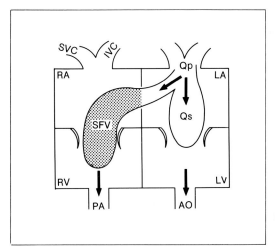

Fig. 12-3 Diagram showing The relation of the shunt flow volume (SFV) to the pulmonary flow (Qp) and the systemic flow (Qs).

$$NSFV = f_1(MSFAI) \quad \cdots\cdots\cdots\cdots\cdots\cdots\cdots\cdots\cdots\cdots\cdots\cdots\cdots (3)$$

Inspection of the distribution of the data obtained suggested that the function f_1 was a power function, and mathematical analysis was employed to derive f_1 from the best-fit curve.

$$NSFV = a \times MSFAI^b = (Qp-Qs)/Qs \quad \cdots\cdots\cdots\cdots\cdots\cdots\cdots\cdots (4)$$

Transformation of this equation yields the equations representing the correlation between MSFAI and Qp/Qs, and MSFAI and the shunt ratio (SR), as follows:

$$Qp/Qs = (Qp-Qs)/Qs + 1 = a \times MSFAI^b + 1 \quad \cdots\cdots\cdots\cdots\cdots (5)$$

$$SR = (Qp-Qs)/Qp \times 100 = 100 - 100/(a \times MSFAI^b + 1) \quad \cdots\cdots\cdots (6)$$

The regression between Qp/Qs and MSFAI (Fig. 12-5 a), and the regression between SR and MSFAI (Fig. 12-5 b) showed a good correlation, having a correlation coefficient (r) of 0.876. The values of a and b for the best-fit regression curves are represented by the following equations:

$$NSFV = 0.025 \times MSFAI^{1.53} \quad \cdots\cdots\cdots\cdots\cdots\cdots\cdots\cdots\cdots\cdots (7)$$

$$Qp/Qs = 0.025 \times MSFAI^{1.53} + 1 \quad \cdots\cdots\cdots\cdots\cdots\cdots\cdots\cdots (8)$$

$$SR = 100 - 100/(0.025 \times MSFAI + 1) \quad \cdots\cdots\cdots\cdots\cdots\cdots (9)$$

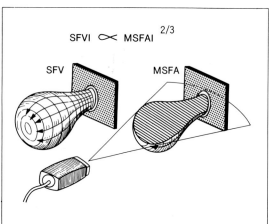

Fig. 12-4 Theoretical relationship between NSFV and MSFAI.

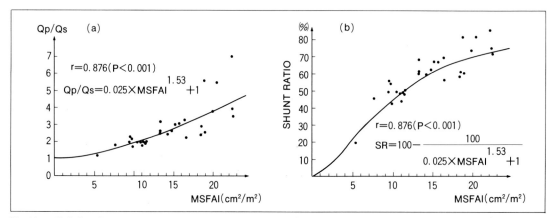

Fig. 12-5 Relations between the maximum shunt flow area index (MSFAI) and the pulmonary/systemic flow ratio (Qp/Qs), and the shunt ratio.

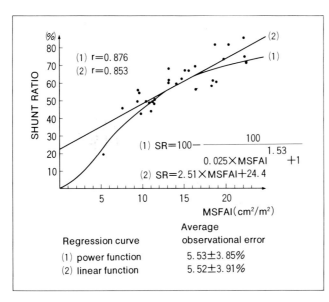

Fig. 12-6 Relation between the maximum shunt flow area index (MSFAI) and shunt ratio. The lines represent the best curves derived from linear and power analyses of the data for patients with atrial septal defect.

(1) r=0.876
(2) r=0.853

$$(1)\ SR = 100 - \frac{100}{0.025 \times MSFAI^{1.53} + 1}$$

$$(2)\ SR = 2.51 \times MSFAI + 24.4$$

Regression curve	Average observational error
(1) power function	5.53±3.85%
(2) linear function	5.52±3.91%

Since flow volume is three-dimensional and the area is a plane concept, NSFV can theoretically be considered to have a linear relationship to the 1.5 power of MSFAI (Fig. 12-4). The exponent of the best-fit curves is 1.53 in the actually observed power regression curves, which is very close to the exponent of the theoretical equation. Linear regression is convenient for the clinical estimation of ASD shunt flow. The linear regression curve between SR and MSFAI also shows a good correlation. Our series of studies gave a correlation coefficient of 0.853 for the linear regression curve. The average observational error of the shunt ratio was about 5% for both linear and power regression curves (Fig. 12-6)

12—3 Ventricular Sptal Defect (VSD)

○ P.183
1. Perimembranous VSD (Kirklin type 2[25]) (Case 62, 11-month-old male) (Tab. 12-5)

Perimembranous VSD located in the membranous infracristal portion of the interventricular septum (Fig. 12-7). The defect can usually be visualized by the apical four-chamber view or the parasternal four-chamber view, or both. **Case 62, B** presents a typical mosaic color flow pattern[2] of the shunt flow through the perimembranous ventricular septal defect in a case with normal pulmonary arterial pressure. Cardiac catheterization of this patient yielded a peak pressure gradient of 79 mm Hg between the right ventricle and the left ventricle. In the scanning of this VSD shunt flow using a 5-MHz transducer with a pulse repetition frequency of 4 KHz (maximum detectable velocity=0.48 m/sec), aliasing can occur in the color flow display of the major part in the VSD shunt flow more than five times.

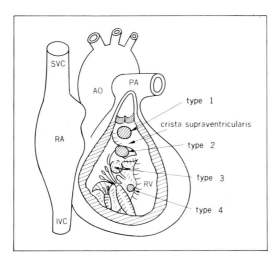

Fig. 12-7 Anatomical position of ventricular septal defects (Kirklin's classification[25])

Tab. 12-5 E. D., 1 year-old male.

	Pressure (mmHg)	Sat. O₂(%)
SVC		78.0
IVC		82.0
RA	mean=4.5	78.0
RV	51/1(edp=10)	86.0
PA	53/17	88.0
LA	mean=9.5	96.0
LV	130/−7.5(edp=12)	96.0
Ao	120/75	96.0
	lt → rt shunt ratio	57.1%

O P.183

2. VSD with pulmonary hypertension (Case 63, 4-year-old female) (Tab. 12-6)

A large ventricular septal defect including the perimembranous septum, in which the posterior margin of the defect is formed by the tricuspid annulus, is seen in **Case 63**. Cardiac catheterization demonstrated a severe degree of pulmonary hypertension with a left-to-right shunt ratio of 34.5% and a reversal shunt ratio of 20.7%. The parasternal long-axis view of the left ventricle reveals a large ventricular septal defect 18 mm in diameter, but the color flow pattern of the shunt flow through the VSD in this case does not have the typical mosaic pattern. Instead, the shunt flow is depicted in a simple red color with a small blue area due to aliasing in the center (**Case 63, A**). Also, reversal of a left-to-right shunt is seen during a very short period of the diastole (**Case 63, B**). The color flow pattern of the VSD shunt is quite different in cases associated with advanced pulmonary hypertension from that of the more usual VSD with normal pulmonary arterial pressure, because the relatively low pressure gradient across the VSD results in a relatively low VSD shunt flow velocity. The peak velocity of the VSD shunt flow determined in this case was 2 m/sec with CW Doppler (Fig. 12-8). We consider that, when the recorded peak velocity of the VSD shunt flow is lower than 2.5 m/sec, and no right ventricular outflow obstruction is detected, the possibiliy of progressive pulmonary hypertension is very high, and so cardiac catheterization should be scheduled as quickly as possible[9]. The results of cardiac catheterization suggested that

Tab. 12-6 M. M., 4-year-old female.

1) Pre-Op

	Pressure (mmHg)	Sat. O₂(%)
SVC		64.0
IVC		73.0
RA	mean=4	67.0
RV	110/0(edp=3)	75.0
PA	115/70(mean=85)	77.0
LV	110/0(edp=1.5)	88.0
Ao	105/72(mean=95)	90.0
	lt → rt shunt ratio	34.5%
	rt → et shunt ratio	20.7%

2) Intra-Op.

	pre-VSD closure	post-VSD closure
Ao	75/45 mmHg	90/60 mmHg
PA	75/45 mmHg	33/17 mmHg
Ao(flow)	1.3 l/min	2.1 l/min
PA(flow)	5.5 l/min	2.0 l/min

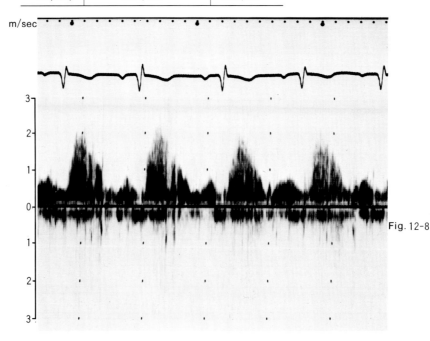

Fig. 12-8 With continuous wave Doppler from the left-parasternal position, the velocity across the VSD is recorded. The decrease in the peak velocity across the VSD can be seen in the case of VSD with pulmonary hypertension.

Case 63 had already developed Eisenmenger syndrome. However, 2-D Doppler demons-trated the dominance of a left-to-right shunt which indicated that the pulmonary resistance was still lower than the systemic pressure. We performed corrective surgery on this patient on the basis of the 2-D Doppler diagnosis, and intraoperative pressure measurement showed a marked reduction in the pulmonary arterial pressure after surgical closure of the VSD, as shown on Tab. 12-6. In this case 2-D Doppler evaluation indicated the hemodynamics of the patient more correctly than cardiac catheterization did[5].

3. Perimembranous outlet type VSD (Case 64, 1-year-old male)

When the ventricular septal defect extends from the membranous septum to the

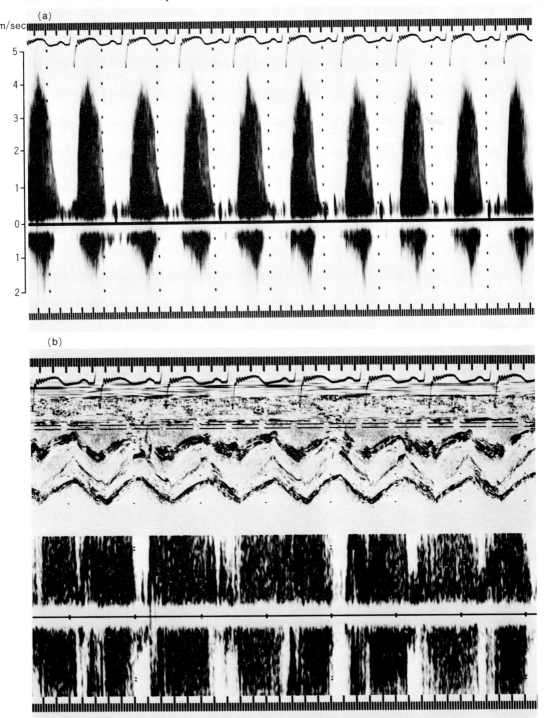

Fig. 12-9 With continuous wave (a), and pulsed Doppler(b), flow through the ventricular septal defect was recorded toward the transducer. The high velocity through the VSD gives a calculated pressure difference of 70 mmHg between the ventricles.

infundibular septum, the entire defect can be visualized in the short-axis view at the aortic valve level, in the parasternal long-axis view of the left ventricle, and in the apical four-chamber view. Anderson[26] termed a ventricular septal defect at this portion as a perimembranous outlet type defect or an infundibular perimembranous defect. The peak velocity of the shunt flow was found by CW Doppler to be 4.3 m/sec (Fig. 12-9 a) and the color flow images B-mode and M-mode are displayed with the typical mosaic pattern (**Case 64, B, C, D, E, F**), which shows a bi-directional, wide-band pattern[27] on pulsed-Doppler spectral analysis (Fig. 12-9 b, **Case 64, F**).

◐ P.184

4. VSD in a premature infant (Perimembranous type) (Case 65, 40-day-old, 2350 g male)

Two-dimensional Doppler diagnosis in premature infants requires a higher spatial resolution and time resolution, because of the small heart size and rapid heart motion. The heart rate in **Case 65** was about 170/min, and so 2-D Doppler scanning at a frame rate (FR) of 10 frames per second on the heart of this patient would yield only about 3.5 images per cardiac cycle, far too few to make possible the precise analysis of intracardiac blood flow patterns indispensable to a reliable diagnosis. Although a 5 MHz transducer offers good spatial resolution for scanning the heart of an infant, in Doppler flow mapping the maximum velocity detectable without aliasing is relatively low with such a transducer, and aliasing can occur even in the observation of normal intracardiac blood flow. In the current model of a 2-Doppler system (Aloka SSD 860), the available maximum pulse repetition frequency is 12 KHz with a scanning depth of 6 cm. Under these conditions the heart of an infant can be scanned at a frame rate of 30 frames per second and a maximum detectable velocity without aliasing of 96 cm/sec, and we can avoid the confusion created by aliasing due to a relatively low maximum detectable velocity (Tab. 12-8)[28].

◐ P.185

Figs. 65 B, C, D and E demonstrate the shunt flow through the perimembranous ventricular septal defect in a premature infant. The jet flow through the defect is more clearly displayed by scanning at a frame rate of 30 than at one of 20 (Tab. 12-7, 12-8).

Tab. 12-7   Characteristics of 2-D Doppler system.

PRF	4 KHz	6 KHz	8 KHz	12 KHz
frame rate	10	15	20	30
depth	18	12	9	6
probe frequency	maximum detectable velocity (m/s)			
2.5 KHz	0.64	0.93	1.23	1.91
3.5 KHz	0.48	0.70	0.93	1.43
5.0 KHz	0.32	0.47	0.62	0.96

$\cos \theta = 1$ PFR = pulse repetition frequency

Tab. 12-8   Normal maximal velocities, Doppler measurements.

	Children		Adults	
	Mean	Range	Mean	Range
Mitral flow	1.00 m/s	0.8~1.3 m/s	0.90 m/s	0.6~1.3 m/s
Tricuspid flow	0.60 m/s	0.5~0.8 m/s	0.50 m/s	0.3~0.7 m/s
Pulmonary artery	0.90 m/s	0.7~1.1 m/s	0.75 m/s	0.6~0.9 m/s
Left ventricle	1.00 m/s	0.7~1.2 m/s	0.90 m/s	0.7~1.1 m/s
Aorta	1.50 m/s	1.2~1.8 m/s	1.35 m/s	1.0~1.7 m/s

(From Hatle, L., Angelsen, B.: Doppler Ultrasound in Cardiology. Second edition, Lea & Febiger, Philadelphia, 1985, p. 93.)

◐ P.185

5. VSD with Eisenmenger syndrome (Case 66, 20-year-old male) (Tab. 12-9)

When the pulmonary/systemic pressure ratio exceeds 0.7, the reversal of a left-to-right shunt flow (in other words, a right-to-left shunt flow) can be observed in 2-D Doppler. However, it does not always indicate that the patient has developed Eisenmenger syndrome as described in **Case 63**. The case presented is diagnosed as Eisenmenger syndrome not only by cardiac catheterization but also by lung biopsy. Cardiac catheterization demonstrates

Tab. 12-9　M. K., 20-year-old male.

	Pressure (mmHg)	Sat. O₂(%)
SVC		59.0
IVC		73.0
RA		68.0
RV in	115/−15(edp=7)	82.0
RV out	115/−15(edp=7)	91.0
PA	110/75(mean=88)	81.0
LV	110/−10(edp=3)	89.0
Ao	110/73(mean=90)	90.0
	lt → rt shunt ratio	44.1%
	rt → lt shunt ratio	17.2%

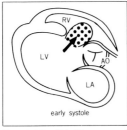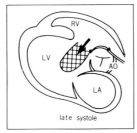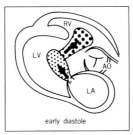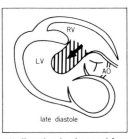

Fig. 12-10　(b) Diagrams of the shunt blood flow through VSD in the long-axis view. The shunt direction is changed four times in one cardiac cycle.

that the left-to-right shunt ratio is 41.1% and the reverse shunt flow ratio is 17.2%. From the cardiac catheterization data, the left-to-right shunt was considered to be dominant in this case, but 2-D Doppler demonstrated that an almost equal time was occupied by each of these shunt flows, as shown in the M-mode flow mapping (**Case 66, D**): the flow mapping M-mode demonstrates a quadriphasic change of direction of the intracardiac shunt flow that is fully compatible with the pressure gradient pattern between the right and left ventricles seen on the simultaneous pressure record of both ventricles.

The quadriphasic shunt flow pattern observed was as follows (Fig. 12-10):
(1) left-to-right shunt in early systole
(2) right-to-left shunt in late systole
(3) left-to-right shunt in early diastole
(4) right-to-left shunt in late diastole

This basically bi-directional, quadriphasic pattern showed variations according to small changes in the pressure balance between the ventricles. Six or eight phasic shunt flow patterns can occasionally be seen in one cardiac cycle of this patient. Despite the complexity of the hemodynamics of the Eisenmenger VSD, it can thus be analyzed by 2-D Doppler alone[5].

6. Residual VSD after surgery (Case 67, 34-year-old male) (Tab. 12-10)

In the early postoperative period, small residual shunt flows from the suture line are often observed around the prosthetic patch used for VSD closure. In some cases, a persistent residual shunt with a relatively high shunt flow volume requires re-operation[29]. The persistent moderate congestive heart failure in **Case 67** could not be controlled with

○ P.186

Tab. 12-10　T. M., 34-year-old male.

	Pressure (mmHg)	Sat. O₂(%)
SVC	mean=11	67.5
IVC	mean=12	76.5
RA	mean=11	76.9
RV	40/1(edp=12)	86.8
PA	34/12(mean=20)	86.5
PV	mean=12	97.7
LV	102/−1(edp=12)	93.6
	lt → rt shunt ratio	56.4%
	rt → lt shunt ratio	15.9%

intensive medication owing to severe pulmonary regurgitation and a residual VSD shunt with a shunt ratio of 56.4%. Although 2-D Doppler can be used to demonstrate two residual shunt flows around the prosthetic patch, as shown in **Case 67, B**, both 2-D echocardiography and a left ventriculogram failed to detect the smaller VSD.

7. Infective endocarditis associated with a small VSD (Case 68, 17-year-old male)

Case 68 is a case of active infective endocarditis associated with a small VSD. Surgery was performed without previous cardiac catheterization, merely on the strength of the 2-D Doppler diagnosis. The vegetation (VGE) is clearly visible on the 2-D echocardiograms ○ P.186 (**Cases 68, A, B**), and moderate tricuspid regurgitation is shown by 2-D Doppler (**Case 68, C**). Infectious endocarditis rarely occurs in the right side of the heart of normal subjects[30], except in drug addicts[31], but the presence of a VSD is one cause of infective endocarditis in the right side of the heart[32].

8. VSD with infundibular pulmonary stenosis (Case 69, 1-month-old male)

The parasternal long-axis view in this boy demonstrates a large perimembranous VSD ○ P.187 (**Case 69, A**), but the VSD shunt flow image displayed by 2-D Doppler does not have the typical mosaic pattern, the color pattern being little more than a plain red field. In such cases, the right ventricular pressure is usually elevated and the pressure gradient between the right and left ventricles is relatively small. The peak velocity of the VSD shunt flow in the present case is 75 cm/sec (**Case 69, C**). When 2-D Doppler suggests an elevation of the right ventricular pressure, the right ventricular outflow tract should be carefully examined. The short-axis view at the aortic valve level reveals a severe infundibular pulmonary stenosis (**Case 69, D**), and the typical mosaic turbulent jet flow pattern is seen in the main pulmonary artery (**Case 69, E**).

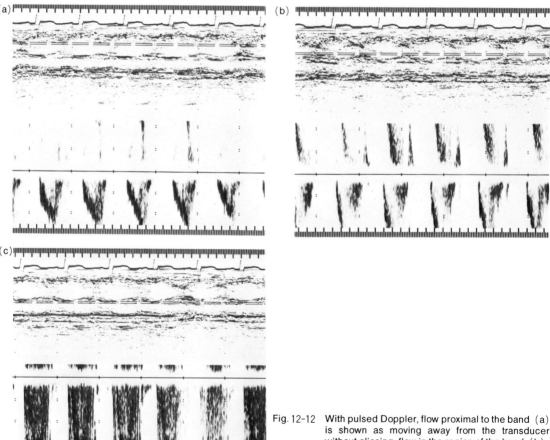

Fig. 12-12 With pulsed Doppler, flow proximal to the band (a) is shown as moving away from the transducer without aliasing, flow in the region of the band (b) is seen moving away from the transducer with aliasing, and flow distal to the band (c) is recorded with a wide-band pattern.

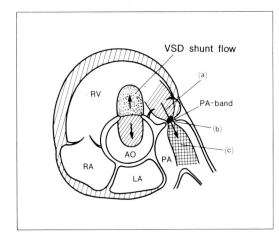

Tab. 12-11 A. S., 1-year-old female.

	Pressure (mmHg)	Sat. O₂(%)
SVC		61.7
IVC		78.3
RA	mean=4.5	63.6
RV	125/0(edp=6)	68.8
main PA	20.5/9.5(mean=13.5)	79.2
et PA	26/10(mean=17)	79.1
rt PA	18.5/10(mean=12.5)	79.3
*Ao(femoral)	125/70	93.0
	lt → rt shunt ratio	34.1%
	rt → lt shunt ratio	14.8%

Fig. 12-12 Diagrammatic representation of pulmonary banding surgery in the case of VSD with pulmonary hypertension.

9. VSD after pulmonary arterial banding surgery (Case 70, 1-year-old female) (Tab. 12-11)

◐ P.188

When pulmonary arterial banding surgery (PA banding)[33] is successfully performed, the right ventricular pressure is elevated almost as far as the left ventricular pressure and the distal pulmonary arterial pressure is decreased to the normal level. In **Case 70**, coarctectomy with subclavian-flap aortoplasty[34] and PA banding was performed 17 days after birth. Two-dimensional Doppler shows a bi-directional, quadriphasic VSD shunt flow pattern after PA banding (Fig. 70, a), and pulsed Doppler spectral analysis indicated a peak velocity of 75 cm/sec (**Cases 70, A, B, C, D**). The pulmonary arterial flow in the flow mapping B-mode is displayed in blue proximal to the band. In the region of the band aliasing has caused a change to red, and distal to the band, this flow is displayed entirely as a mosaic pattern (**Case 70, E, F**). The pulsed Doppler spectral analysis of the pulmonary arterial flow distal to the band demonstrates a bi-directional, wide-band pattern (**Case 70, a3**), and its peak velocity was given as 5 m/sec by CW Doppler, a figure that is compatible with the result of cardiac catheterization (105 mmHg).

12—4 Patent Ductus Arteriosus (PDA) (Case 71, 4-year-old male) (Tab. 12-12)

◐ P.189

A patent ductus arteriosus can be detected in the parasternal long-axis view of the main pulmonary artery. In premature and other infants and in the newborn, it is usually easy to detect the anatomical orientation of a PDA in relation to the descending aorta[10] and the main pulmonary artery (**Case 71, A**), but in some cases of PDA in adults 2-D Doppler fails to demonstrate the PDA shunt flow owing to poor echo penetration via the transthoracic approach. PDA shunt flow is usually observed as a continuous flow depicted in red (i.e., approaching the transducer) along the anterior wall of the main pulmonary artery (**Case 71, B**). In a case with a shunt flow that is more than moderate in degree through the PDA, the shunt jet reaches the pulmonary valve and turns in the posterolateral direction (**Case 71, D**). Thus, the PDA shunt jet assumes a swirling pattern in the main pulmonary artery. A continuous shunt flow pattern with a peak velocity of 4.4 m/sec was recorded with CW

Tab. 12-12 Y. Y., 4-year-old male.

	Pressure (mmHg)	Sat. O₂(%)
SVC	mean=4	75.4
IVC		84.3
RA	mean=4.5	76.6
RV	34/2.5(edp=6)	74.3
main PA	34/15(mean=23)	82.0
lt PA	34/13(mean=23)	82.9
rt PA	29/13(mean=20)	80.7
Ao	110/55(mean=80)	97.5
	lt → rt shunt ratio	37.1%

Doppler (**Case 71, E**) which gives a peak pressure drop of 77 mmHg, which is very close to the result of cardiac catheterization.

12—5 PDA in a Premature Infant (Case 72, 3-week-old, 1450 g female) (Case 73, 2-week-old, 1280 g male)

O P.190

In the treatment of premature infants with respiratory failure, it is important to differentiate between infant respiratory distress syndrome (IRDS) and a patent ductus arteriosus[35], and, if the latter is present, to evaluate the grade of the shunt flow through it. Continuous turbulent flow, usually depicted by 2-D Doppler as a mosaic pattern in the main pulmonary artery, is diagnostic for PDA (**Case 72, D**), but to confirm this diagnosis it is essential to demonstrate the exact anatomical orientation of the ductus between the descending aorta and the main pulmonary artery. For this purpose the aortic arch view from the suprasternal or the higher parasternal approach is often useful in a premature infant. The aortic arch view can more easily demonstrate the continuous shunt flow pattern of PDA shown in **Case 72, B** (diastole) and **Case 72, C** (systole). The peak velocity of the shunt flow was found to be 3.5 m/sec, which indicates a pressure drop of 49 mmHg (**Case 72, F**).

The shunt flow through a patent foramen ovale (PFO) is also commonly observed in 2-D Doppler examinations of newborn or premature infants (Fig. 12-13)[36]. A shunt flow through the PFO was observed in all of the 15 premature infants with PDA and in 8 of the

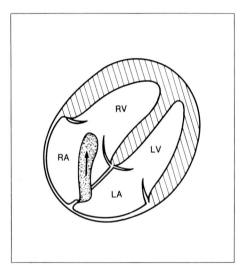

Fig. 12-13 Diagrammatic representation of **Case 71, G**. In 2-D Doppler a shunt flow through the patent foramen ovale is often observed in newborn or premature infants.

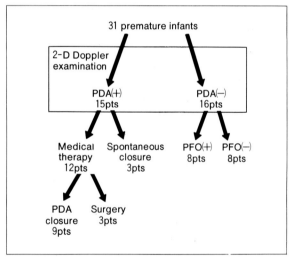

Fig. 12-14 Therapeutic approach to the PDA in premature infant.

16 premature infants without PDA in our early series (Fig. 12-14). **Cases 72, F** and **G** demonstrate PFO and the shunt flow through it in one premature infant.

The majority of premature infants do not develop severe respiratory failure, and the patent ductus usually closes spontaneously, generally within 2 to 3 months after birth. However, once premature infants develop severe respiratory or left ventricular failure, or both, an aggressive form of therapy should be initiated. Fig. 12-14 presents the results of 2-D Doppler evaluation of 31 premature infants with respiratory failure in our early series. PDA was seen in 15 patients (48.4%) and in 3 of them the PDA closed spontaneously. Sulindac[37] was administered to 12 patients, in 9 PDAS was successfully closed. In 3 patients, however, this treatment was unsuccessful and the ductus was surgically ligated. **Case 73** is a typical case showing the results of Sulindac administration, and Fig. 12-15 demonstrates the typical clinical course of a patient requiring surgical ligation of a PDA, in whom all therapeutic management was based on 2-D Doppler examinations.

O P.190

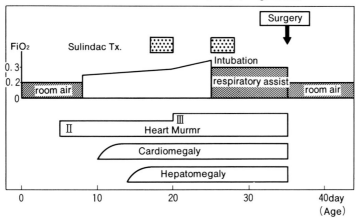

SURGICAL CASE
CLINICAL COURSE OF CASE Y.K(38W, 2,500g, MALE)

Fig. 12-15　Typical clinical course of a patient requiring surgical ligation of a PDA.

12—6　Coarctation of the Aorta (Case 74, 9-month-old female)

○ P.191

The great majority of coarctations in infants are usually associated with other cardiac anomalies, as coarctation complexes, and so it is very important to check for associated lesions. **Case 74** is a moderate case of coarctation with a small PDA, so that clinically differential cyanosis was not seen (Fig. 12-16). The coarctation, 3 mm in diameter, can be observed by the parasternal approach on the postero-lateral aspect of the descending aorta just distal to the left subclavian artery. In this view the anatomical relationship between the PDA and the pre-ductal coarctation can be clearly appreciated (**Case 74, A**). The color flow mapping B-mode depicts the stenotic jet flow through the coarctation as a mosaic pattern (**Case 74, B**) and the peak velocity in systole was 3.2 m/sec with CW Doppler (**Case 74, C**). **Case 74, D, E**, and **F** demonstrate postoperative echo evaluation of the reconstructed descending aorta two weeks after subclavian flap aortoplasty. No residual stenosis was found in the 2-D echocardiogram (**Case 74, E**), and no stenotic jet flow was seen with 2-D Doppler (**Case 74, F**). Pulsed Doppler spectral analysis demonstrated a laminar blood flow pattern in the descending aorta at a peak velocity of 1.2 m/sec (**Case 74, D**).

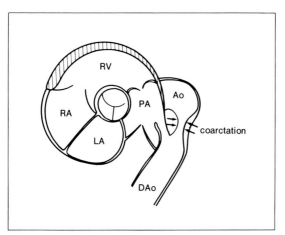

Fig. 12-16　Diagrammatic representation of Case 73, A. In 2-D echo a moderate coarctation and a small PDA are seen.

12—7　Tetralogy of Fallot with Aortic Regurgitation (Case 75, 11-year-old female) (Tab. 12-13)

○ P.192

Fallot's tetralogy can be diagnosed echocardiographically from the presence of a large perimembranous ventricular septal defect, overriding of the aorta (**Case 75, A, B**), and the stenosis of the right ventricular outflow tract or the pulmonary artery or both (**Case 75, F, G**). Two-dimensional Doppler shows that the systolic flow is ejected from both ventricles simultaneously into the aorta (**Case 75, C**). In diastole, the parasternal long-axis view demonstrates aortic regurgitant flow due to associated aortic insufficiency passing through the aortic valve into both ventricles (**Case 75, D**). The flow mapping M-mode and pulsed Doppler spectral analysis demonstrate the typical turbulent pattern of an aortic regurgitant jet (**Case 75, E**). The severity of symptoms of the tetralogy of Fallot will depend on the severity of the right ventricular outflow obstruction. **Case 75, G** demonstrates a typical infundibular pulmonary stenosis of the tetralogy of Fallot and the stenotic turbulent jet flow, depicted as a mosaic pattern, is seen in the main pulmonary artery (**Case 75, H**). The peak velocity of the jet flow through the infundibular stenosis was measured with CW Doppler as 4.3 m/sec, which indicates a peak pressure drop of 74 mmHg. However, Doppler measurement often underestimates the pressure drop across the infundibular pulmonary stenosis because the direction of the stenotic jet through the infundibular pulmonary stenosis is almost perpendicular to the Doppler beam in the parasternal view.

The associated aortic insufficiency in **Case 75** is perforation of the non-coronary aortic cusp due to infective endocarditis[38] at the age of 5(**Case 75, J, K**). Catheterization data(Tab. 12-6) shows a left-to-right shunt ratio of 69.3%, but when the aortic regurgitation is taken into account the calculated shunt ratio is unreliable, because the arterial blood regurgitates directly from the aortic root into the right ventricle, as demonstrated by 2-D Doppler (**Case 75, D**).

Tab. 12-13 K. S., 11-year-old female.

	Pressure (mmHg)	Sat. O$_2$(%)
SVC		70.4
IVC		72.5
RA	mean=2.0	72.0
RV	110/0(edp=4.5)	76.5
PA	18/7(mean=12)	90.2
lt PA	24/7(mean=14)	88.6
rt PA	23/5(mean=12)	88.4
LV	115/0(edp=7)	—
Ao(Fem A)	120/60(mean=85)	95.6
	lt → rt shunt ratio	69.3%
	rt → lt shunt ratio	5.5%

12—8 Tetralogy of Fallot with a Gore-Tex Shunt (Case 76, 4-month-old female)

○ P.193

Following a palliative shunt operation, 2-D Doppler is effective not only for the evaluation of the patency of the shunt but also for the evaluation of the increased pulmonary arterial flow supplied through the shunt as opposed to the shunt flow through the PDA. In **Case 76** a Gore-Tex shunt was inserted between the ascending aorta and the right pulmonary artery at the age of 1 month. **Case 76, A** and **D** demonstrate the patency of the Gore-Tex shunt at 3 months. The size of right pulmonary artery is well maintained, and both shunt flows, through the Gore-Tex shunt and through the PDA are depicted in red in the pulmonary trunk and the right pulmonary artery.

12—9 Double Outlet Right Ventricle (DORV) (Case 77, 4-year-old male) (Tab. 12-14)

In cases of double outlet right ventricle, both great arteries arise from the anatomical right ventricle, and the large VSD usually associated with this condition is generally the only outlet of the left ventricle[39-41]. Two-dimensional echocardiography shows both great vessels arising anterior to the interventricular septum and the bulboventricular flange (or conus tissue) between the anterior mitral leaflet and the aorta[40]. However, since it is not in most cases easy to demonstrate the bulboventricular flange, it is more advantageous from the clinical point of view to define DORV so that it covers conditions in which more than 50% of both great arteries arise from the anatomical right ventricle[43]. Although a bi-directional and

◯ P.193
quadriphasic VSD shunt flow pattern is seen in the flow mapping M-mode and pulsed Doppler spectral analysis (**Case 77, B**), the dominant direction of the VSD shunt flow is from left to right (**Case 77, D**). Thus, VSD is the only outflow available to the anatomical left ventricle.

Tab. 12-14 K. W., 4-year-old male.

	Pressure (mmHg)	Sat. O_2(%)
SVC	mean＝4	33.9
IVC	mean＝6.5	57.5
RA	mean＝3	47.7
RV	105 2(edp＝5.5)	45.4
PA	10/6.5(mean＝8.5)	53.3
LA	mean＝4	97.7
LV	110/0(edp＝5)	—
Ao	112/75(mean＝90)	74.4
	lt → rt shunt ratio	18.7%
	rt → lt shunt ratio	42.7%

12−10 Transposition of the Great Arteries (TGA)

◯ P.194
1. TGA Type 1 (Case 78, 1-month-old male) (Tab. 12-15)

In transposition of the great arteries the aorta originates from the anatomic right ventricle and the pulmonary artery originates from the anatomic left ventricle, so that the normal anatomical orientation of the two great arteries is reversed (ventriculo-arterial discordance). In the parasternal long-axis view, the great arteries exhibit a parallel orientation[44,45]. It is essential in a critical case of TGA with severe cyanosis to establish the diagnosis and to evaluate the degree of intracardiac communication between the parallel systemic and pulmonary circulations[46]. With 2-D echocardiography, the size of an interatrial or interventricular communication, or of a PDA, can be evaluated, but it is impossible to evaluate the degree of mixing that takes place between the arterial and venous blood flows through these orifices. The grade of an intracardiac shunt flow can be evaluated with 2-D Doppler from the size of an intracardiac communication. **Case 78, D, F** demonstrate the mixing of the arterial and venous blood flows through the interatrial opening created by balloon atrioseptostomy (BAS). In diastole the direction of the shunt flow is from left to right (**Case 78, C**) and in systole, from right to left (**Case 78, E**) and bi-directional shunt flow can be observed at the point when the shunt direction reverses (**Case 78, D**).

Tab. 12-15 A. T., 1-month-old male.

	BAS 前			BAS 後	
	Pressure (mmHg)	Sat. O_2(%)		Pressure (mmHg)	Sat. O_2(%)
SVC		14.8	SVC		32.2
IVC		23.7	IVC		42.1
RA	mean＝3	25.0	RA	mean＝4	67.1
LA	mean＝4	88.0	LA	mean＝4	85.7
RV	60/5(edp＝7)	40.3	RV	60/5(edp＝7)	65.9
LV	56/4(edp＝4)	96.1	LV	34/1(edp＝5)	82.8
Ao	60/45(mean＝52)	41.1	Ao	60/40(mean＝50)	57.9

Shunt ratro at the atrcal leuel

	lt → rt shunt ratio	22.6%		lt → rt shunt ratio	35.1%
	rt → lt shunt ratio	0 %		rt → lt shunt ratio	23.3%

2. TGA Type 1 (Case 79, female)
Operative balloon atrioseptostomy (age 2 months)
Mustard operation (age 6 months)

◯ P.195
In **Case 79**, balloon atrioseptostomy was first performed at 16 days after birth and the subsequent clinical course was uneventful until the end of the second month. At this point,

there was a rapid advance in the patient's cyanosis as a result of re-narrowing of the interatrial opening, detected with 2-D Doppler. Two dimensional echocardiography failed almost completely to demonstrate the interatrial opening (**Case 79, B**) and 2-D Doppler demonstrated only a very small shunt flow image in the right atrium originating from the center of interatrial septum (**Case 79, C** Fig. 12-17). A second balloon atrioseptostomy was tried at 2 months via both femoral veins, but this failed because the inferior vena cava and both iliac veins were completely occluded after the first operation. Then, an operative attempt was made at a second BAS through the right atrial wall by means of a small thoracotomy using blade and balloon catheters[46-48]. With the assistance of 2-D Doppler echocardiography the catheters were easily introduced through the narrowed interatrial opening into the left atrium (**Case 79, F, G, H** Fig. 12-19). This operation was successful, and created an interatrial opening of sufficient size that permitted a considerable increase of shunt flow (**Case 79, D, E** Fig. 12-18). BAS can be safely performed with the help of 2-D Doppler without the need for bedside fluoroscopy in an intensive care unit or an operating theater.

Subsequently, at 6 months of age, this patient underwent a Mustard operation using an atrial baffle, for the purpose of long-term palliation of the transposition of the great arteries. Two-dimensional echocardiography with or without contrast medium has been utilized to evaluate the efficacy of the procedure and to assess the presence or absence of stenosis in the inflow tracts of the right and left ventricles[49-51]. Two-dimensional echocardiography clearly demonstrates the anatomical structure of the atrial baffle (**Case 79, I**), and contrast echocardiography can show the blood inflow from the inferior vena cava into the left

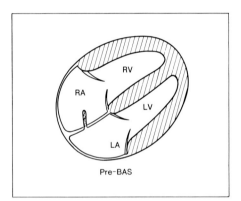

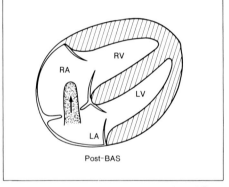

Fig. 12-17 Diagrammatic representation of **Case 79 D**. In 2-D Doppler only a small shunt flow seen owing to the re-narrowing of the interatrial opening (IAO) 2 months after 1st BAS.

Fig. 12-18 Diagrammatic representation of **Case 79, E**. An IAO of considerable size and the shunt flow through IAO are demonstrated in 2-D Doppler.

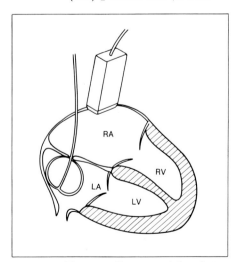

Fig. 12-19 Diagrammatic representation of operative balloon atrioseptostomy.

ventricle (**Case 79, J**). The blood inflow into the left ventricle may also be visualized using 2-D Doppler without contrast material. Two-dimensional Doppler can, moreover, simultaneously indicate the velocity of the flow through the atrial baffle. In cases of stenosis of the inflow tract the color flow pattern makes detection easy. In **Case 79** the blood inflow from both the inferior vena cava (**Case 79, K**) and the superior vena cava (**Case 79, L**) are depicted in a simple red color without aliasing, so that the peak velocities of both inflows are less than 46 cm/sec, which is the maximum detectable velocity without aliasing using a 5 MHz transducer with a pulse repetition frequency of 8 KHz. After palliative surgery, for long-term follow-up, 2-D Doppler in the outpatient clinic is considered to be the most effective diagnostic tool for the pediatric patient.

3. TGA (type 2) with aortic arch interruption (Case 80, 19-day-old male)

Aortic arch interruption rapidly becomes fatal and is often associated with other congenital anomalies. In Case 80 aortic arch interruption is associated with TGA type 2. Before being transferred to our hospital, the patient was intubated with mechanical ventilation support and cardiac resuscitation was performed twice. Two-dimensional echocardiography performed on admission revealed a parallel disposition of the great

○ P.196

arteries, together with a large VSD, 13 mm in diameter (**Case 80, A**). In the aortic arch view, the aortic arch is abruptly terminated just distal to the branch of left subclavian artery (**Case 80, C**), and the large patent ductus arteriosus, smoothly continuous with the descending aorta can also be seen. Two-dimensional Doppler shows no continuity of the blood flow between the aortic arch (♯ 1) and the descending aorta (♯ 2). The flow in the descending aorta is simply supplied through the patent ductus arteriosus (**Case 80, E, F**). Pulsed Doppler spectral analysis demonstrates the bounding pulse pattern of the descending aortic flow with diastolic regurgitation into the pulmonary artery (**Case 80, F**).

As a first step in the surgical palliation of this condition, end-to-end anastomosis of the aorta and pulmonary arterial banding were performed, since the large VSD was considered capable of maintaining the blood mixing between the systemic and pulmonary circulations. However, even after surgery, severe hypoxia persisted with the arterial blood oxygen level at 15% of saturation. Accordingly, the patient was examined again by 2-D Doppler, which demonstrated poor blood mixing through the ventricular septal defect. Balloon atrioseptostomy was then performed in order to obtain better blood mixing between the systemic and

○ P.197

pulmonary circulations with the aid of 2-D Doppler in the intensive care unit (**Case 80, H**)[46-48]. Balloon atrioseptostomy was performed without difficulty using 2-D Doppler, and the excellent results obtained are shown in **Case 80, I, J, K, L, M**, and **N**. The arterial blood oxygen saturation was increased to 87%.

4. TGA Type 1 (Case 81, 14-month-old female) (Tab. 12-16)

After a Jatene operation

In Case 81, a Jatene operation was performed at 12 months using the Lecompte technique[52]. Postoperative cardiac catheterization and 2-D Doppler examination 3 months later demonstrated the successful anastomosis of the switched great arteries. The findings of

○ P.198

2-D Doppler observation of the reconstructed great arteries (**Case 81, C, D**) were fairly compatible with the roentgenographic evaluation (**Case 81, A, B**). Ten months after the Jatene operation, 2-D Doppler demonstrated moderate tricuspid regurgitation (grade 2)

Tab. 12-16 Y. G, 2-year-old female

	Pressure (mmHg)	Sat. O$_2$(%)
SVC	mean=8	61.0
IVC	mean=7.5	56.2
RA	mean=7	54.9
RV	117/0(edp=7)	51.3
PA	117/43(mean=72)	53.5
LV	110/−7(edp=1.5)	94.3
Ao	105/50(mean=72)	92.2

with a peak velocity of 5 m/sec, indicating that the right ventricular pressure was at the systemic level. We lost this patient 18 months after the Jatene operation through postoperative aggravation of pulmonary hypertension with severe right ventricular failure.

5. TGA Type 3 (Case 82, 3-year-old male)

○ P.199

A palliative Mustard operation[53] was performed in **Case 82** at the age of 2 years old. The associated VSD was not closed at this time because of the increasing pulmonary hypertension (pulmonary resistance = 1271 dyne.m^2). The mild pulmonary stenosis present was also left untouched. Two-dimensional Doppler one year after the Mustard operation revealed a bi-directional shunt flow through the untouched VSD, but the major direction of the shunt was from right to left, as displayed in blue from mid-systole (**Case 82, A**) to the end of diastole (**Case 82, C**). A reversal of the right-to-left shunt is seen for a very short period in early systole (**Case 82, D**). The main pulmonary flow in systole appears as a mosaic pattern, and has a peak velocity of 2.5 m/sec as measured with CW Doppler, which indicates a pressure drop of 25 mmHg. No stenosis was seen in the blood inflow through the atrial baffle into the ventricles (**Case 82, E, F**, Fig. 12-20), and the patient's clinical condition was stable.

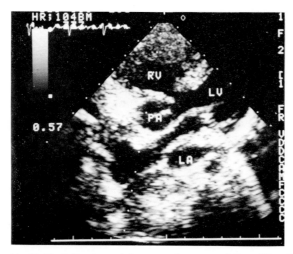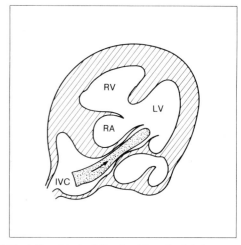

Fig. 12-20 2-D echo and diagrammatic representation of **Case** 82, **E**. The left ventricular inflow tract from the inferior vena cava (IVC) is clearly observed.

12—11 Total Anomalous Pulmonary Venous Connection (TAPVC)

1. TAPVC Supracardiac type[54] (Case 83, 1-year-old male)

Total anomalous pulmonary venous connection is an anomaly in which all the pulmonary veins connect directly to the right atrium or to one of the systemic veins. In about one-third of cases, the pulmonary veins are anomalously connected to the left innominate vein (supracardiac TAPVC)[55]. In this type, a cardiac shadow of a figure-of-eight or snowman-like appearance is one of the diagnostic signs, the upper portion of the shadow being composed of the anomalous vertical vein on the left, the left innominate vein superiorly, and the superior vena cava at the right (**Case 83, A**). In **Case 83**, the parasternal

○ P.200

short-axis view demonstrates the common pulmonary venous chamber (CC), which is connected with the innominate vein (IV) through the vertical vein (VV). By means of several parasternal approaches, the entire abnormal pulmonary circulation can be visualized, as shown in **Case 83, B**. In addition, superior vena cava is enlarged due to the increased venous return flowing to it. The presence of an interatrial opening is essential for maintaining life in TAPVC, and **Case 83** also has a large ASD with diameters of 2.0 and 2.5 cm.

In the corrective surgery for TAPVC, an opening of considerable size between the common chamber and the left atrium is important. Intraoperative epicardial 2-D Doppler demonstrates that a sufficiently large opening was created between the common chamber and the left atrium (**Case 83, C**) as indicated by the * mark, and also demonstrates the non-stenotic blood inflow from the common chamber into the left atrium (**Case 83, F**).

2. TAPVC cardiac type (Case 84, 2-month-old male)

○ P.201

In Darling type 2-a TAPVC[54], all the pulmonary veins join a common chamber which is connected to the coronary sinus in the region of the atrio-ventricular groove. The parasternal long-axis view reveals a common pulmonary chamber behind the left atrium (**Case 84, A**), with a mosaic color pattern within it (**Case 84, B**). When this abnormal mosaic pattern is followed by rotation, tilting and shifting of the transducer, the abnormal drainage of the pulmonary venous flow into the coronary sinus can be seen in the subcostal four-chamber view. The peak velocity of the abnormal pulmonary drainage is 2.0 m/sec, as recorded with pulsed Doppler spectral analysis (**Case 84, F**), which indicated a stenosis in the connection between the pulmonary vein and the common drainage chamber. Also, a moderate tricuspid regurgitation (group 2) with a peak velocity of 3.5 m/sec was found with CW Doppler. The increased velocity of the pulmonary venous flow and the elevated pulmonary arterial pressure are important signs suggesting obstruction of the pulmonary venous drainage.

12—12 Pure Pulmonary Atresia (Case 85, 2-month-old female)

○ P.202

In pure pulmonary atresia or pulmonary atresia with an intact ventricular septum, an infundibular stenosis or atresia is often present, and the right ventricular cavity is often hypoplastic, having a small cavity and a thickened ventricular wall[57,58]. The right ventricular cavity in **Case 85** is so small that it can hardly be seen in the apical four-chamber view (**Case 85, A**). In systole a small area of blue is seen between the hypertrophied trabeculae in the right ventricle (**Case 85, B**) indicating a flow away from the transducer from the right ventricle into the right atrium. A short-axis view at the aortic valve level shows this small cavity in the right ventricular outflow tract, as well as a completely obstructed pulmonary valve in which a swirling flow pattern is seen during isometric contraction (**Case 85, C**). The presence of both an interatrial opening and a patent ductus arteriosus is necessary to sustain life. Balloon atrioseptostomy was performed just after birth. The subcostal four-chamber view reveals a large interatrial opening with a right-to-left shunt in diastole which is depicted in blue (**Case 85, D**, Fig. 12-21). Moderate tricuspid regurgitation is seen in the right atrium in systole (**Case 85, E**), and the to-and-fro flow pattern associated with atrial contraction is seen in the hepatic vein (**Case 85, G**). Opening of the ductus arteriosus

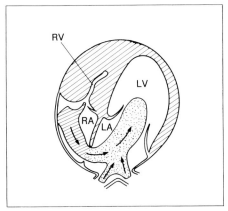

Fig. 12-21 Diagrammatic representation of **Case 85, D**.
2-D Doppler demonstrates the right-to-left shunt flow through the interatrial opening in diastole.

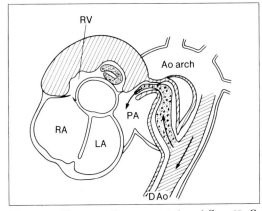

Fig. 12-22 Diagrammatic representation of **Case 85, C, and I**.
The pulmonary artery is completely occluded and a swirling flow is seen in the right ventricular outflow tract. The pulmonary blood flow is supplied by the PDA shunt flow.

is necessary for survival in the neonatal stage and it is maintained with the administration of prostaglandin E1. A parasternal long-axis view of the main pulmonary artery demonstrates the wide opening of the ductus arteriosus (**Case 85, H**) with an obvious shunt flow from the descending aorta (**Case 85, I**, Fig. 12-22). In the neonatal stage, the size of the ductus arteriosus and the amount of flow through it are changeable, and so occasional 2-D Doppler evaluation of the PDA is very important for patient management. At 2 months, 2-D Doppler revealed a rapid reduction of the shunt flow through the PDA, and palliative right ventricular outflow tract reconstruction using a patch was consequently performed. After surgery the right ventricular ejection flow started to supply the pulmonary arterial flow (**Case 85, J, K**), and the enlarged right ventricular cavity can be seen at 40 days after surgery (**Case 85, L, M**). This enlargement indicates growth of the right ventricle after opening of the right ventricular outflow tract.

◯ P.203

12—13 Congenital Valvular Aortic Stenosis (Case 86, 1-month-old male)

◯ P.204

In congenital valvular aortic stenosis, the valve is often bicuspid, with a commissural fusion. The aortic valve ring may be relatively underdeveloped in infants and young children. The parasternal long-axis view demonstrates the typical dome-shaped ballooning of the stenosed valve (**Case 86, A**) and the stenotic jet flow, depicted as a mosaic pattern, is seen in the dilated ascending aorta (**Case 86, D**). The marked thickening of the left ventricular wall is also seen: the thickness in diastole is 6 mm, and that in systole, 9 mm. The peak velocity of the stenotic jet was shown by CW Doppler to be 4 m/sec, which indicates a pressure drop of 64 mmHg between the left ventricle and the aortic root. Other cardiac anomalies are associated with about 20% of congenital valvular aortic stenoses[56], and in **Case 86** a mild mitral regurgitation (grade 1) is seen in systole in the left atrium from the parasternal long-axis view (**Case 86, D**).

12—14 Valvular Pulmonary Stenosis (Case 87, 3-year-old male)

◯ P.204

The prevalence of valvular pulmonary stenosis with an intact ventricular septum is reported in 8 to 10% of all cases of congenital heart disease. The short-axis view at the aortic valve level shows the stenotic pulmonary valve both in systole and diastole. The thickening of the pulmonary valve prevents its full movement to the pulmonary artery wall in systole (**Case 87, A**). From the center of the stenotic pulmonary valve, the jet flow is seen along the anterior wall of the main pulmonary artery in systole (**Case 87, C**). The jet flow then turns at the bifurcation of the left and right pulmonary arteries, forming a swirling flow pattern. The peak velocity of the stenotic jet was found with CW Doppler to be 2 m/sec, representing a pressure drop of 16 mmHg, and leading to a diagnosis of mild valvular pulmonary stenosis (**Case 87, D**).

12—15 Ruptured Valsalva Sinus Aneurysm

1. Rupture of Valsalva sinus aneurysm into right atrium (Konno type 4)[59] (Case 88, 62-year-old male) (Tab. 12-17)

◯ P.205

In some cases of ruptured Valsalva sinus aneurysm, severe congestive heart failure advances very rapidly, often making it difficult to perform cardiac catheterization in the acute stage. In this stage, non-invasive diagnosis using echocardiography, including Doppler echocardiography, has been considered to be the most effective and safest diagnostic approach. According to Konno's classification, **Case 88** is of type 4, since the aneurysm originated from the sinus of Valsalva of the non-coronary aortic cusp and ruptured into the right atrium (**Case 88, A**). On admission the clinical condition of the

Tab. 12-17 O. G., 62-year-old male

	Pressure (mmHg)	Sat. O₂(%)
SVC		69.0
IVC		72.0
RA		85.0
RV	47/−3(edp=3)	90.0
PA	44/15(mean=24)	90.0
LV	105/−5(edp=7)	—
Ao	108/38(mean=60)	97.0
	lt → rt shunt ratio	73.6%

patient was NYHA class 4. Two-dimensional Doppler shows that the shunt flow through the aneurysm is directed toward the center of the right atrium in systole (**Case 88, B**), and that it changes direction in diastole to feed into the right ventricle along the septal leaflet of the tricuspid valve (**Case 88, C**). This directional change of the shunt flow through the aneurysm is also seen in the aortogram (Fig. 12-23, 12-24, 12-25).

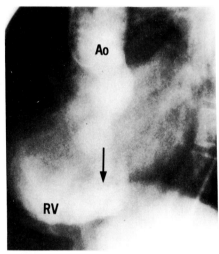

Fig. 12-23 Aortogram in Case 88. The shunt flow through the aneurysm is directed to the right ventricle in diastole.

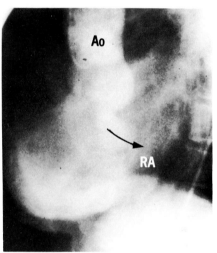

Fig. 12-24 Aortogram in Case 88. The shunt flow through the aneurysm is directed to the right atrium in systole.

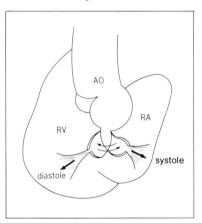

Fig. 12-25 Diagrammatic representation of the aortogram in Case 88 demonstrates changes of the shunt direction in the cardiac cycle.

2. Rupture of Valsalva sinus aneurysm into right ventricle (Konno type 1) with VSD (type 1) and AR (grade 3) (Case 89, 32-year-old male)

Ruptures of Valsalva sinus aneurysms frequently lead to acute symptoms when there is severe aortic valve incompetence. **Case 89** developed very severe congestive heart failure with septicemia due to infective endocarditis after rupture of the aneurysm. The parasternal long-axis view by 2-D echocardiography demonstrates a large Valsalva sinus aneurysm with a perforation 10 mm in diameter in its center (**Case 89, A**). Two-dimensional Doppler

○ P.206

clearly shows a continuous shunt flow through the ruptured aneurysm and the associated aortic regurgitation (grade 3) in the parasternal long-axis view of the left ventricle (**Case 89, B**). The parasternal long-axis view of the right ventricular outflow tract indicates the anatomical orientation of the subpulmonic VSD (type 1) and shows that the aneurysm originated from the right-coronary aortic cusp (**Case 89, C**). **Case 89, D** illustrates the shunt flow pattern of the ruptured aneurysm in diastole, but it is very complicated to analyze. The moderate tricuspid regurgitation also present (grade 2) can be seen in the short-axis view at the aortic valve level.

12—16 Ebstein's Anomaly

1. Ebstein's anomaly with severe tricuspid regurgitation (grade 3) (Case 90, 36-year-old male)

In this anomaly, the septal and posterior leaflets or all leaflets of the tricuspid valve are deformed and arise from the wall of the right ventricle below the normal tricuspid annulus[60-62]. The deformity and displacement of the tricuspid valve leaflets cause various grades of tricuspid regurgitation, as well as right ventricular failure due to the poor functioning of this ventricle.

○ P.207   In **Case 90** the apically displaced septal leaflet and the elongated anterior leaflet tethered to the free wall of the right ventricle are seen in the apical four-chamber view (**Case 90, A**).

Marked incompetence of the tricuspid valve leaflet in systole causes severe tricuspid regurgitation in the atrialized right ventricle and in the right atrium (**Case 90, B**). The large atrialized right ventricle and the severe tricuspid regurgitation associated with the large ASD in **Case 90** can become a cause of severe right ventricular failure with cyanosis in the later stages of life.

2. Ebstein's anomaly with mild tricuspid regurgitation (grade 2) (Case 91, 47-year-old female)

○ P.207   Although the apical displacement of the septal leaflet of tricuspid valve in **Case 91** is of the same grade as **Case 90**, the grade of the elongation of the anterior leaflet and its tethering to the free wall are rather mild. As a result, incompetency of the tricuspid regurgitation is fairly small. In this case, no associated ASD was detected by 2-D Doppler and the patient's condition was fairly good until her present age.

12—17 Hypertrophic Obstructive Cardiomyopathy (Case 92, 78-year-old female)

Hypertrophic obstructive cardiomyopathy (HOCM) is characterized by asymmetrical septal hypertrophy[63,64] of the left ventricular outflow tract and by obstruction of the ejected

○ P.208   systolic blood flow (**Case 92, A, C**). The pattern of the systolic anterior motion of the anterior mitral valve leaflet (SAM)[65,66] is important for M-mode echocardiographic diagnosis (Fig. 12-26), which can indicate the degree of obstruction. The distensibility of the left ventricular wall is markedly impaired, and this diminishes the compliance of the left ventricle[67]. Therefore, in diastole it takes longer in the area of the lesion than in the normal heart to reach the maximum inflow velocity and volume (**Case 92, E**). In early systole, laminar flow towards the aorta is seen in blue, and, in accordance with the degree of muscular protrusion of the septum in mid-systole, it forms a typical turbulent mosaic flow pattern in the left ventricular outflow tract and at the aortic root (**Case 92, C**). CW Doppler demonstrates a gradual, and then a more abrupt, increase in maximal velocity[68] to 3.9 m/sec in systole, representing a pressure drop of 61 mmHg.

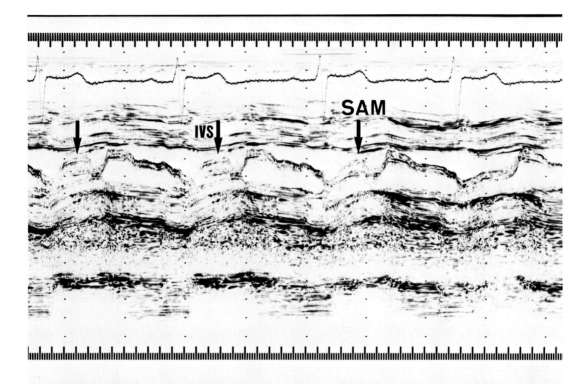

Fig. 12-26 A representative M-mode echocardiographic record of the systolic anterior motion of the anterior mitral valve leaflet (SAM).

References

1) Kyo, S., Omoto, R., Takamoto, S., Ueda, K., Emoto, H., Asano, H., and Yokote, Y. : Real-time two-dimensional Doppler echocardiography (2-D Doppler) in congenital heart disease. Its clinical significance. J. Cardiogr., 14 : 785, 1984.

2) Kyo, S., Takamoto, S., Ueda, K., Emoto, H., Tamura, F., Yokote, Y., and Omoto, R. : Clinical significance of newly developed real-time two-dimensional Doppler echocardiography (2-D Doppler) in congenital heart disease. With special reference to the assessment of intracardiac shunts. Proceedings of the 43rd Meeting of the Japan Society of Ultrasonics in Medicine, 43 : 465, 1983.

3) Kyo, S., Omoto, R., Takamoto, S., and Takanawa, E. : Clinical significance of color flow mapping real-time two-dimensional Doppler echocardiography (2-D Doppler) in congenital heart disease. Circulation, (Suppl. II), 70 : 37, 1984. (Abstract)

4) Kyo, S., Omoto, R., Takamoto, S., and Takanawa, E. : Quantitative estimation of intracardiac shunt flow in atrial septal defect by real-time two-dimensional color flow Doppler. Circulation, (Suppl. II), 70 : 39, 1984. (Abstract)

5) Kyo,S., Omoto, R., Takamoto, S., and Yokote, Y. : Noninvasive analysis of bi-directional multi-phasic intracardiac shunt flow by real-time two-dimensional Doppler echocardiography. Circulation, (Suppl. II), 70 : 365, 1984. (Abstract)

6) Sahn, D.J. : Real-time two-dimensional Doppler echocardiographic flow mapping. Circulation, 71 : 849 1985.

7) Talano, J.V., and Gardin, J.M. : Textbook of two-dimensional echocardiography, N.Y.,Grune & Stratton, 1983.

8) Rice, M.J., Seward, J.B., Hagler, D.J., Mair, D.D., Feldt, R.H., Puga, F.J., Danielson, G.K., William, D.E., and Tajik, A.J. : Impact of 2-dimensional echocardiography on the management of distressed newborns in whom cardiac disease is suspected. Am. J. Cardiol., 51 : 288, 1983.

9) Kyo, S., Takamoto, S., Takanawa, E., Matsumura, M., Yokote, Y., and Omoto, R. : Does color flow mapping Doppler echocardiography allow the cath. lab. to be bypassed in surgery of congenital heart disease ? *In* Color Doppler Flow Imaging. Edited by J. Roelandt. Dordrecht, Martinus Nijhoff Publishers, 1986.

10) Kyo, S., Shime, H., Omoto, R., and Takamoto, S. : Evaluation of intracardiac shunt flow in premature infants by color flow mapping real-time two-dimensional Doppler echo. Circulation, (Suppl. II), 70 : 456, 1984. (Abstract)

11） Takamoto, S., Kyo, S., Adachi, H., Matsumura, M., Yokote, Y., and Omoto, R. : Intraoperative color flow mapping by real-time two-dimensional Doppler echocardiography for evaluation of valvular and congenital heart disease, and vascular disease. J. Thorac. Cardiovasc. Surg., 90 : 802, 1985.

12） Ikeda, Y., Sugawara, M., Homma, M., Atak, Y., Bando, M., Sudo, H., Ono, H., Miura, M., and Kanazawa, T. : A study of shunt flow in atrial septal defect using pulsed Doppler echocardiography and contrast echocardiography. Proceedings of the 42 nd Meeting of the Japan Society of Ultrasonics in Medicine, 42 : 473, 1983.

13） Nakamura, Y., Suzuki, S.,Sasaki, T., Miyazawa, S., and Arai, T. : A study of shunt flows on atrial septal defect with use of the ultrasonic pulsed Doppler echocardiography. Proceedings of the 41 st Meeting of the Japan Society of Ultrasonics in Medicine : 737, 1982.

14） Murata, M., Kyo, S., Asano, H., Adachi, H., Takamoto, S., Yokote, Y., and Omoto, R. : 2-D Doppler evaluation for residual mitral and/or tricuspid regurgitation after surgery in the case of advanced atrial septal defect (ASD). Proceedings of the 45th Meeting of the Japan Society of Ultrasonics in Medicine : 229, 1984.

15） Kronik, G., Slany, J., and Moesslacher, H. : Contrast M-mode echocardiography in diagnosis of atrial septal defect in acyanotic patients. Circulation, 59 : 372, 1979.

16） Lange, L.W., Sahn, D.J., Allen, H.D., and Goldberg, S.J. : Subxyphoid cross-sectional echo cardiography in infants and children with congenital heart disease. Circulation, 59 : 513, 1979.

17） Shub, C., Dimopoulos, I.N., Seward, J.B., Callahan, J.A., Tancredi, R.G., Schattenberg, T.T., Reeder, G.S., Hagler, D.J., and Tajik, A.J. : Sensitivity of two-dimensional echocardiography in the direct visualization of atrial septal defect utilizing the subcostal approach : experience with 154 patients. J. Am. Coll. Cardiol., 2 : 127, 1983.

18） Hanrathe, P., Schluter, M., Langenstein, B.A., Polster, J., Engel, S., Kremer, P., and Krebber, H.J. : Detection of ostium secundum atrial septal defects by transoesophageal cross- sectional echocardiography. Br. Heart J., 49 : 350, 1983.

19） Isaji, F. : Diagnosis of atrial septal defect (secundum type) with transesophageal echocardiography : special reference to size and type of ASD. J. Jpn. Assoc. Thorac. Surg., 32 : 37, 1984.

20） Valdes-Cruz, L.M., Pieroni, D.R., Roland, J.M.A., and Shematek, J.P. : Recognition of residual postoperative shunts by contrast echocardiographic technique. Circulation, 55 : 148, 1977.

21） Santoso, T., Meltzer, R.S., Castellanos, S., Serruys, P.W., and Roelandt, J. : Contrast echocardiographic shunts may persist after atrial septal defect repair. Eur. Heart J., 4 : 129, 1983.

22） Kutcher, M.A., King, B.B., Alimurung, B.N., Craver, J.M., and Logue, R.B. : Constrictive pericarditis as a complication of cardiac surgery : Recognition of an entity. Am. J. Cardiol., 50 : 742, 1982.

23） Cohen, M.V., and Greenberg, M.A. : Constrictive pericarditis : Early and late complication of cardiac surgery. Am. J. Cardiol., 43 : 657, 1979.

24） Nasser, F.N., Tajik, A.J., Seward, J.B., and Hagler, D.J. : Diagnosis of sinus venosus atrial septal defect by two- dimensional echocardiography. Mayo Clin. Proc., 56 : 568, 1981.

25） Kirklin,J.W., Harshbarger, H. G., Donald, D.E., and Edwards, J.E. : Surgical correction of ventricular septal defect : Anatomic and technical consideration. J. Thorac. Cardiaovasc. Surg., 33 : 45, 1957.

26） Becker, A.E., and Anderson, R.H. : Pathology of congenital heart disease. London, Butterworths, 1981.

27） Stevenson, J.G., Kawabori, I., Dooley, T., and Guntheroth, W.G. : Diagnosis of ventricular septal defect by pulsed Doppler echocardiography : Sensitivity, specificity and limitations. Circulation, 58 : 322, 1978.

28） Miura, K., Katoh, K., Hirosawa, K., Katabami, T., Yoshikawa, Y., Matsumura, M., Kyo, S., and Omoto, R. : Processing of color Doppler information on 2-D Doppler echography system. Proceedings of the 48th Meeting of the Japan Society of Ultrasonics in Medicine : 613, 1986.

29） Rein, J.G., Freed, M.D., Norwood, W.I., and Castaneda, A.R. : Early and late results of closure of ventricular septal defect in infancy. Ann. Thorac. Surg., 24 : 19, 1977.

30） Roberts, W.C., and Buchbinder, N.A. : Right-sided infective endocarditis. Am. J. Med., 53 : 7, 1972.

31） Corone, P., Doyan, F., Gaudeau, S., Guerin, F., Vernant, P., Ducam, H., Rumeau-Rouquette, C., and Gaudeul, P. : Natural history of ventricular septal defect : A study involving 790 cases. Circulation, 55 : 908, 1977.

32) Agathangelou, N.E., Santos, L.A.D., and Lewis, B.S. : Real- time 2-dimensional echocardiographic imaging of right-sided cardiac vegetations in ventricular septal defect. Am. J. Cardiol., 52 : 420, 1983.

33) Muller, W.H., Jr., and Dammann,J.F. : The treatment of certain congenital malformation of the heart by the creation of pulmonic stenosis to reduce pulmonary hypertension and excessive pulmonary blood flow. Surg. Gynecol, Obstet., 95 : 213, 1952.

34) Waldhausen, J.A., and Nahrwold, D.L. : Repair of coarctation of the aorta with a subclavian flap. J. Thorac. Cardiovasc. Surg., 51 : 533, 1966.

35) Bhat, R., Raju, T.N.K., and Vidyasagar, D. : Patent ductus arteriosus : Recent advances in diagnosis and management. Ped. Cli. Nor. Am., 29 : 1117, 1982.

36) Shime, H., Kyo,S., Omoto,R., Takanawa, E., Kobayashi, T., and Miyaji, T. : Clinical significance of real-time two- dimensional Doppler echocardiography (2-D Doppler) in premature infants. Proceedings of the 44 rd Meeting of the Japan Society of Ultrasonics in Medicine : 283, 1984.

37) Bunning, R., and Barth, W.F : Sulindac : Apotentially renal-sparing nonsteroidel anti-inflammatory drug. J.A.M.A., 248 : 2864, 1982.

38) Emanuel, R., Somerville, J., Prusty, S., and Ross, D.N. : Aortic regurgitation from infective endocarditis in Fallot's tetralogy and pulmonary atresia. Br. Heart J., 37 : 365, 1975.

39) DiSessa, T.G., Hagan, A.D., Pope, C., Samtoy, L., and Friedman, W.F. : Two-dimensional echocardiographic characteristics of double outlet right ventricle. Am. J. Cardiol., 44 : 1146, 1979.

40) Yeh, H.C., Wolf, B.S., Steinfield, L., and Baron, M.G. : Echo cardiography of double outlet right ventricle : new diagnostic criteria. Radiology, 123 : 435, 1977.

41) Hagler, D.J., Tajik, A.J., Seward, J.B., Mair, D.D., and Ritter, D.G. : Double-outlet right ventricle : wide-angle two- dimensional echocardiographic observations. Circulation, 63 : 419, 1981.

42) Henry, W.L., Maron, B.J., Griffith, M., Redwood, D.R., and Epstein, S.F. : Differential diagnosis of anomalies of the great arteries by real-time two-dimensional echocardiography. Circulation, 51 : 283, 1975.

43) Anderson, R.H., Allwork, S.P., Ho, S.Y., Lenox, C.C., and Zuberbuhler, J.R. : Surgical anatomy of tetralogy of Fallot. J. Thorac. Cardiovasc. Surg., 81 : 887, 1981.

44) Daskalopoulos, D.A., Edwards, W.D., Driscoll, D.J., Seward, J.B., Tajik, A.J., and Hagler, D.J. : Correlation of two- dimensional echocardiographic and autopsy findings in complete transposition of the great arteries. J. Am. Coll. Cardiol., 2 : 1151, 1983.

45) Houston, A.B., Gregory, N.L., and Coleman, E.N. : Echocardiographic identification of aorta and main pulmonary artery in complete transposition. Br. Heart J., 40 : 377,1978.

46) Kyo, S., Omoto, R., Takamoto, S., Yokote, Y., and Takanawa, E. : Echo guide balloon atrioseptostomy by color flow mapping real-time two-dimensional Doppler echo. J. Am. Coll. Cardiol., 5 : 453, 1985. (Abstract)

47) Perry, L.W., Ruckman, R.N., Galioto, F.M., Jr., Shapiro, S.R., Potter, B.M., and Scott, L.P.III : Echocardiographically assisted balloon atrial septostomy. Pediatrics, 70 : 403, 1982.

48) Allan, L.D., Leanage, R., Wainwright, R., Joseph, M.C., and Tynan, M. : Balloon atrial septostomy under two dimensional echocardiographic control. Br. Heart J., 47 : 41, 1982.

49) Thompson, K., and Serwer, G.A. : Echocardiographic features of patients with and without residual defects after Mustard's procedure for transposition of the great vessels. Circulation, 64 : 1032, 1981.

50) Silverman, N.H., Snider, R., Colo, J., Ebert, P.A., and Turley, K. : Superior vena caval obstruction after Mustard's operation : detection by two-dimensional contrast echocardiography. Circulation, 64 : 392, 1981.

51) Aziz, ., Paul, M.H., Bharati, S., Cole, R.B., Muster, A.J., lev, M., and Idriss, F.S. : Towdimensional echocardiographic evaluation of Mustard operation for D-transposition of the great arteries. Am. J. Cardiol., 47 : 654, 1981.

52) Lecompte, Y., Neveux, J.Y., Leca, F., Zannini, L., Tran Viet, T., Duboys, Y., and Jarreau, M.M. : Reconstruction of the pulmonary outflow tract without prosthetic conduit. J Thorac. Cardiovasc. Surg., 84 : 727, 1982.

53) Mair, D.D., Ritter, D.J., Danielson, G.K., Wallace, R.B., and McGoon, D.C. : The palliative Mustard operation : Rationale and results. Am. J. Cardiol., 37 : 762, 1976.

54) Darling, R.C., Rothney, W.B., and Craig, J.M. : Total pulmonary venous drainage into the right side of the heart : report of 17 autopsied cases not associated with other major cardiovascular anomalies. Lab. Invest., 6 : 44, 1957.

55) Burroughs, J.T., and Edwards, J.E. : Total anomalous pulmonary venous connection. Am. Heart J. 59 : 913,1960.

56) Braunwald, E., Goldblatt, A., Aygen, M.M., Rockoff, S.D., and Morrow, A.G. : Congenital aortic stenosis, clinical and hemodynamic findings in 100 patients. Circulation, 27 : 426, 1963.

57) Morgan, B.C., Stacy, G.S., and Dillard, D.H. : Pulmonary valvular and infundibular atresia with intact ventricular septum. Am. J. Cardiol., 16 : 246, 1965.

58) Kirklin, J.W., and Barratt-Boyes, B.G. : In Cardiac Surgery, page 844, N.Y., John Willey & Sons, 1986.

59) Sakakibara, S., and Konno, S. : Congenital aneurysm of the sinus of Valsalva : anatomy and classification. Am. heart J., 63 : 405, 1962.

60) Giuliani, E.R., Fuster, V., Brandenburg, R.O., and Mair, D.D. : Ebstein's anomaly : the clinical features and natural history of Ebstein's anomaly of tricuspid valve. Mayo Clin. Proc., 54 : 163, 1979.

61) Daniel, W., Rathsack, P., Walpurger, G., Kahle, A., Gisbertz, R., Schmitz, J., and Lichtlen, P.R. : Value of M-mode echocardiography for non-invasive diagnosis of Ebstein's anomaly. Br. Heart J., 43 : 38, 1980.

62) Gussenhoven, W.J., Spitaels, S.F.C., Bom, N., and Becker, A.E. : Echocardiographic criteria for Ebstein's anomaly of tricuspid valve. Br. Heart J., 43 : 31, 1980.

63) Henry, W.L., Clark, C.E., and Epstein, S.E. : A symmetric septal hypertrophy : the unifying link in IHSS disease spectrum : observation regarding its pathogenesis, pathophysiology, and course. Circulation, 47 : 827, 1973

64) Henry, W.L., Clark, C.E., Roberts, W.C., Morrow, A.G., and Epstein, S.E. : Differnce in distribution of myocardial abnormalities in patients with obstructive and non- obstructive asymmetric septal hypertrophy (ASH) : echocardiographic and gross anatomic findings. Circulation, 50 : 477, 1974.

65) King, J.F., Demaria, A.N., Reis, R.L., Bolton, M.R., Dunn, M.I., and Mason, D.T. : Echocardiaographic assessment of idiopathic hypertrophic subaortic stenosis. Chest, 64 : 723, 1973.

66) Popp, R.L., and Harrison, D.C. : Ultrasound in the diagnosis and evaluation of therapy of idiopathic hypertrophic subaortic stenosis. Circulation, 40 : 905, 1969.

67) Sanderson, J.E., Traill, T.A., St. John Sutton, M.G., Brown, D.J., Gibson, D.G., and Goodwin, J.F. : Left ventricular relaxation and filling in hypertrophic cardiomyopathy : an echocardiographic study. Br. Heart J., 40 : 596, 1978.

68) Hatle, L., and Angelsen, B. : In Doppler Ultrasound in Cardiology, page 207, Philadelphia, Lea & Febiger, 1985.

Case 56 ASD (secundum type) 8-year-old male

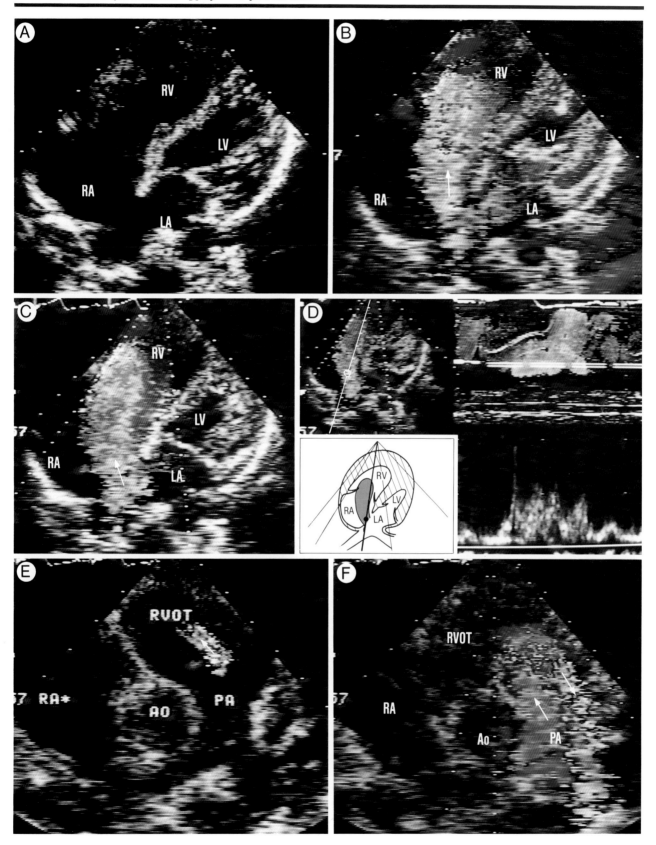

2-D Doppler images in ASD.

ⒶⒷⒸ Apical four-chamber view demonstrates the atrial septal detect Ⓐ and the ASD shunt flow through the defect with the normal left atrial blood flow Ⓑ. Tilting the transducer the ASD shunt flow is more clearly seen Ⓒ. Ⓓ Flow Mapping M-mode and spectral analysis demonstrate the "four peak" turbulent ASD shunt flow pattern. **ⒺⒻ** Short-axis view at the aortic valve level demonstrates the pulmonary regurgitant flow in diastole Ⓔ and the turbulent ejection flow in systole Ⓕ.

Case 57 ASD (secundum type) + MR (grade 2) + TR (grade 1) + Pulmonary Hypertension 52-year-old female

2-D Doppler Images in ASD accompanied with advanced pulmonary hypertension.
A B C Apical four-chamber view demonstrates the large atrial septal defect **A**, the ASD shunt flow through the defect in diastole **B**, and the moderate mitral regurgitation (grade 2) and the mild tricuspid regurgitation (grade 1) in systole. **D E F G** Subcostal four-chamber view more clearly demonstrates the bi-directional and bi-phasic ASD shunt flow pattern. The left to right shunt flow is depicted with red color in diastole **D**, the right to left shunt flow is depicted with blue color in the early systole **E**, and the bi-directional shunt flow is observed simultaneously at the end of diastole **F**. Flow Mapping M-mode demonstrates the bi-directional and bi-phasic shunt flow pattern **G**.

Case 58   ASD (secundum type)   52-year-old female

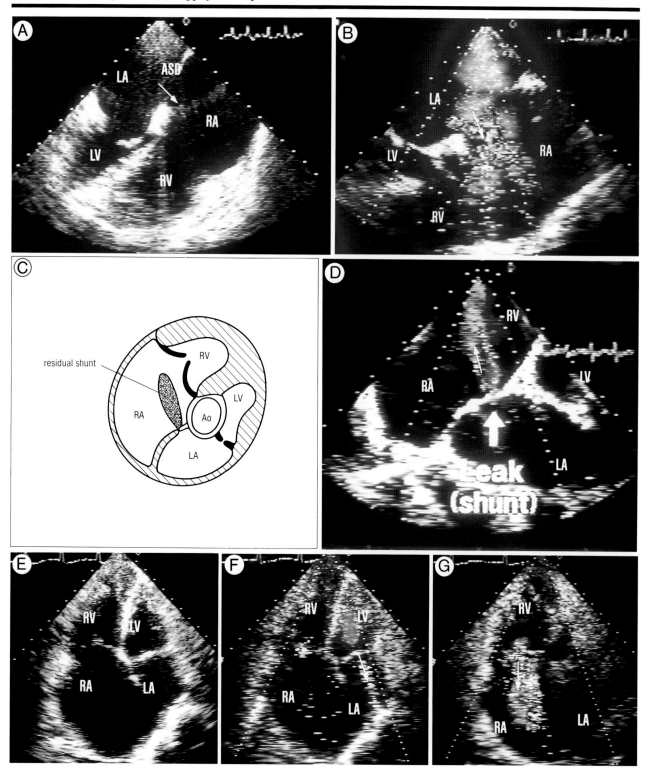

Preoperative 2-D Doppler transesophageal diagnosis and intra-and post-operative 2-D Doppler evaluation.
Ⓐ Ⓑ Transesophageal four-chamber view demonstrates the atrial septal defect **Ⓐ** and the ASD shunt flow through the defect. **Ⓒ**
Ⓓ Intra-operative epicardial evaluation demonstrates the mild residual shunt flow through the suture line of the defect **Ⓓ** and its schematic
diagram **Ⓒ**. **Ⓔ Ⓕ Ⓖ** This case has developed post-operative constrictive pericarditis 3 months after surgery. Apical four-chamber view
demonstrates the impaired distensibility in two ventricles in diastole **Ⓔ**, and the moderate mitral **Ⓕ** (grade 2) and tricuspid regurgitation **Ⓖ** (grade
2) in systole.

180

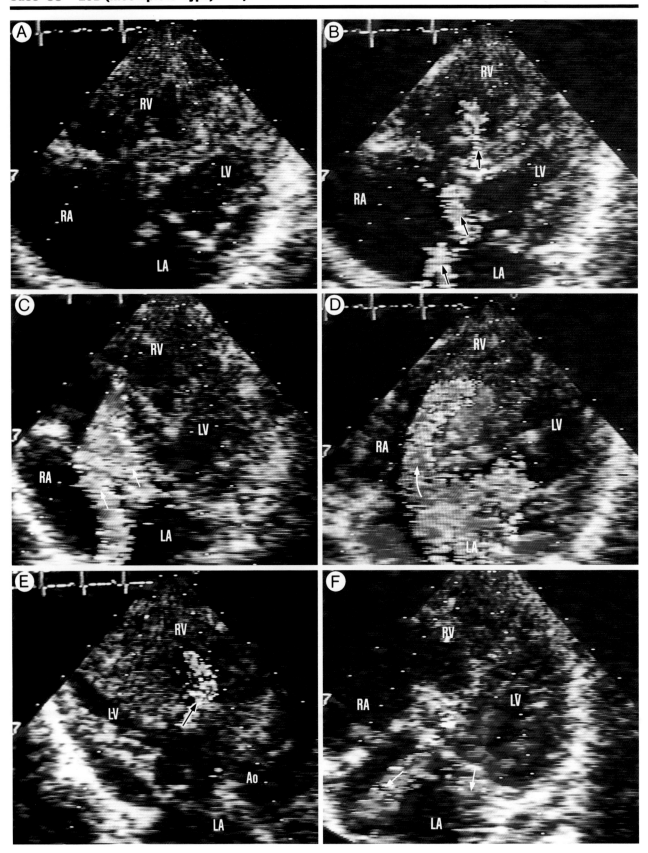

2-D Doppler images in ECD (incomplete type).

ABCDF Apical four-chamber view demonstrates the two channels of ASD shunt flow though the primum and secundum ASD **BC** and the small VSD shunt flow **B** in early diastole. The two channels of ASD shunt flow cannot be differentiated clearly in the middle of diastole **D**. Also the apical four-chamber view demonstrates the moderate mitral regurgitation (grade 2) in systole **F**. To detect these three septal defects is not easy in the apical-four chamber view of 2 DE. **E** Parasternal long-axis view also demonstrates the small VSD shunt flow in systole.

Case 60　ECD (incomplete type)　36-year-old male

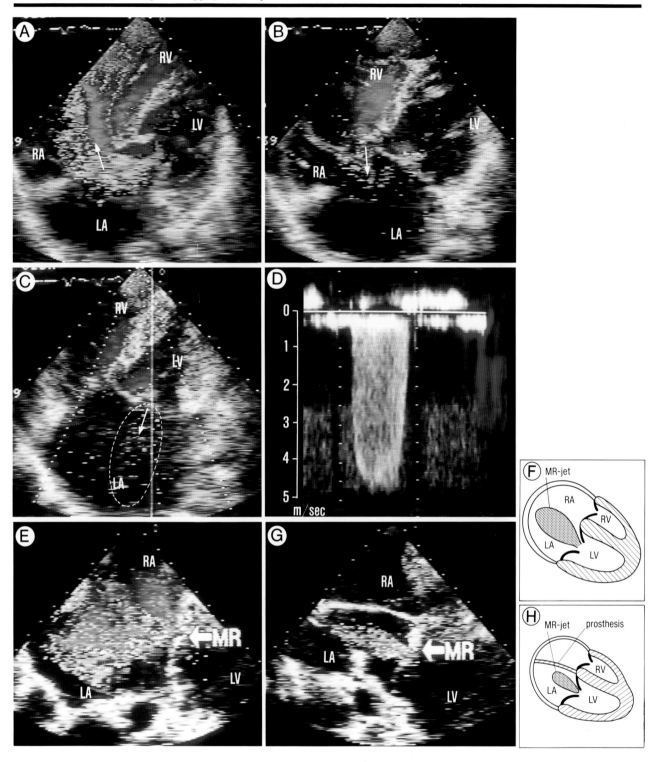

2-D Doppler images in ECD (incomplete type).
A B C D Apical four-chamber view demonstrates the shunt flow through the primum ASD in diastole **A**, the mild tricuspid regurgitation(grade 1) **B**, and the severe mitral regurgitation　(grade 3)　**C** as indicated by the dotted line. Although CW Doppler demonstrates the definite presence of the mitral regurgitation **D**, in some cases with the cardiomegaly the mitral regurgitation located in the deeper area of the scanning field may be underestimated as to grade by standard precordial echo with normal gain adjustment **C**. **E G** Intraoperative epicardial 2-D Doppler is useful for correct evaluation in such a case with cardiomegaly which clearly demonstrates the severe mitral regurgitation　(grade 3)**E**. Intraoperative evaluaton is also effective for confirmation of the result of surgery, after mitral annuloplasty the mitral regurgitation has reduced to grade 1 **F**.

Case 61 ASD (sinus venosus type) 28-year-old female

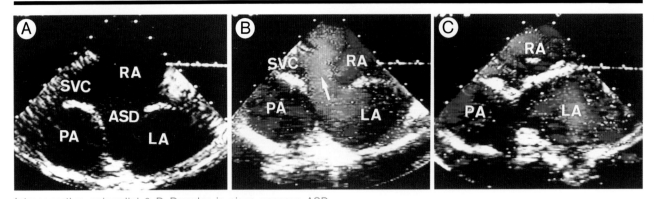

Intraoperative epicardial 2-D Doppler in sinus venosus ASD.
Ⓐ Ⓑ Ⓒ The sinus venosus ASD is often difficult to visualize by transthoracic approach in adults, but intraoperative epicardial echo can clearly visualize the defect **Ⓐ** and the ASD shunt flow through the sinus venosus defect **Ⓑ** surgical result after patch closure can be confirmed **Ⓒ**.

Supplement Correlation between the MSFAI (Maximum Shunt Flow Area Index) and the Shunt Ratio in atrial septal defect (See text pp.153)

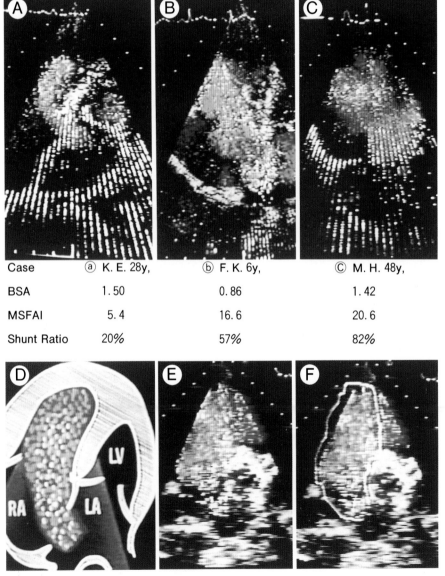

Case	ⓐ K. E. 28y,	ⓑ F. K. 6y,	ⓒ M. H. 48y,
BSA	1. 50	0. 86	1. 42
MSFAI	5. 4	16. 6	20. 6
Shunt Ratio	20%	57%	82%

Supplement   Correlation between the MSFAI (Maximum Shunt Flow Area Index) and the Shunt Ratio in atrial septal defect. (See text pp. 153).
Ⓐ Ⓑ Ⓒ The maximum shunt flow area (MSFA) of the visualized ASD shunt flow image in apical or parasternal four-chamber view correlates with the grade of shunt flow volume through the ASD. To normalize the body size we use the maximum shunt flow area index (MSFAI) which can correlate the shunt ratio of ASD ($\gamma=0. 86$). **Ⓐ** The mild ASD shunt flow. **Ⓑ** The moderate ASD shunt flow. **Ⓒ** The severe ASD shunt flow. MSFAI =MSFA/BSA ; BSA=Body Surface Area. **Ⓓ Ⓔ Ⓕ** Measurement of MSFA using the caliper system of the scanner.

Case 62 VSD (Kirklin type II) 1-year-old male

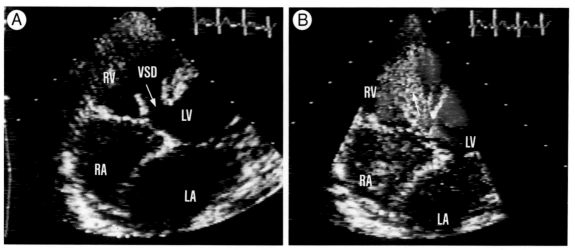

2-D Doppler images in perimembranous VSD.

A B Apical four-chamber view demonstrates the typical perimembranous ventricular septal defect (Kirklin type II) just below the septal leaflet of the tricuspid valve **A**, and the shunt flow through the defect is depicted with a typical mosaic pattern **B**.

Case 63 VSD (Kirklin type II +III) with Pulmonary Hypertension 4-year-old female

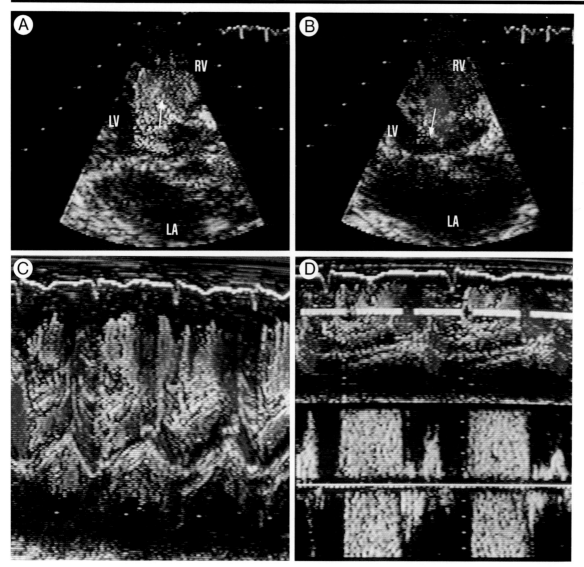

A B Parasternal long-axis view demonstrates the large ventricular septal defect extending from the perimembranous area to the RV inflow area. The shunt flow is depicted with a simple red color in systole **A** and blue color in the short period of early diastole **B**. This color pattern and the bi-directional VSD shunt flow pattern indicate the increased right ventricular pressure. Color Flow Mapping M-mode **C** and pulsed Doppler **D** also demonstrate the bi-directional shunt flow pattern of VSD with pulmonary hypertension.

184

Case 64 VSD (perimembranous outlet type) 1-year-old male

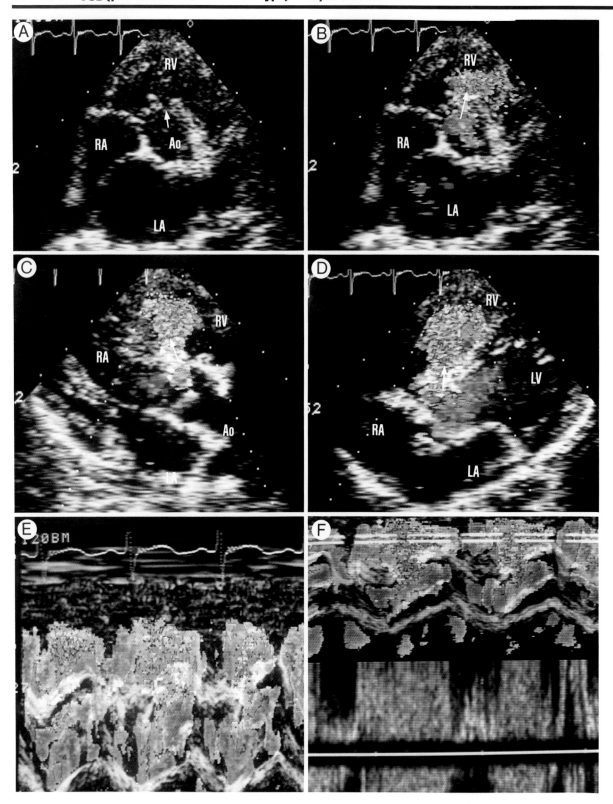

2-D Doppler images in perimembranous outlet type VSD.
A B Short-axis view at the aortic valve level demonstrates the perimembranous outlet type defect of ventricular septum **A** and the mosaic color pattern of VSD shunt flow through the defect **B**. **C D** The mosaic color flow pattern and the ventricular septal defect are also observed in the parasternal long-axis view **C** and in the apical four-chamber view **D**. **E F** Color Flow Mapping M-mode and pulsed Doppler of the VSD shunt flow also demonstrate the mosaic color pattern **E** and the bi-directional and wide-band pattern **F**.

185

Case 65   VSD in Premature Infant (Kirklin type II)   40-day-old 2350g male

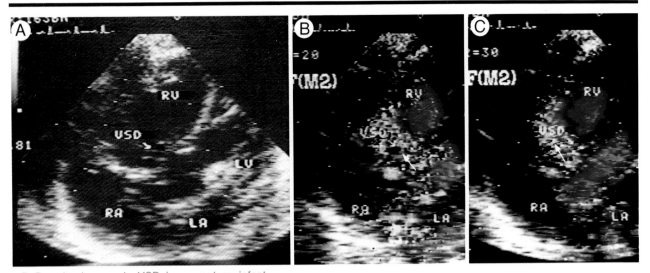

2-D Doppler images in VSD in premature infant.
Ⓐ Ⓑ Ⓒ Apical four-chamber view demonstrates the perimembranous ventricular septal defect Ⓐ and the shunt flow through the defect Ⓑ Ⓒ in premature infant using 5 MHz transducer. The color flow image of shunt flow is more clearly visualized in the scan with 30 frame rate (FR) and 12 KHz pulse repetition frequency (PRF) Ⓒ than in the scan with 20 FR and 8 KHz PRF Ⓑ.

Case 66   VSD with Eisenmenger Syndrome   20-year-old male

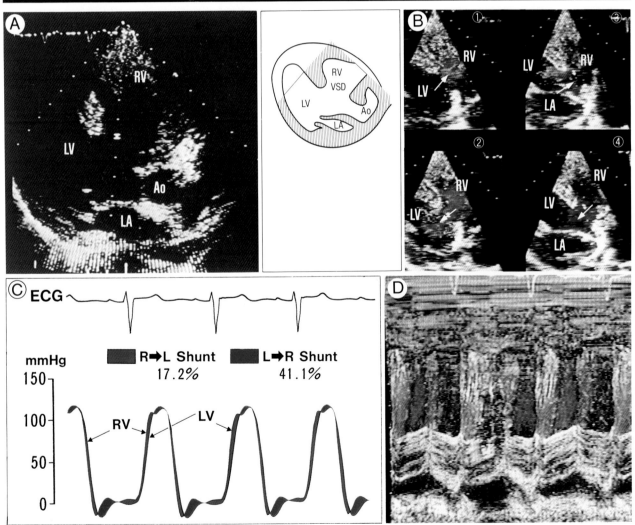

Ⓐ Ⓑ Parasternal long-axis view demonstrates the large ventricular septal defect Ⓐ and the quadriphasic shunt flow pattern through the defect Ⓑ : ① The flow towards the prensaducer in early systole, ② The flow away from the transducer in late systole, ③ The flow towards the transducer in early diastole, ④ The flow away from the transducer in late diastole. Ⓒ The simultaneous record of left ventricular and right ventricular pressure demonstrates four inversions in one cardiac cycle which is compatible with the quadriphasic VSD shunt flow pattern in Flow Mapping B-mode Ⓑ and M-mode Ⓒ. Ⓓ Flow Mapping M-mode also demonstrates the quadriphasic VSD shunt flow pattern in Eisenmenger syndrome.

Case 67   Residual VSD after Surgery in Tetralogy of Fallot   34-year-old male

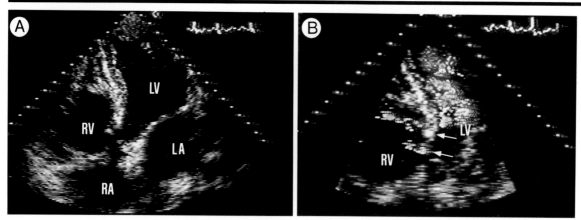

2-D Doppler images in residual VSD.
Ⓐ Ⓑ Apical four chamber view of 2 DE fails to demonstrates the small dehiscences around the Teflon patch closing the ventricular septal defect Ⓐ, but the apical four-chamber view of 2-D Doppler clearly demonstrates the two streams of leakage around the Teflon patch Ⓑ.

Case 68   Infective Endocarditis as a complication of Small VSD   17-year-old male

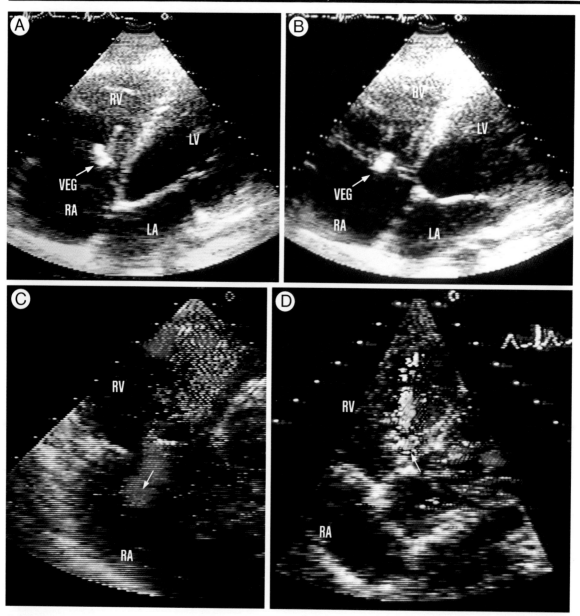

Ⓐ Ⓑ Ⓒ Ⓓ Apical four-chamber view demonstrates the vegetation (VGE) in the septal leaflet of tricuspid valve in diastole Ⓐ and systole Ⓑ. Color Flow Mapping demonstrates the associated mild tricuspid regurgitation (grade 2) Ⓒ and the small shunt flow through the ventricular septal defect which is not easy to be detected by 2 DE.

Case 69　VSD with Infundibular Pulmonary Stenosis　1-month-old male

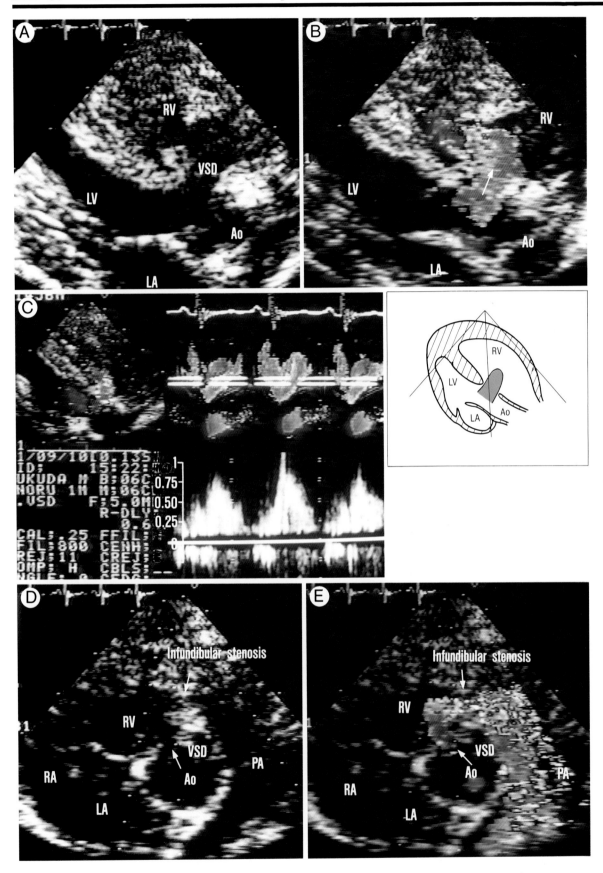

2-D Doppler images in VSD with infundibular PS.
A B Parasternal long-axis view demonstrates the large perimembranous ventricular septal defect **A** and the shunt flow through the defect **B**. However, color flow pattern is not the typical mosaic pattern but a simple red color **B**. **C** Color Flow Mapping M-mode and pulsed Doppler demonstrate the low velocity of the VSD shunt flow : The peak velocity of VSD shunt flow is 75 cm/sec. **D E** Short-axis view at the aortic valve level demonstrates the severe infundibular stenosis **D** and the stenotic jet flow is depicted as a mosaic pattern in the right ventricular outflow tract in systole **E**.

188

Case 70 VSD with Pulmonary Hypertension, after Pulmonary Arterial Banding Surgery 1-year-old female

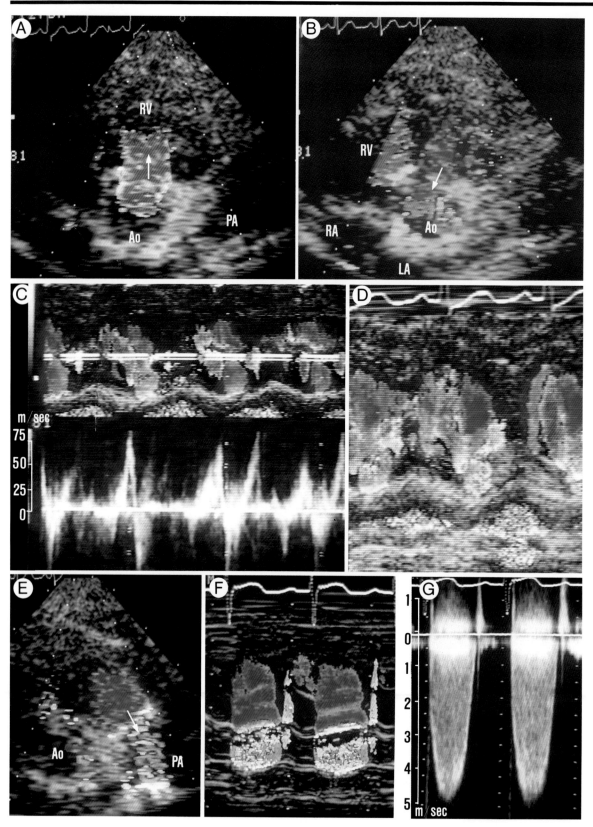

2-D Doppler images in VSD with pulmonary hypertension after palliative surgery (PA-banding).
Ⓐ Ⓑ Short-axis view at the aortic valve level demonstrates the subpulmonary ventricular septal defect (Kirklin type Ⅰ) and the VSD shunt flow depicted with simple red and blue color **Ⓐ Ⓑ**. **Ⓒ Ⓓ** Flow Mapping M-mode and pulsed Doppler demonstrate the low velocity of VSD shunt flow (peak velocity=75 cm/sec), and bi-directional and quadriphasic shunt flow pattern. **Ⓔ Ⓕ** Long-axis view of pulmonary artery demonstrates the supra-valvular pulmonary stenosis produced by pulmonary arterial banding surgery and the stenotic jet flow depicted as a mosaic pattern **Ⓔ**. Flow Mapping M-mode demonstrates the mosaic pattern distal to the stenosis **Ⓕ**.
Ⓖ The peak velocity of stenotic jet flow is measured as 5 m/sec by CW Doppler and the pressure gradient across the stenosis is estimated as 100 mmHg.

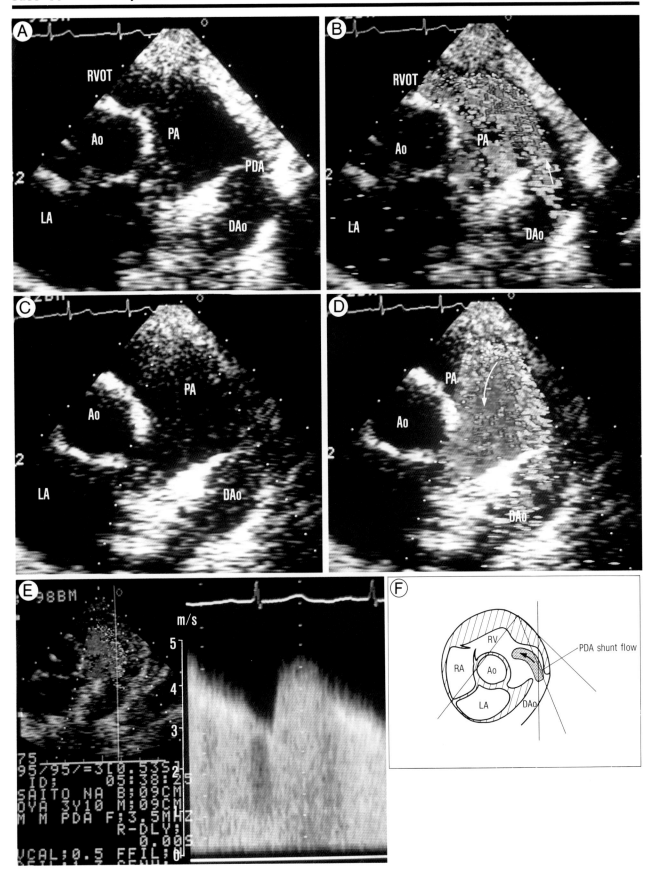

Case 71 **PDA** 4-year-old male

2-D Doppler images in PDA.

A B Short-axis view at the aortic valve level demonstrates the patent ductus arteriosus **A** and the PDA shunt flow depicted with mosaic pattern going upward along the anterior wall of the main pulmonary artery **B**. **C D** Standard short-axis view at the aortic valve level often fails to demonstrate the anatomical structure of patent ductus arteriosus with moderate shunt flow **C**, but the turbulent mosaic color flow pattern is usually demonstrated in the main pulmonary artery **D**. **E** CW Doppler demonstrates the continuous shunt flow pattern of PDA with peak velocity of 4.5 m/sec.

Case 72 PDA in Premature Infant with Patent Foramen Ovale   3-week-old 1450g female

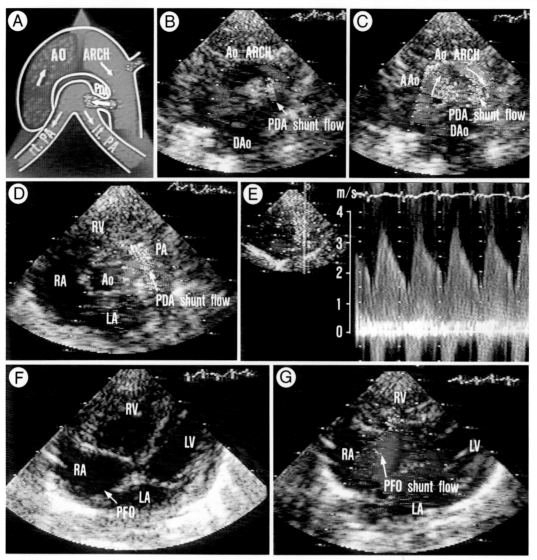

2-D Doppler images in PDA and PFO in premature infant.

A B C Schematic presentation of PDA shunt flow in aortic arch view **A** the flow in the ascending aorta is depicted in red and the flow in the descending aorta is depicted in blue. Aortic arch view demonstrates the PDA shunt flow as a mosaic pattern in both diastole **B** and systole **C**. **D E** Short-axis view at the aortic valve level demonstrates the PDA shunt depicted as a mosaic pattern in the main pulmonary artery **D**, and the continuous shunt flow pattern with a peak velocity of 3.3 m/sec is demonstrated by continuous wave Doppler **E**. **F G** Apical four-chamber view demonstrates the patent foramen ovale (PEO) **F** and the PFO shunt flow depicted with red color **G**.

Case 73 PDA in Premature Infant: Effects of sulindac administration
Pre-administration at 5 days, and post-administration at 13 days ; 1280g male

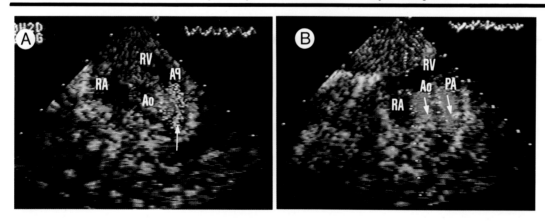

A B Subcostal long-axis view demonstrates the PDA shunt flow as a mosaic pattern in the main pulmonary artery before Sulindac (Prostaglandin antagonist) administration **A**, and no PDA shunt flow is observed after Sulindac administration **B**.

Case 74 Coarctation of Aorta 9-month-old female

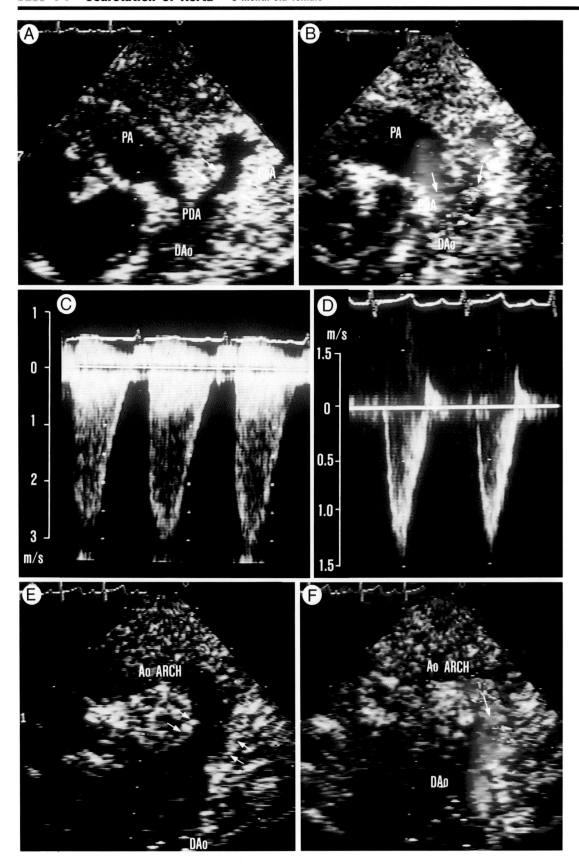

2-D Doppler images in coarctation of aorta.

A B Parasternal view observing the main pulmonary artery and the descending aorta demonstrates the PDA and the stenosis (coarctation) in the proximal descending aorta (DAO) **A**. In systole the stenotic (coarctation) jet flow is depicted as a mosaic pattern in the descending aorta distal to the stenosis **B**. **C D** The velocity of the stenotic jet flow through the coarctation is estimated as 3 m/sec before surgery **C** and as 1. 3 m/sec after surgery **C D**. **E F** The stenosis (coarctation) in the descending aorta has disappeared **E** and almost normal systolic flow pattern has been restored in the descending aorta **F** after subclavian flap aortoplasty.

Case 75　Tetralogy of Fallot with AR (grade 3)　11-year-old female

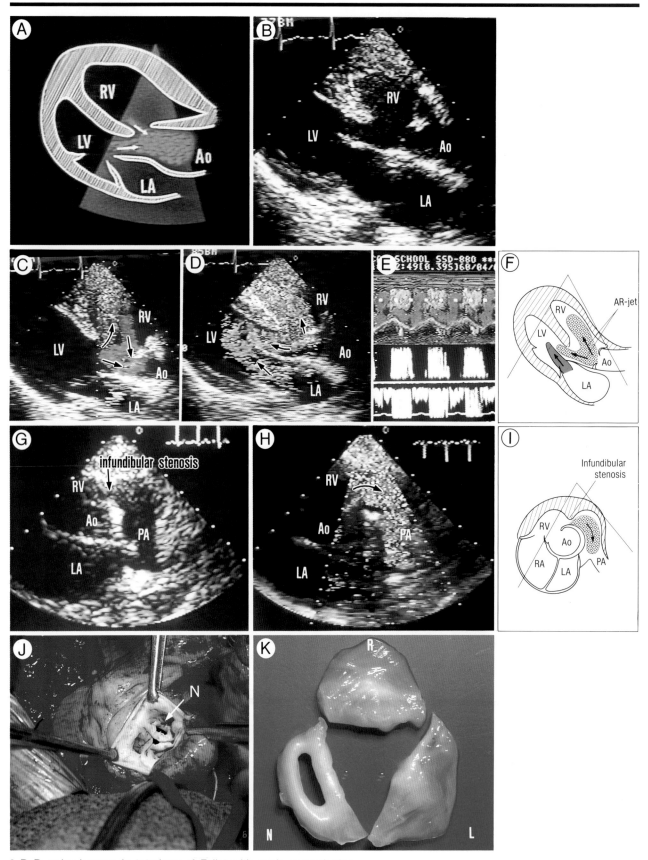

2-D Doppler images in tetralogy of Fallot with aortic regurgitation.
ⒶⒷⒸⒹⒻ The large VSD and the aorta overriding on the interventricular septum are demonstrated in the parasternal long-axis view **Ⓑ**. The systolic aortic flow ejected from the ventricles is depicted with blue color in the parasternal long-axis view **ⒶⒸ**. Parasternal long-axis view in diastole demonstrates the severe aortic regurgitation (grade 3) in the right and left ventricular outflow tracts **ⒹⒻ**. **Ⓔ** Pulsed Doppler in the outflow tract demonstrates the diastolic aortic regurgitant flow signal. **ⒼⒽⒾ** Short-axis view at the aortic valve level demonstrates the infundibular stenosis in the right ventricular outflow tract **Ⓖ** and the stenotic right ventricular ejection flow depicted as a mosaic pattern **ⒽⒾ**. **Ⓙ** **Ⓚ** Intraoperative observation **Ⓙ** and the resected specimen **Ⓚ** of the aortic valve demonstrate the perforation in non-coronary cusp (N) of the aortic valve. N=non-coronary cusp; R=right-coronary cusp; L=left-coronary cusp.

Case 76 Tetralogy of Fallot after Gore-Tex Shunt Surgery 4-month-old female

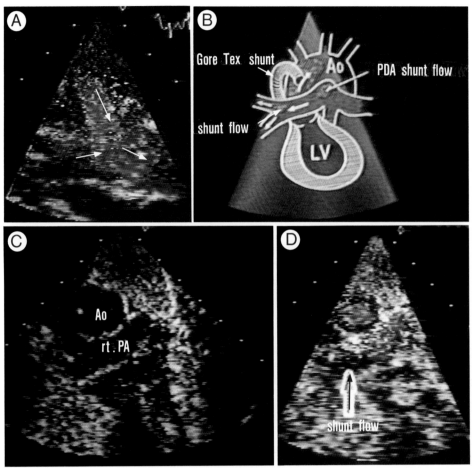

2-D Doppler images in Gore-Tex shunt flow.
Ⓐ Parasternal long-axis view demonstrates the typical blood flow pattern of tetralogy of Fallot, the large VSD and the aorta overriding on the interventricular septum. ⒷⒸ Ⓓ After Gore-Tex shunt between the ascending aorta and the right pulmonary artery Ⓑ the diameter of the right pulmonary artery has increased to 10 mm Ⓒ and the Gore-Tex shunt flow is demonstrated in the distal right pulmonary artery with red color Ⓓ.

Case 77 DORV (Double Outlet Right Ventricle) 4-year-old male

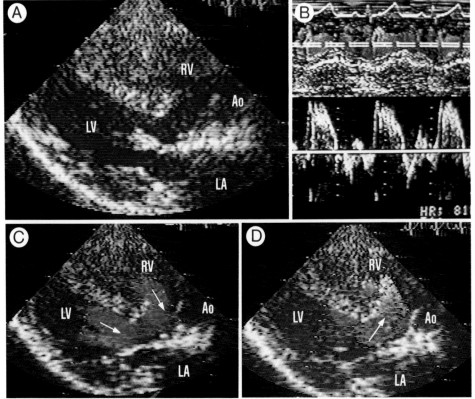

2-D Doppler images in DORV.
ⒶⒸⒹ Parasternal long-axis view demonstrates the aorta overriding more than 50% to the right side on the interventricular septum Ⓐ, the right-to-left shunt flow depicted with blue color in systole Ⓒ and the left-to-right shunt flow depicted with red color in diastole Ⓓ. Ⓑ Color Flow Mapping M-mode and pulsed Doppler demonstrate the bi-directional shunt flow pattern.

Case 78　TGA(Transposition of Great Arteries)(type Ⅰ)　1-month-old male

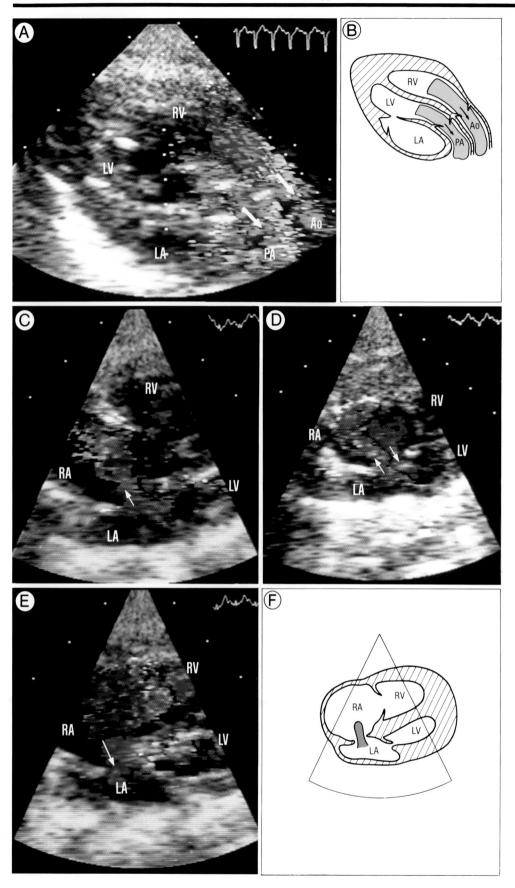

2-D Doppler images in d-TGA.

Ⓐ Ⓑ Parasternal long-axis view demonstrates the parallel orientation of the two great vessels : The aorta originates from the right ventricle and the pulmonary artery originates from the left ventricle **Ⓐ**. **Ⓒ Ⓓ Ⓔ** Subcostal four-chamber view demonstrates the bi-directional shunt flow pattern through the created interatrial opening : **Ⓒ** left-to-right shunt flow in systole **Ⓓ** bi-directional shunt flow at the end of systole **Ⓔ** right-to-left shunt flow in diastole.

Case 79　TGA　(A—H, operative BAS at age 2-months ; 1-L, Mustard operation at 6-months, female

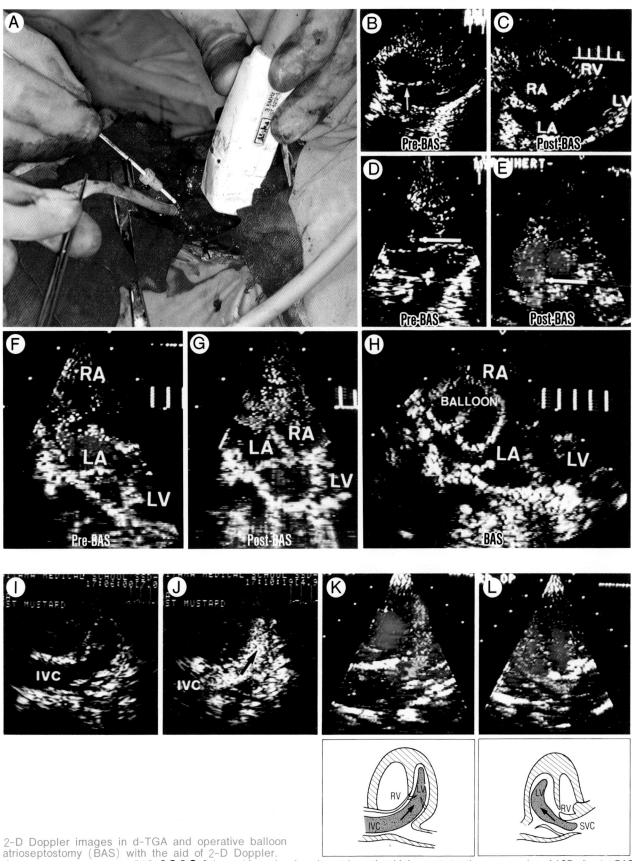

2-D Doppler images in d-TGA and operative balloon
atrioseptostomy (BAS) with the aid of 2-D Doppler.
Ⓐ Snap picture of operative BAS. ⒷⒸⒹⒺ Subcostal four-chamber view at 2 months old demonstrates the re-narrowing of ASD after 1st BAS
performed at 16 days old ⒷⒸ. The sufficient size of ASD has obtained by 2nd BAS ⒹⒺ. ⒻⒼⒽ Intra-operative epicardial 2-D Doppler before
BAS Ⓕ and after BAS Ⓖ. Inflated balloon catheter is seen in the left atrium (LA) Ⓗ.
2-D Doppler evaluation after Mustard operation.
Ⓘ 2-D Echo observing inferior vena cava (IVC). Ⓙ Contrast echo demonstrates the blood inflow from IVC into LV. Ⓚ 2-D Doppler
demonstrates the blood inflow from IVC into LV. Ⓛ 2-D Doppler demonstrates the blood inflow from superior vena cava (SVC) into LV.

Case 80 (1) TGA (type II) with Interruption of Aortic Arch (Celoria type A) 19-day-old male

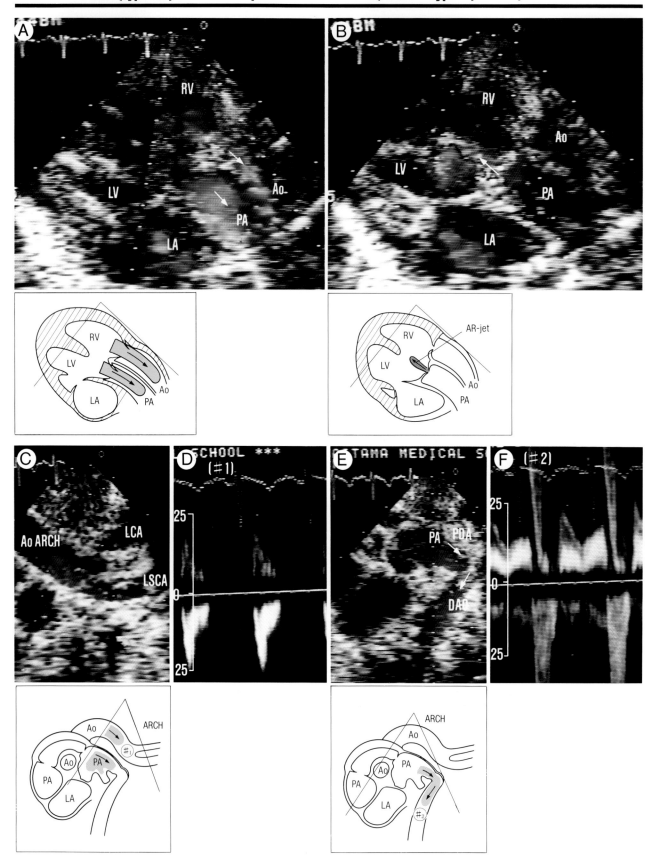

2-D Doppler images in d-TGA with interruption of aortic arch.
ⒶⒷ Parasternal long-axis view demonstrates the parallel orientation of the two great vessels Ⓐ and the mild pulmonary regurgitation in diastole
Ⓑ. ⒸⒹⒺⒻ The aortic arch is interrupted at the origin of the descending aorta Ⓒ and the descending aortic flow is supplied through PDA Ⓓ.
Pulsed Doppler shows the quite different flow pattern in the aortic arch (♯1) and in the descending aorta (♯2).

Case 80 (2) BAS Using 2-D Doppler   19-day-old male

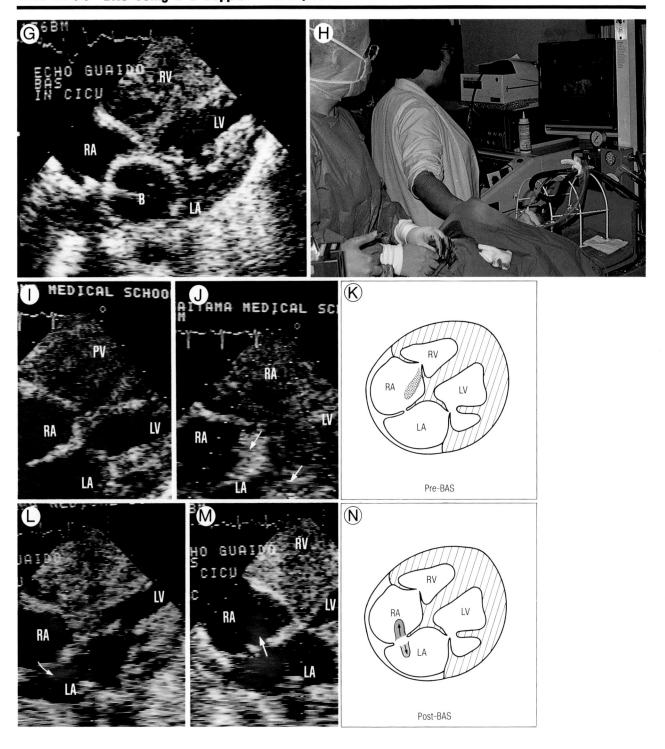

G The balloon catheter is inflated in the left atrium （LA） with the aid of 2-D Doppler. **H** Snap picture of BAS with the aid of 2-D Doppler. **I** **J** Although the moderate tricuspid regurgitation is seen **I** in the apical four-chamber view no effective interatrial communication is seen **H** before BAS. **L M N** Apical four-chamber view after BAS demonstrates the bi-directional and bi-phasic shunt flow through the created interatrial opening. **L** Right-to-left shunt flow. **M** Left-to-right shunt flow.

Case 81 TGA after Jatene Operation 1-year-old female

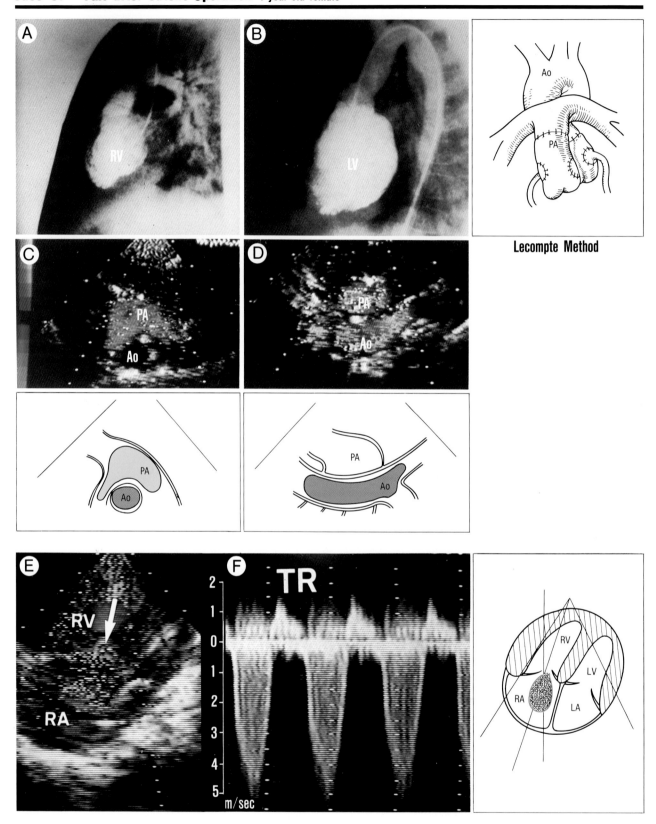

Lecompte Method

2-D Doppler images and cardiac angiograms in d-TGA after Jatene operation.
Ⓐ Right ventriculogram. Ⓑ Left ventriculogram. Ⓒ Right and left pulmonary arterial flow. Ⓓ Ascending aortic flow. ⒺⒻ Apical four-chamber view demonstrates the severe tricuspid regurgitation (grade 3) Ⓔ and the peak velocity of TR is 5 m/sec assessed by continuous-wave Doppler Ⓕ.

Case 82 TGA (type III) after Palliative Mustard Operation   3-year-old male

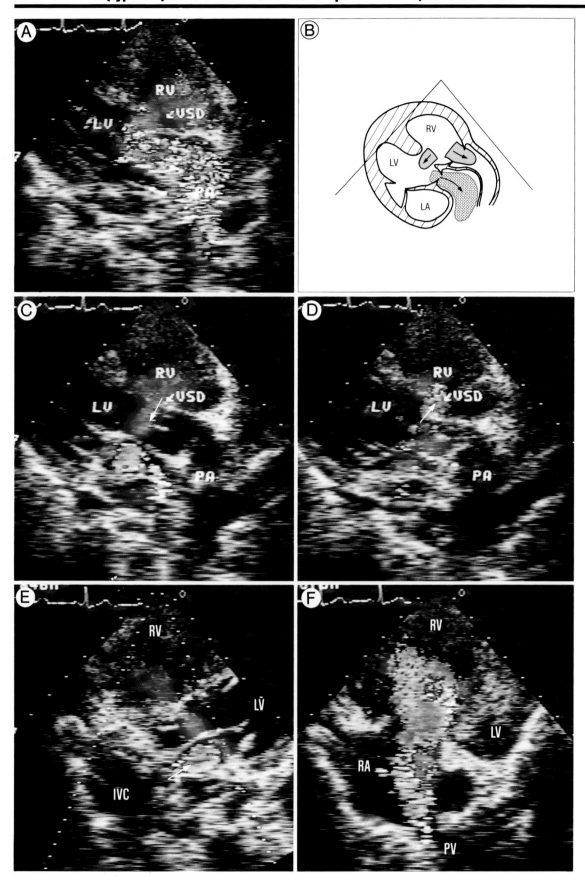

2-D Doppler images in d-TGA (type III) after palliative Mustard surgery.

Ⓐ Ⓑ Ⓒ Ⓓ Parasternal long-axis view demonstrates the parallel orientation of the two great vessels with mosaic stenotic flow pattern in the pulmonary trunk **Ⓐ**. The VSD shunt flow pattern is bi-directional **Ⓒ Ⓓ**. **Ⓔ Ⓕ** Apical four-chamber view demonstrates the left ventricular inflow from the inferior vena cava (IVC) **Ⓔ** and the right ventricular inflow from the pulmonary (PV) **Ⓕ**.

Case 83 Total Anomalous Pulmonary Venous Connection (TAPVC) (supracardiac type) 1-year-old male

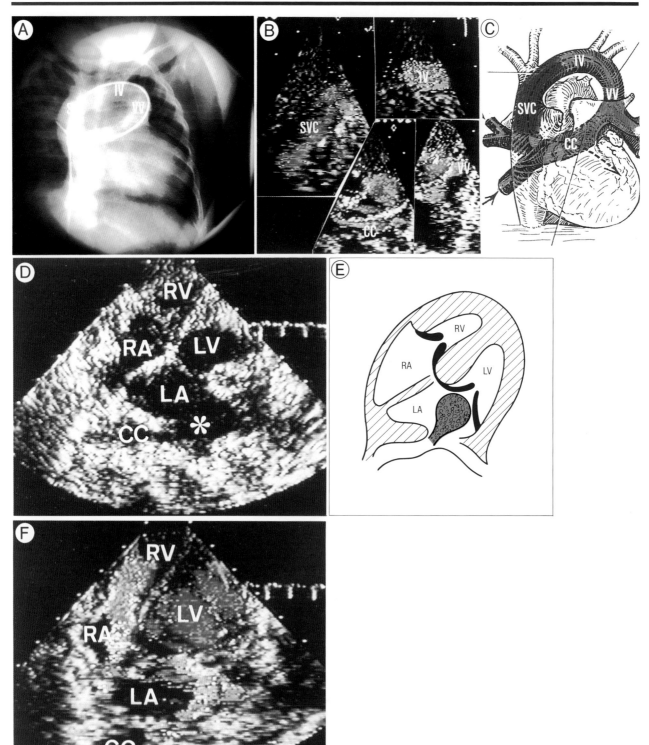

2-D Doppler images in TAPVC (supracardiac type)

Angiogram Ⓐ of abnormal pulmonary venous return [contrast material is injected from the common chamber (CC)] is compatible with 2-D Doppler images of abnormal pulmonary venous flow Ⓑ. VV=vertical vein ; IV=innominate vein ; SVC=superior vena cava. Ⓒ Schematic diagram of TAPVC (supracardiac type).

Intraoperative 2-D Doppler evaluation in TAPVC (supracardiac type).

ⒹⒺⒻ Apical four-chamber view after anastomosis of CC and LA. Note the wide anastomosis and the blood inflow from CC into LA without stagnancy.

Case 84 Total Anomalous Pulmonary Venous Connection (cardiac type) 2-month-old male

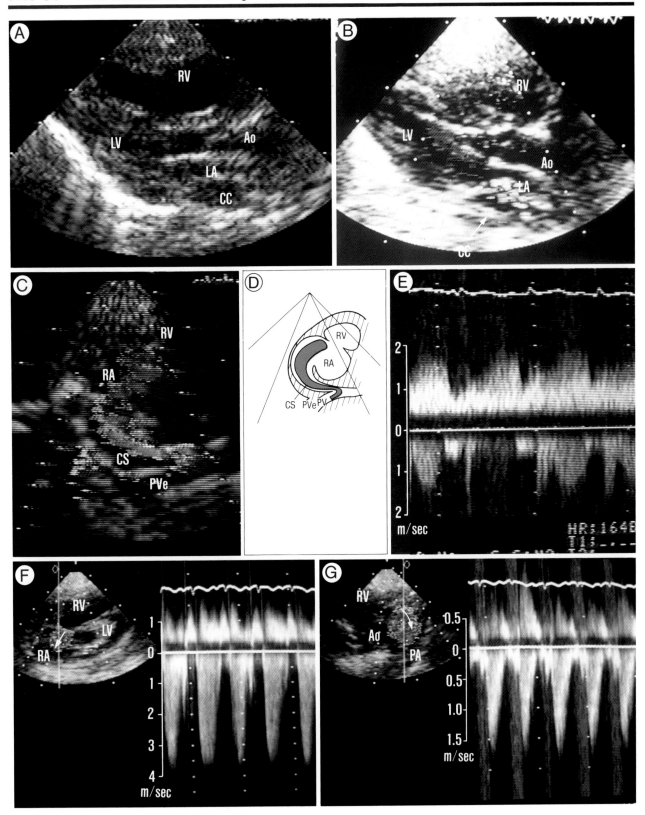

2-D Doppler images in TAPVC (cardiac type).

A B Parasternal long-axis view demonstrates the abnormal chamber (CC) behind LA **A** and the abnormal mosaic blood flow pattern in CC **B**.
C D E Subcostal four-chamber view demonstrates the abnormal pulmonary venous return from pulmonary vein (PVe) through coronary sinus (CS) into right atrium (RA). **D** Schematic diagram of subcostal four-chamber view. **E** Pulsed Doppler demonstrates the turbulent flow pattern of CS flow. **F** 2-D Doppler and CW Doppler images of the associated tricuspid regurgitation (grade 2). The velocity of TR (3.5 m/sec) indicates the moderately elevated pulmonary arterial pressure. **G** 2-D Doppler and CW Doppler images of the pulmonary arterial flow. Note the increased velocity and the turbulent flow pattern of the pulmonary arterial flow.

Case 85 (1) Pure Pulmonary Atresia 2-month-old famale

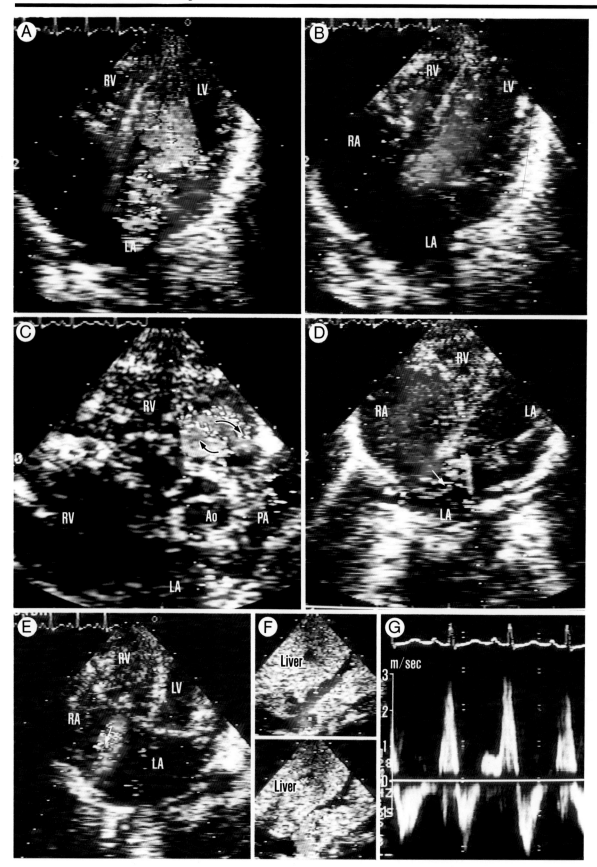

2-D Doppler images in pure pulmonary atresia.

Ⓐ Ⓑ Apical four-chamber view demonstrates little blood flow in the right ventricle both in diastole **Ⓐ** and in systole **Ⓑ**. **Ⓒ** Short-axis view at the aortic valve level demonstrates the complete atresia of the pulmonary valve and the swirling flow is seen in the right ventricular outflow tract. **Ⓓ** **Ⓔ** Subcostal four-chamber view demonstrates the right to left shunt flow through the atrial septal defect **Ⓓ** and the moderate tricuspid regurgitation (grade 2) in systole **Ⓔ**. **Ⓕ Ⓖ** The regurgitant blood flow in the hepatic vein is demonstrated by 2-D Doppler and pulsed Doppler.

Case 85 (2) Pure Pulmonary Atresia   2-month-old female

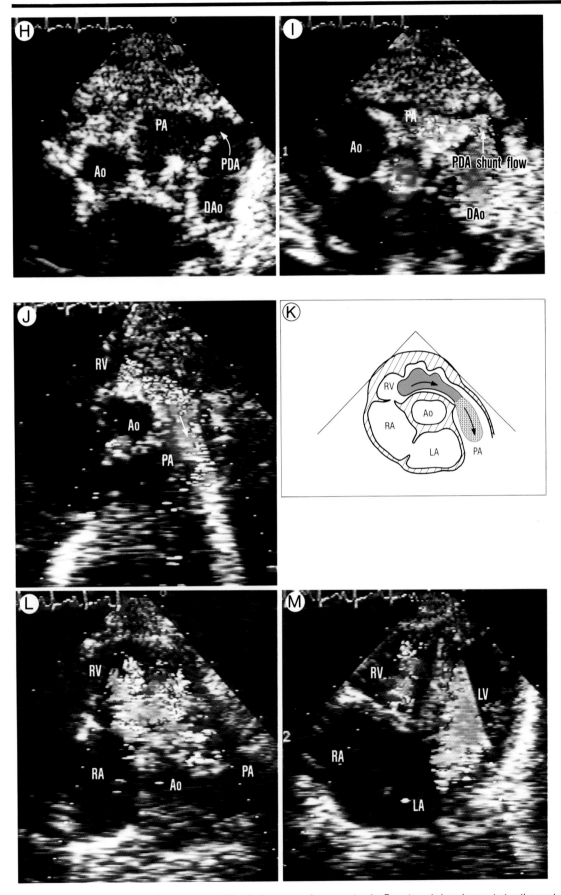

H I 2-D Doppler images of pulmonary arterial flow in the pure pulmonary atresia. Parasternal view demonstrates the anatomical connection of the main pulmonary artery, the patent ductus arteriosus, and the descending aorta **H** and the shunt flow through PDA **I**. **J K L M** 2-D Doppler evaluation of the effect of the prosthetic patch enlargement of the right ventricular outflow tract. Short-axis view at the aortic valve level demonstrates the right ventricular ejection flow in systole **J** and the increased right ventricular inflow in diastole **L**. **K** Schematic diagram. Apical four-chamber view also demonstrates the increased right ventricular inflow **M**.

Case 86 Congenital Valvular Aortic Stenosis 1-month-old male

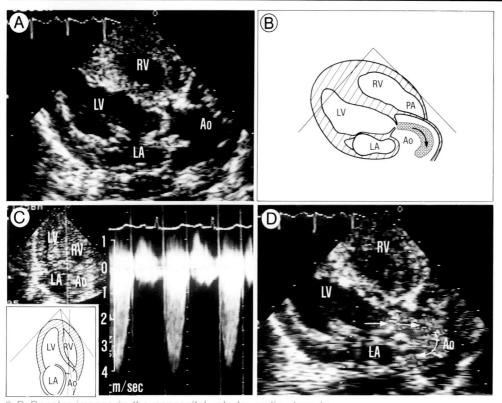

2-D Doppler images in the congenital valvular aortic stenosis.
Ⓐ Ⓑ Ⓓ Parasternal long-axis view demonstrates the stenosis and ballooning of the aortic valve **Ⓐ** and the turbulent stenotic aortic blood flow image. **Ⓓ**. **Ⓑ** Schematic diagram. **Ⓒ** The peak velocity of 4 m/sec is recorded with CW Doppler.

Case 87 Valvular Pulmonary Stenosis 3-year-old male

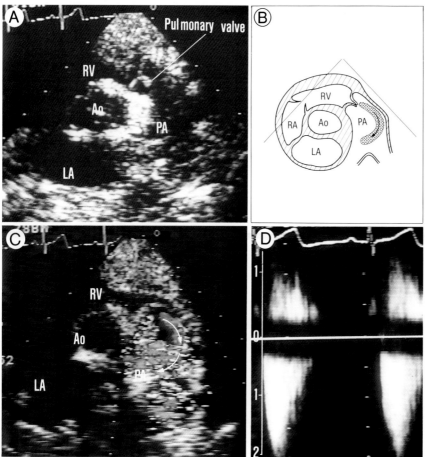

2-D Doppler images in valvular pulmonary stenosis.
Ⓐ Ⓑ Ⓒ Short-axis view at the aortic valve level demonstrates the stenosis of the pulmonary valve **Ⓐ** and the stenotic jet flow through the pulmonary valve **Ⓒ**. **Ⓑ** Schematic diagram. **Ⓓ** Continuous wave Doppler demonstrates 2 m/sec of peak velocity of pulmonary jet flow.

Case 88   Rupture of Valsalva Sinus Aneurysm into Right Atrium (Konno type IV)   62-year-old male

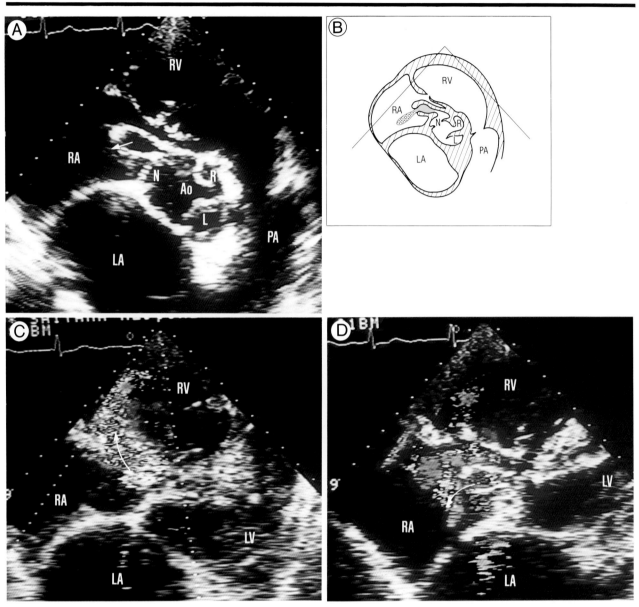

2-D Doppler images in ruptured Valsalva sinus aneurysm.
A B Short-axis view at the aortic valve level demonstrates the ruptured Valsalva sinus aneurysm **A**. **B** Schematic diagram. **C D** Parasternal four-chamber view demonstrates the shunt flow through the ruptured aneurysm in diastole **C** and in systole **D**.

Case 89 Rupture of Valsalva Sinus Aneurysm (Konno type IV) + VSD (type I) + AR (grade 3)
32-year-old male

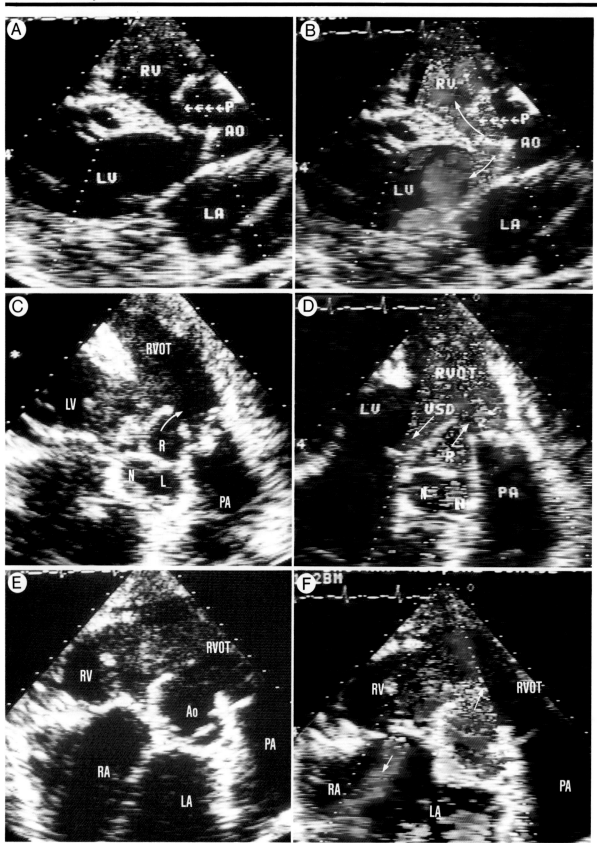

2-D Doppler images in ruptured Valsalva sinus aneurysm associated with VSD and AR.
A B Parasternal long-axis view demonstrates the ruptured Valsalva sinus aneurysm **A**, and the shunt flow through the perforation (P) and the severe aortic regurgitation (grade 3) **B**. **C D** Parasternal long-axis view of the pulmonary artery demonstraes the ruptured Valsalva sinus aneurysm and VSD **C**, and the shunt flow through them in diastole **D**. **E F** Short-axis view at the aortic valve level also demonstrates the subpulmonary VSD **E** and the associated tricuspid regurgitation (grade 2) in systole **F**.

Case 90 Ebstein's Anomaly + TR (grade 3)   36-year-old male

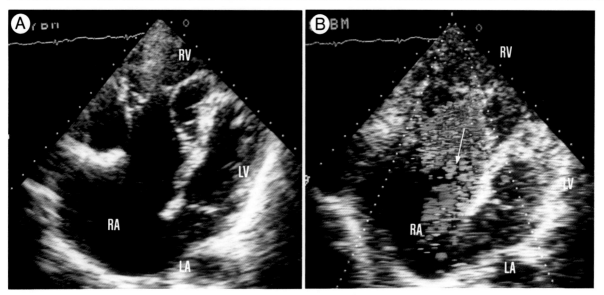

2-D Doppler images in Ebstein's anomaly associated with severe tricuspid regurgitation.
Apical four-chamber view demonstrates the apically displaced septal leaflet and the elongated anterior leaflet of the tricuspid valve Ⓐ, and the severe tricuspid regurgitation (grade 3) in the atrialized right ventricle and the right atrium Ⓑ.

Case 91 Ebstein's Anomaly + TR (grade 2)   47-year-old male

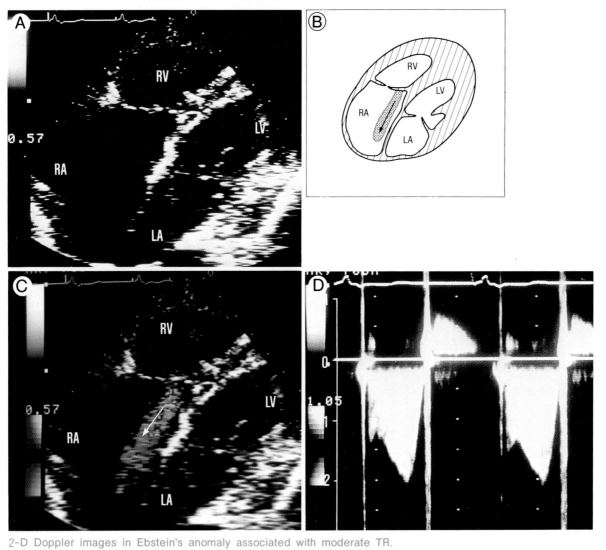

2-D Doppler images in Ebstein's anomaly associated with moderate TR.
Apical four-chamber view demonstrates the apically displaced septal leaflet of tricuspid valve and the atrialized right ventricle Ⓐ, and the moderate tricuspid regurgitation in systole Ⓒ. Ⓑ Schematic diagram. Ⓔ The maximum velocity of TR is 2 m/sec estimated by CW Doppler.

Case 92 Hypertrophic Obstructive Cardiomyopathy (HOCM)   78-year-old female

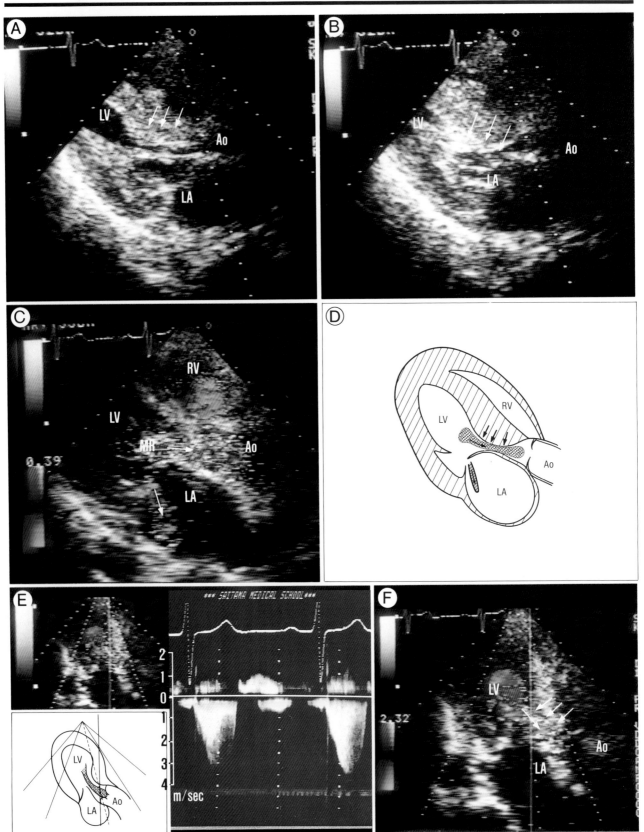

2-D Doppler images in hypertrophic obstructive cardiomyopathy.
Ⓐ Ⓑ Ⓒ Parasternal long-axis view demonstrates the septal hypertrophy and the stenosis in the left ventricular outflow tract in both diastole Ⓐ and systole Ⓑ, and the turbulent stenotic ejection flow and moderate mitral regurgitation (grade 2) in systole Ⓒ. Ⓓ Ⓕ Apical long-axis view more clearly demonstrates the obtruction of the left ventricular outflow tract Ⓕ. Ⓓ Schematic diagram. Ⓔ The peak velocity of the stenotic jet flow is estimated as 3.9 m/sec by CW Doppler.

Index